Charity and Mutual Aid in Europe and North America Since 1800

Routledge Studies in Modern British History

Charity and Mutual Aid in Europe and North America Since 1800

Edited by
Bernard Harris and Paul Bridgen

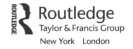
Routledge
Taylor & Francis Group
New York   London

First published 2007
by Routledge
711 Third Avenue, New York, NY 10017

Simultaneously published in the United Kingdom
by Routledge
2 Park Square, Milton Park, Abingdon, Oxon OX14 4RN

Routledge is an imprint of the Taylor & Francis Group, an informa business

First issued in paperback 2012

© 2007 Paul Bridgen and Bernard Harris

Typeset in Sabon by IBT Global

l

Library of Congress Cataloging-in-Publication Data
Charity and mutual aid in Europe and North America since 1800 / edited by Bernard Harris and Paul Bridgen.
p. cm. — (Routledge studies in modern history)
Includes bibliographical references and index.
ISBN-13: 978-0-415-36559-8 (hardback : alk. paper)
1. Public welfare—History. 2. Welfare economics. 3. Public welfare administration.
I. Harris, Bernard, 1961– II. Bridgen, Paul.

HV51.C43 2008
361.7094--dc22   2007031877

ISBN13: 978-0-415-36559-8 (hbk)
ISBN13: 978-0-415-54105-3 (pbk)
ISBN13: 978-0-203-93240-7 (ebk)

Contents

List of Tables

1   Introduction

The "Mixed Economy of Welfare" and the Historiography of Welfare Provision

Bernard Harris and Paul Bridgen

University of Southampton

After 1945, it was often assumed that the "rise" of state welfare provision was both desirable and inevitable, and that the task of welfare-state historians was to locate the origins of public welfare provision and explain its growth. However, during the 1970s and 1980 these assumptions were called into question by critics on both sides of the political spectrum, and this led to major changes in the pattern of welfare provision and the relationship between the state and other welfare providers.[1] These changes have also had a major effect on the historiography of welfare provision. Historians have been forced to pay much more attention to other sources of welfare, including individuals and families, neighbours and communities, mutual-aid organisations, charities and commercial organisations, and to treat them seriously in their own right, instead of simply regarding them as "precursors" of state welfare.[2] The reasons why different forms of welfare provision have been chosen at different points in time have also been subjected to greater scrutiny.[3]

As Norman Johnson has remarked, there is nothing inherently new in the concept of a "mixed economy of welfare," because "welfare states have always been mixed and the same four sectors [the state, the commercial sector, the voluntary sector, and the informal sector] have always been present," even though the boundaries between them have often been blurred.[4] However, the term itself does not appear to have been widely used before the 1980s. In 1983, Sheila Kamerman used the phrase "the new mixed economy of welfare" to describe the relationship that was beginning to emerge between the statutory and voluntary sectors in the United States, and Ken Judge and Mike Reddin prepared a briefing paper on "the mixed economy of welfare" for a conference of social-policy academics in the UK.[5] They argued that the term was less ideologically loaded than the alternative concept of "welfare pluralism," which had become increasingly popular among those who not only wished to highlight the existence of a plurality of welfare-providers but also to advocate their use.[6]

Although the terminology of the "mixed economy of welfare" originated in debates about the evolution of social policy in contemporary societies, it has become increasingly popular in the historical literature. In 1994, Geoffrey Finlayson argued (with respect to Britain) that "there was always what is now often called a 'mixed economy of welfare', and within that mixed economy, the state was only one element—and, arguably, for much of the nineteenth and even the twentieth century—it was not the most important."[7] Jane Lewis has also argued that both Britain and other European countries have "always . . . had a mixed economy of welfare, in which the state, the voluntary sector, the family, and the market have played different parts at different points in time,"[8] and Joanna Innes has claimed that "a mixed economy of welfare" has persisted in western Europe from the sixteenth century onwards.[9] Michael Katz and Christoph Sachße used the phrase "the mixed economy of social welfare" to describe the relationship between public and private welfare provision in England, Germany, and the United States between the 1870s and the 1930s,[10] and David Green and Alastair Owens made the concept of a "mixed economy" one of the main organising themes of their introduction to a series of essays on family welfare in Europe and America since the mid-seventeenth century.[11]

Although the development of historical interest in the concept of a mixed economy of welfare owed much to the emergence of new attitudes to welfare provision in the 1980s and 1990s, it also reflected the application of new approaches and methods on the part of historians themselves. One important dimension of this was the desire expressed by many historians to move away from a focus on organisations and institutions and to strengthen their efforts to reconstruct the experiences of "ordinary people" from below.[12] An important example of this kind of work was Olwen Hufton's pathbreaking study of *The Poor of Eighteenth-Century France*. Hufton examined the full range of strategies employed by peasant households under the *ancien régime* to make ends meet, including not only subsistence production but also begging and migration.[13] Hufton was responsible for introducing the phrase "economy of makeshifts" to the study of early-modern welfare and her work has recently been described as "the first systematic historical analysis" of informal relief in early-modern societies.[14]

The desire to reconstruct the history of "informal welfare" has not been confined to the early-modern period. In Britain, both Michael Anderson and Marguerite Dupree have argued that the first call for individuals who were experiencing distress was on their own families, and this principle remained at the heart of much public-welfare policy for much of the nineteenth and twentieth centuries.[15] However, as Catharina Lis and Hugo Soly have argued, many individuals were likely to find themselves in situations in which they were unable to call on their families for assistance, and in these situations they often found it necessary to rely on their friends and neighbours.[16] In imperial Russia, it was customary for the members of peasant communities to help one another by providing food and shelter, together with other forms of assistance.[17] In London, during the late-nineteenth and early-twentieth centuries, poor women helped each other by providing gifts of food and clothing, contributing to funeral expenses, assisting with childbirth, and offering accommodation to battered wives and evicted families.[18]

Although it is important not to underestimate the extent of the informal ties that help to bind working-class communities, these were not the only factors that helped to sustain poor families in times of need. As Paul Johnson has shown, working-class families also sought to maintain and improve their living standards and protect themselves against misfortune by taking out private insurance, joining mutual-aid organisations, acquiring credit, and accruing small amounts of personal savings. Although such activities have often been seen as an integral part of working-class community life during the late-nineteenth and early-twentieth centuries, Johnson argued that they also had a strongly individualistic motivation and that they tended "as much to strengthen the particularism of local communities as to mould a national working-class consciousness."[19]

Among the different types of organisations studied by Johnson, one of the most important was the fraternal or friendly society. As David Neave has shown, friendly societies have existed in Britain since at least the seventeenth century,[20] but their numbers increased significantly in the late-eighteenth and early-nineteenth centuries, and they grew most rapidly after 1850. Although there were some female friendly societies and some "mixed" societies admitted female members, the majority of friendly societies drew the bulk of their membership from the male working class.[21] They often had a rich associational culture, which was reflected in their colourful titles and rituals, and this played a crucial role in establishing the bonds of trust that helped to maintain organisational solidarity.[22] However, their most important contribution to the maintenance of material well-being was to provide a range of welfare benefits, including sickness insurance, medical care, old-age pensions, and death benefits. By 1914, there were just under 29,000 "true" friendly societies in the United Kingdom, with a combined membership of just over 7.6 million.[23]

These were not the only mutual-aid organisations that sought to provide welfare benefits for their members. In Britain, many trade unions also provided welfare services, including not only sickness and accident insurance but also unemployment benefits.[24] The second half of the nineteenth century also witnessed the development of a range of other initiatives, including cooperative and building societies, together with hospital contributory schemes.[25] These were designed to enable working-class people to obtain free medical treatment in charitable, or "voluntary," hospitals, without the need for a subscriber's recommendation, in return for a regular subscription.[26]

There has also been a significant increase in the amount of interest shown in the history of mutual aid in other parts of the world. In 1989, Michael Sibalis published a pioneering study of the mutual-aid societies of Paris between 1789 and 1848,[27] and Allan Mitchell subsequently published an overview of the development of mutual-aid societies in the whole of France during the second half of the nineteenth century.[28] In 1996, Marcel van der Linden edited a collection of essays on the development of mutual-aid organisations in 26 different countries, including contributions dealing not only with Europe but also with different parts of Asia, Australasia, and both North and South America.[29] A number of important monographs have also been published, including Alan Baker's analysis of fraternity in the French countryside, George and Herbert Emery's study of the Independent Order of Odd Fellows and the evolution of sickness insurance in the United States and Canada, David Beito's account of the history of mutual aid in the United States, and David Green's account of the history of friendly societies in Australia.[30]

Although membership of the majority of mutual-aid organisations was usually voluntary, this was not necessarily the case. Between 1845 and 1876, the Prussian authorities passed a series of laws that enabled municipal authorities to compel "journeymen, assistants, apprentices and industrial workers" to join local sickness insurance funds, or *Hilfskassen*, and many local authorities in industrial areas decided to implement this power as a way of reducing the cost of poor relief, especially in the Rhine provinces and around Berlin.[31] However, these powers were much less likely to be adopted in other parts of the country. According to Peter Hennock, only 226 local authorities had adopted local compulsion by 1854, and fewer than 769,000 workers belonged to state-supervised provident funds for industrial workers offering sickness benefit in 1872. This figure compares quite poorly with the number of workers who belonged to voluntary friendly societies providing sickness insurance in England and Wales in the same year.[32]

In his account of the relationship between voluntarism and the state in twentieth-century Britain, Geoffrey Finlayson drew an important distinction between what he described as the "self-regarding" nature of self-help and mutual-aid organisations and the "other-regarding" nature of private charities,[33] but this distinction can be overdrawn.[34] As Simon Cordery has explained, one of the largest British friendly societies, the Manchester Unity of Oddfellows, originally provided assistance on the basis of need, and it was only later that it decided to establish a direct link between the receipt of benefits and the payment of contributions.[35] This was not the only way in which friendly societies could sometimes blur the boundaries between "self-help" and helping others. During the early-nineteenth century, a number of "patronised" friendly societies were established by members of the local gentry for the benefit of agricultural workers in the rural counties of southern England, although these societies never achieved the popularity of more conventional organisations.[36] The friendly societies might also be expected to perform charitable activities within their own communities. According to Audrey Fisk, the Ancient Order of Foresters often called upon its members to make donations to people affected by mining disasters, and they contributed to appeals launched on behalf of those affected by the Lancashire "cotton famine" in the 1860s. They also responded to appeals launched on behalf of fellow Foresters in the wake of the Chicago fire in 1871 and the San Francisco earthquake in 1906.[37] In the United States, the Independent Order of Foresters also launched an appeal on behalf of members affected by the San Francisco earthquake, and in 1927 the Improved Benevolent and Protective Order of the Elks donated more than US$4000 to members affected by the Mississippi floods and the Florida hurricanes.[38]

The friendly societies were not the only mutual-aid organisations in which the boundaries between self-help and charity could sometimes be blurred. As we have already seen, a large number of contributory insurance schemes were established to raise money for voluntary hospitals in Britain during the second half of the nineteenth century. The individuals who joined the schemes contributed a small weekly payment, which meant that they would not have to pay for any treatment they might subsequently receive. However, the schemes did not provide members with an automatic right to be treated,[39] and they were careful to couch their appeals for funds in the language of charity as well as personal self-interest. This is reflected in the following verse, which accompanied a cartoon showing the reasons why it was in the worker's own interest to subscribe to the Hospital Saturday Fund in Birmingham during the 1880s:

> Now don't turn away, but remember today
> Is the day of all days in the year
> When the true working man says "I'll do all I can
> The sorrowing sick ones to cheer."
> Then don't turn aside, with a false sort of pride,
> Since you cannot give dollars or crowns!
> But *do what you can*, like a brave-hearted man,
> And give us a handful of "browns."[40]

If historians of friendly societies and contributory insurance schemes have challenged the idea that mutual-aid organisations are either necessarily or exclusively "self-regarding," historians of charity and philanthropy have often questioned the assumption that charities are necessarily "other-regarding."[41] In nineteenth-century Britain, philanthropic activity was regarded as compensation for childlessness (Frederic Mocatta), a way of coping with the consequences of bereavement (Josephine Butler and Olive Malvery), and as a way of escaping "inner conflicts of personality" (the seventh Earl of Shaftesbury).[42] It offered opportunities for the cultivation of useful social contacts and provided middle-class women with opportunities for participation in public life that were otherwise denied them.[43] During the twentieth century, charitable organisations became an increasingly important source of paid employment.[44] Charity was often regarded as an important mechanism for the establishment of social ties and the maintenance of social harmony. As one contributor to a Moscow religious journal wrote in 1862:

> The parish community . . . has long attracted the attention of many
> as the most suitable form of moral-social activity; to use the parish to
> draw the well-to-do and the poor together morally and economically
> and to stop the evil that inequality of social conditions produces, is an
> excellent idea, fully worthy of a society based on Christian principles.[45]

Although historians have often argued about the motives behind philanthropy, and will doubtless continue to do so,[46] it is also important to
recognise the contributions that charity and philanthropy did make towards
meeting social needs. In Florence, the Congregation of San Giovanni Bat-
tista played a leading role in the provision of outdoor relief and employment
opportunities during the occupation of Tuscany between 1808 and 1814,
and also took responsibility for the licensing of beggars and the accommodation and training of orphans.[47] During the hungry years of the 1840s,
the city council of Lyon launched a public appeal for donations to assist
the town's unemployed workers, and two-thirds of the additional aid provided in the Netherlands came from private foundations and individual
donors.[48] In nineteenth-century Germany, "a local culture of associations
became established, especially in the cities, which encompassed all areas of
civil life and also formed the organisational backbone for private—both
confessional and nonconfessional—initiatives for the poor and needy."[49] In
England and Wales, charity trusts played an important part in the relief of
poverty in rural areas, and several towns and cities launched appeals for
emergency relief during periods of high unemployment during the 1840s,
1860s, and 1880s, as well as during the 1920s.[50] In the United States, private
philanthropists had traditionally attached more importance to the preven-
tive role of charity than to its ameliorative functions, but that did not prevent them from launching a series of appeals for the relief of distress caused
by unemployment before the introduction of the New Deal.[51]

Charity also made an important contribution to the development of other
welfare services. In post-Emancipation Russia, voluntary societies provided
soup kitchens and homeless shelters for people migrating to cities in search
of jobs and played a leading role in the provision of subsidised and model
housing for the poor.[52] In the United States, almost every American community possessed its complement of "well-to-do citizens [who] contributed to
the founding and support of churches, hospitals and orphanages," and private philanthropists took the lead in providing financial support for schools
and colleges.[53] In England and Wales, voluntary organisations contributed
to the development of social housing and provided the majority of the country's elementary-school places before 1900, whilst more than 20 per cent
of all hospital beds were located in voluntary institutions on the eve of the
First World War.[54]

During the last thirty years, a number of historians have attempted to
express the contribution made by charity to the "mixed economy of welfare" in quantitative terms. In France, it has been estimated that "outlays of

charity represented twenty per cent of a bourgeois family's expenditures" and that "private aid to the poor equalled that provided by official municipal organs" at the end of the nineteenth century.[55] Adele Lindenmeyr has argued that "along with individual almsgiving, organised private charity constituted the major source of poor relief in the [Russian] Empire.[56] In Britain, it has often been claimed that unofficial exertion "far outweighed official exertion" during the mid-nineteenth century and that "eleemosynary contributions were greater by far than the whole national expenditure on poor relief" at the beginning of the 1870s.[57] However, these comparisons should be interpreted with a certain amount of care. One of the main problems is that a substantial proportion of recorded charity was used for purposes which would have stood far outside any contemporary definition of the legitimate scope of the poor law, such as missionary activity.[58] This is without taking account of the fact that significant amounts of money were embezzled, whilst large sums were devoted to the organisation of social activities and the construction of lavish buildings that may have had little direct bearing on the lives of those in whose name they were organised.[59]

Despite these difficulties, a number of historians have attempted to compare levels of charitable expenditure in different countries. According to Frank Prochaska, no nation (or country) on earth can lay claim to a richer philanthropic past or a greater philanthropic tradition than (Great) Britain.[60] However, the economic historian Peter Lindert has calculated that the amount distributed by private charities to the poor in England and Wales fell from 0.4 per cent of GNP in 1790 to less than 0.1 per cent between 1861 and 1876. These figures compare relatively poorly with the figures for France (≤0.5% of GNP in 1880), Italy (≤0.5% of GNP in 1868), and the Netherlands (between 0.67 and 1.49% of GNP at the end of the eighteenth century).[61] On the other hand, Lindert's figures for England and Wales are confined to those charities that filed their accounts with the Charities Commission and may therefore be an underestimate. He estimated that these charities earned an annual average income of £2.2 million between 1861 and 1876, of which £0.9 million was devoted to the relief of the poor. In contrast, Thomas Hawksley estimated that London's charities alone had a total income of £6.9 million at the end of the 1860s, including £1.7 million for "the ordinary necessaries of life" and a further £1.6 million donated from various sources for the relief of the poor.[62]

During the 1990s, Lester Salamon and Helmut Anheier embarked on an ambitious attempt to define the voluntary or "nonprofit" sector. They argued that the nonprofit sector "is a set of organisations that are formally-constituted, non-governmental in basic structure, self-governing, non-profit distributing, and voluntary to some meaningful extent."[63] However, as Susannah Morris has argued, it can be difficult to apply this definition to particular historical circumstances. During the second half of the nineteenth century, joint-stock companies were established on both sides of the Atlantic to provide model housing for the residents of large cities. Although these organisations were designed to yield a small profit for their shareholders, their primary purpose was "to provide a more salubrious standard of accommodation for the working-classes at an affordable cost," and they achieved this by charging "below-market rents which were in many cases equivalent to those charged by the non-profit distributing organisations in the field."[64]

Morris's work also highlights the importance of the role played by commercial organisations in the provision of welfare services more generally. As Paul Johnson has shown, some of the most successful "welfare" organisations in Britain during the late-nineteenth and early-twentieth centuries were the commercial life assurance companies, such as the Prudential Assurance Company, which was responsible for approximately 21 million paid-up policies on the eve of the First World War.[65] These organisations continued to expand throughout the twentieth century, as individuals took out an increasing range of insurance policies to protect themselves against an ever-expanding selection of risks. The expansion of these forms of provision, alongside the growth of personal and occupational pension plans and the increasing involvement of commercial organisations in the provision of public services, is likely to provide fertile ground for future historians.[66]

Although this review has concentrated on those aspects of welfare provision that often seemed to be underresearched by earlier generations of welfare historians, it is important to recognise that the most important feature of welfare history over the last two hundred years has been the expanding role of the state. In Britain, the earliest poor-law legislation was introduced in the sixteenth and early-seventeenth centuries. The Elizabethan Poor Laws of 1597 and 1601 allowed the churchwardens and overseers of each parish to levy a tax, or poor rate, on the inhabitants and occupiers of land and made them responsible for "setting the poor on work," maintaining those who were unable to work, and making arrangements for the apprenticeship of pauper children. The cost of the poor law rose substantially during the late-eighteenth and early-nineteenth centuries, and this led to a major change in the system of poor law administration in 1834, but it continued to play a major role in the development of public welfare provision in England and Wales until 1948.[67]

In a famous paper, the British sociologist T. H. Marshall drew an important distinction between three different sorts of rights—civil rights, political rights, and social rights. He defined civil rights as "the rights necessary for individual freedom—liberty of the person, freedom of speech, the right to own property and to conclude valid contracts, and the right to justice." Political rights included "the right to participate in the exercise of political power, as a member of a body invested with political authority and as an elector of the members of such a body"; and social rights covered "the whole range from the right to a modicum of economic welfare and security to the right to share to the full in the social heritage and . . . live the life of a civilised being according to the standards prevailing in the society."[68] In principle, the establishment of the Poor Law gave individuals the opportunity to assert a limited version of their "social rights" by giving them the right to a "modicum of economic welfare," but they might find that they were only able to exercise this right by relinquishing some of their other rights (e.g., by being required to enter a workhouse, or being denied the right to vote in either Parliamentary or local elections). Consequently, although the Poor Law enabled individuals to make claims upon the community, it also excluded them from full membership of the community. One of the most important "badges" of membership, the right to vote, was only extended to paupers in 1918.[69]

During the nineteenth and twentieth centuries, Parliament introduced a number of different measures that extended the boundaries of state welfare intervention without subjecting those affected by them to the "disabilities" associated with the Poor Law. Some of the earliest examples of such measures were the introduction of acts to limit the working hours of children and young persons and establish minimum standards in factories and workplaces. These measures were followed by the introduction of parliamentary grants to support the provision of public education after 1833 and the acceptance of state responsibility for the provision of education after 1870. However, some of the most significant changes in public-welfare policy followed the election of the Liberal government in 1906. This government expanded the state's role in the prevention of individual poverty by introducing such measures as old-age pensions in 1908, minimum-wage legislation in 1909, and insurance against sickness and unemployment in 1911. Although many of these measures were quite limited, they helped to lay the foundations for further changes in state welfare policy, such as the introduction of subsidised local authority housing in 1919 and the creation of the National Health Service in 1948.[70]

Although the precise details of this chronology may vary from country to country, virtually all industrialised countries have witnessed significant increases in the role of state welfare over the past two centuries, even though there have also been significant differences in the pattern of welfare provision and the entitlements that this entails.[71] However, this development has often been associated with fierce controversy. During the 1970s and 1980s, a growing army of critics claimed that welfare state regulations were stifling innovation and initiative and that national economies were being hampered by excessive levels of public expenditure, but in spite of these criticisms, there has been relatively little change in the total share of national wealth that is consumed by public welfare spending since the 1980s.[72] However, within the context of the welfare state, major changes have occurred in the relationship between public and private welfare providers, and this has led to further changes in the size of the contributions that each sector makes to the overall "welfare mix."[73] The question of how this relationship may continue to evolve is likely to remain at the heart of social-policy debates for many years to come.

* * *

The essays in this volume are primarily concerned with two elements of the mixed economy of welfare—charity and mutual aid. They emphasise the close relationship between these two elements and the often blurred boundaries between each of them and commercial provision, and they reinforce the impression of fluidity and hybridity in the organisation of welfare provision before 1945. They also illustrate the dynamic nature of the mixed economy and highlight the "messy" negotiated process of state growth, in which social and political factors, as well as performance, made a significant contribution to sectoral change. Finally, the essays also raise important questions about the relationship between rights and responsibilities within the mixed economy of welfare and the ties that bind both the donors and recipients of charity and the members of voluntary organisations. Three of the chapters are primarily concerned with England and Wales, one with the Netherlands, one with Sweden and Norway, and one with the United States of America. Thomas Adams' chapter ranges more widely across more than six centuries of European history, and Thomas Adam examines the process of policy transfer between Britain, Germany, and North America.

In Chapter 2, Bernard Harris starts by exploring the role played by charity in debates over the reform of the Poor Law in England and Wales before 1834. He argues that critics of the "Old Poor Law" drew a distinction between the idea of a statutory entitlement to welfare, which they believed the Poor Law had come to represent, and the much more conditional, or discretionary, entitlement associated with a system of charitable relief. He then goes on to examine the extent of the assistance provided by charity following the introduction of the "New Poor Law" in 1834. In the final section of the chapter, he discusses the changing boundary between voluntary and statutory welfare after 1870. Although groups such as the Charity Organisation Society campaigned for further restrictions on the provision of poor relief and the establishment of a more "scientific" relationship between charity and the Poor Law, their efforts were largely undermined by the development of new forms of state welfare from the 1870s onwards. These developments paved the way for the emergence of what subsequently became known as the "new philanthropy" after the First World War.

Although Harris's chapter is particularly concerned with the concept of changes in the relationship between charity and the poor law, Thomas Adams's chapter uses the concept of a "mixed moral economy of welfare" to highlight the existence of some striking continuities. He argues that there are strong similarities between the sense of obligation that underpinned the idea of charity in continental Europe before 1800 and some of the ideas associated with the concept of "social citizenship" after 1945. He also identifies strong similarities between the ways in which traditional forms of welfare support sought to discipline the poor and the concerns of welfare states today. However, although Adams emphasises the extent to which the welfare state has built on earlier ideas, he also acknowledges the extent to which some modern observers have criticised the ways in which it does this. In the final section of his chapter, he explores the ways in which politicians such as Helmut Kohl, the former German Chancellor, have utilised the concept of "subsidiarity" to argue that the welfare state needs to find a way of restoring responsibility to the lowest level at which it can reasonably be exercised, whether this is the individual, the family, the local community, or the national state.

In Chapter 4, Daniel Weinbren examines the complex relationship between "philanthropy" and "mutual aid." Although many previous authors have tended to place philanthropy and mutual aid in separate and often unrelated compartments, he argues that they have often been closely related. He begins by examining the extent to which charities and friendly societies in England and Wales could both trace their origins to the medieval guilds. He then draws on Marcel Mauss's concept of "the gift"[74] to argue that they also shared a common understanding of the importance of reciprocity in social relationships. In the third and fourth sections of the chapter, he explores the practical implications of this insight. On the one hand, the friendly societies encouraged their members to behave charitably towards each other and their local communities; on the other hand, they often relied on "élite" members to provide financial support, administrative expertise, and social patronage. Although Weinbren does not seek to diminish the differences between charities and friendly societies, he is also concerned to highlight "their common roots . . . their continuing common interest in institutionalising benevolence . . . and their interest in transcending economic transfers . . . by extending them to involve emotional and social relationships."[75]

In contrast to Weinbren's chapter, Marco van Leeuwen is much more directly concerned with the financial benefits provided by mutual-aid organisations and their relationship to other kinds of insurance schemes in the Netherlands during the nineteenth century. To facilitate this, he distinguishes between five types of insurance scheme—those provided by factory schemes, mutual-aid organisations, trade unions, commercial organisations, and general-practitioner schemes—and six varieties of "risk"—loss of income due to sickness, the cost of medical treatment, childbirth, old-age and widowhood, unemployment, and death. Table 1.1 shows that there was at least some form of provision for each type of risk in the Netherlands by the end of the nineteenth century, but the extent of this provision should not be exaggerated. Van Leeuwen estimates that less than 1 per cent of the Dutch population was insured against the financial risks of unemployment, widowhood, or old age at the start of the last decade of the nineteenth century, fewer than 10 per cent were insured against loss of income due to ill-health, and fewer than sixteen percent were insured for medical costs. The only form of benefit which could really be said to be widely available was funeral benefit, which covered more than half the population.[76]

Table 1.1 Mutual Aid and Private Insurance in the Netherlands During the Nineteenth Century

Type/Risk	Sickness Insurance (Income Replacement)	Sickness Insurance (Cost of Treatment)	Childbirth	Old Age and Widows' Pensions	Unemployment	Death
Factory	✓	✓	✓	✓		✓
Mutual (excluding trade unions)	✓			✓	✓	✓
Commercial	✓			✓		✓
Trade union	✓	✓			✓	✓
General Practitioner	✓	✓				

Source: Chapter 5.

In view of the limited extent of this form of welfare provision, it is perhaps not surprising that so many European governments should have been considering the introduction of some form of statutory intervention. In Chapter 6, Peter Johansson examines the different ways in which governments responded to this challenge in Sweden and Norway. During the mid-1880s, the governments of both countries viewed the threat of industrial and social unrest with considerable alarm, and this led them to establish commissions to investigate the possibility of introducing new forms of sickness insurance; but there were still important differences in the nature of the schemes they introduced. In Sweden, the government was able to build on the foundations of existing schemes and introduce its own voluntary system in 1891, but the Norwegian government determined upon a mandatory scheme, which was only introduced in 1907. The main aim of Johansson's chapter is to explain the reasons for these differences. Although he recognises the importance of farmers' interests in the two countries, he argues that the most important factor in explaining the differences between them was that the existing voluntary schemes appeared to have made much greater inroads in Sweden than in Norway, and this meant that they generated a much greater capacity for "third-sector growth."

Thomas Adam's chapter also has a multinational focus, but it is more concerned with the question of housing than health; and it utilises ideas drawn from the "policy-transfer" literature to explore the ways in which different ideas about the problem of housing reform flowed between Britain, Germany, and North America.[77] During the second half of the nineteenth century, British housing reformers pursued a number of different strategies for the improvement of working-class housing conditions, including the letting of existing properties to model tenants (Octavia Hill) and the construction of new housing under the guise of "five-per-cent philanthropy."[78] Adam shows how German and North American investigators travelled to Britain to study these schemes and explore the possibility of transplanting them to their own countries. However, there were also important differences in the ways in which the ideas were applied. In the United States, the concept of five-per-cent philanthropy attracted considerable interest, but its proponents were never able to demonstrate that it provided a viable method of meeting housing needs. In Germany, reformers were able to combine the concept of five-per-cent philanthropy with ideas borrowed from the British cooperative movement, and this provided a much firmer foundation for subsequent development.

Adam's chapter also raises further issues about the location and clarity of the boundaries between different forms of welfare provision. As we have just seen, Adam argues that it was easier to transplant the concept of five-per-cent philanthropy to Germany because it became absorbed within the cooperative movement, and this helps to blur the boundaries between philanthropy and mutual aid.[79] However, the concept of five-per-cent philanthropy (or the limited-dividend company) also blurs the boundary between charity and commercial welfare. As Adam points out, several modern commentators have argued that limited dividend companies were commercial organisations because they were designed to yield a dividend for their investors, but these organisations should also be regarded as charitable institutions because the dividends they offered were lower than those that investors might have obtained elsewhere.

In Chapter 8, Andrew Morris explores the relationship between voluntary and statutory welfare provision in the United States before the Great Depression. He argues that even before 1929, voluntary agencies were beginning to argue that the public sector should assume a greater share of responsibility for meeting material needs. He attributes this to the emergence of new psychoanalytic theories which encouraged voluntary social workers "to focus on the psychological and emotional roots of their clients' 'maladjustment' to society," and to the increasing financial difficulties that the voluntary agencies themselves were facing. He also examines the ways in which leading figures within the voluntary sector sought to define a new role for themselves within the context of an expanding public welfare sector. Rather like their counterparts in the United Kingdom, they argued that the voluntary sector could support the public sector by showing greater sensitivity in its relationships with welfare clients, scrutinising the work of public agencies, representing the interests of disadvantaged groups, and pioneering the development of new forms of welfare activity.

The spotlight returns to the UK in Chapter 9. In this chapter, Paul Bridgen examines the reasons for the "demise" of the voluntary hospital system in Britain after the Second World War. The voluntary hospitals have received an increasing amount of attention in recent years, with much of it focusing on their performance.[80] However, Bridgen argues that sectoral change can only be understood properly if greater attention is given to the social and political context within which change occurred, particularly the relationship between the voluntary hospitals and the middle classes. During the nineteenth century, the majority of middle-class patients were most likely to receive medical treatment in their own homes; but the emergence of new forms of treatment, allied to the introduction of more hygienic operating environments, meant that an increasing number of patients were likely to seek hospital treatment. Bridgen argues that the voluntary hospitals failed to respond to this demand by providing sufficient accommodation on terms that middle-class patients found acceptable. This meant that when the government proposed to bring the voluntary hospitals under some form of state control during the first half of the 1940s, the hospitals lacked the kind of middle-class support that might have enabled them to maintain their independence.

NOTES

1. See, e.g., Martin Powell and Martin Hewitt, *Welfare state and welfare change*, Buckingham: Open University Press, 2002.
2. See Susannah Morris, "Changing perceptions of philanthropy in the voluntary housing field in nineteenth- and early-twentieth century London," in Thomas Adam, ed., *Philanthropy, patronage and civil society: Experiences from Germany, Great Britain and North America*, Bloomington: Indiana University Press, 2004, pp. 138–78, at p. 140.
3. *Ibid.*, "Organisational innovation in Victorian social housing," *Nonprofit and Voluntary Sector Quarterly*, 31 (2002), 186–206.
4. Norman Johnson, *Mixed economies of welfare: A comparative perspective*, Hemel Hempstead: Prentice Hall, 1999, p. 22.
5. Sheila Kamerman, "The new mixed economy of welfare: Public and private," *Social Work*, 28 (1983), 5–10; Ken Judge and Mike Reddin, "Notes prepared for the 1983 Social Administration Conference on the Mixed Economy of Welfare." Cited in Norman Johnson, *The welfare state in transition: The theory and practice of welfare pluralism*, Brighton: Wheatsheaf, 1987, p. 55.
6. See also Johnson, *The welfare state in transition*, p. 55. The concept of welfare pluralism was also discussed in Peter Beresford and Suzy Croft, "Welfare pluralism: The new face of Fabianism," *Critical Social Policy*, 9 (1984), 19–39.
7. Geoffrey Finlayson, *Citizen, state and social welfare in Britain, 1830–1990*, Oxford: Clarendon Press, 1994, p. 6.
8. Jane Lewis, "The voluntary sector in the mixed economy of welfare," in David Gladstone, ed., *Before Beveridge: Welfare before the welfare state*, London: Institute of Economic Affairs, 1999, pp. 10–17, at p. 11; see also ibid., *The voluntary sector, the state and social work in Britain: The Charity Organisation Society/Family Welfare Association since 1869*, Aldershot: Edward Elgar, 1995, p. 3; "Voluntary and informal welfare," in Robert Page and Richard Silburn, eds., *British social welfare in the twentieth century*, Basingstoke: Palgrave Macmillan, 1999, pp. 249–70, at p. 249.

9. Joanna Innes, "The "mixed economy of welfare in early-modern England: Assessments of the options from Hale to Malthus (*c.* 1683–1803)," in Martin Daunton, ed., *Charity, self-interest and welfare in the English past*, London: UCL Press, 1996, pp. 139–80, at p. 140.
10. Michael Katz and Christoph Sachße, eds., *The mixed economy of social welfare: Public/private relations in England, Germany and the United States, the 1870s to the 1930s*, Baden Baden: Nomos Verlagsgesellschaft, 1996.
11. David R. Green and Alastair Owens, eds., "Introduction: Family welfare and the welfare family," in David R. Green and Alastair Owens, eds., *Family welfare: Gender, property and inheritance since the seventeenth century*, Wesport: Praeger, 2004, pp. 1–30 (see esp. pp. 5–8).
12. See, e.g., Jim Sharpe, "History from below," in Peter Burke, ed., *New perspectives on historical writing*, Oxford: Polity Press, 1991, pp. 24–41. Sharpe argues that the first "serious statement" of the possibility of such an approach was made by Edward Thompson in an article published in the *Times Literary Supplement* in 1966 (see ibid., p. 25).
13. Olwen Hufton, *The poor of eighteenth-century France, 1750–1789*, Oxford: Clarendon Press, 1974.
14. Steve Hindle, *On the parish: The micropolitics of poor relief in rural England, c. 1550–1750*, Oxford: Oxford University Press, 2004, pp. 17–18.
15. Michael Anderson, *Family structure in nineteenth-century Lancashire*, Cambridge: Cambridge University Press, 1971, p. 137; Marguerite Dupree, *Family structure in the Staffordshire Potteries*, Oxford: Oxford University Press, 1995, p. 334; Anne Crowther, "Family responsibility and state responsibility in Britain before the welfare state," *Historical Journal*, 25 (1982), 131–45.
16. Catharina Lis and Hugo Soly, "Neighbourhood social change in west European cities: Sixteenth to nineteenth centuries," *International Review of Social History*, 38 (1993), 1–30, at p. 13.
17. Adele Lindenmeyr, *Poverty is not a vice: Charity, society and the state in Imperial Russia*, Princeton: Princeton University Press, 1996, p. 53.
18. Ellen Ross, "Survival networks: Women's neighbourhood sharing in London before World War 1," *History Workshop Journal*, 15 (1983), 4–27, at pp. 6–8; see also ibid., *Love and toil: Motherhood in outcast London, 1870–1914*, Oxford: Oxford University Press, 1993.
19. Paul Johnson, *Saving and spending: The working-class economy in Britain, 1870–1939*, Oxford: Oxford University Press, 1985, p. 10. See also ibid., "Private and public social welfare in Britain, 1870–1939," in Michael Katz and Christoph Sachße, eds., *The mixed economy of social welfare: Public/private relations in England, Germany and the United States, the 1870s to the 1930s*, Baden-Baden: Nomos Verlagsgesellschaft, 1996, pp. 129–47; "Risk, redistribution and social welfare in Britain from the Poor Law to Beveridge," in Martin Daunton, ed., *Charity, self-interest and welfare in the English past*, London: UCL Press, 1996, pp. 225–48.
20. David Neave, "Friendly societies in Great Britain," in Marcel van der Linden, ed., *Social security mutualism: The comparative history of mutual benefit societies*, Bern: Peter Lang, pp. 41–64, at p. 46; see also Simon Cordery, *British friendly societies, 1750–1914*, Basingstoke: Palgrave, 2003, p. 22.
21. Neave, "Friendly societies in Great Britain," p. 45; Cordery, *British friendly societies*, pp. 24–5. In Paris, "women formed only six per cent of all mutualists in 1848." See Michael Sibalis, "The mutual aid societies of Paris, 1789–1848," *French History*, 3 (1989), pp. 1–30, at p. 12.
22. See, e.g., Cordery, *British friendly societies*.
23. Bernard Harris, *The origins of the British welfare state: Social welfare in England and Wales, 1800–1945*, Basingstoke: Palgrave, 2004, pp. 79–84. There

were also 55 "collecting societies," which were large national organisations specialising in burial insurance. They were responsible for 7,554,266 policies in 1914.

24. Harris, *Origins of the British welfare state*, pp. 84–7.
25. Ibid., pp. 87, 193–5. See also Peter Gosden, *Self-help: Voluntary associations in nineteenth-century Britain*, London: Batsford, 1973; Johnson, *Saving and spending*, esp. Chs. 2, 3, and 5; Eric Hopkins, *Working-class self-help in nineteenth-century England*, London: UCL Press, 1995.
26. Martin Gorsky and John Mohan, with Tim Willis, *Mutualism and health care: British hospital contributory schemes in the twentieth century*, Manchester: Manchester University Press, esp. Ch. 2.
27. Sibalis, "The mutual aid societies of Paris."
28. Allan Mitchell, "The function and malfunction of mutual-aid societies in nineteenth-century France," in Jonathan Barry and Colin Jones, eds., *Medicine and charity before the welfare state*, London: Routledge, 1991, pp. 172–89. See also ibid., *The divided path: The German influence on social reform in France after 1870*, Chapel Hill: University of North Carolina Press, 1991, esp. Ch. 10 (pp. 223–51).
29. Marcel van der Linden, ed., *Social security mutualism: The comparative history of mutual benefit societies*, Bern: Peter Lang, 1996.
30. Alan Baker, *Fraternity among the French peasantry: Sociability and voluntary associations in the Loire valley, 1815–1914*, Cambridge: Cambridge University Press, 1999; George Emery and J. C. Herbert Emery, *A young man's benefit: The Independent Order of Odd Fellows and sickness insurance in the United States and Canada, 1860–1929*, Montreal: McGill-Queen's University Press; David Beito, *From mutual aid to the welfare state: Fraternal societies and social services, 1890–1967*, Chapel Hill: University of North Carolina Press, 2000; David G. Green, *Mutual aid or welfare state: Australia's friendly societies*, London: Allen and Unwin, 1984.
31. Gunnar Stollberg, "*Hilfskassen* in nineteenth-century Germany," in Marcel van der Linden, ed., *Social security mutualism: The comparative history of mutual benefit societies*, Bern: Peter Lang, pp. 309–28, at p. 311.
32. Peter Hennock, *The origin of the welfare state in England and Germany, 1850–1914*, Cambridge: Cambridge University Press, 2007, pp. 151–60, 172–8.
33. Geoffrey Finlayson, "A moving frontier: Voluntarism and the state in British social welfare 1911–1949," *Twentieth Century British History*, 1 (1990), pp. 183–206, at pp. 183–4.
34. See also Brett Fairbairn, "Self-help and philanthropy: The emergence of cooperatives in Britain, Germany, the United States and Canada from mid-nineteenth to mid-twentieth century," in Thomas Adam, ed., *Philanthropy, patronage and civil society: Experiences from Germany, Great Britain and North America*, Bloomington: Indiana University Press, 2004, pp. 55–78; and Daniel Weinbren's contribution to this volume (Ch. 4 below).
35. Cordery, *British friendly societies*, p. 108.
36. Peter Gosden, *The friendly societies in England, 1815–75*, Manchester: Manchester University Press, 1961, pp. 52–5; Hopkins, *Self-help*, p. 15; Cordery, *British friendly societies*, pp. 49–50.
37. Audrey Fisk, *Mutual self-help in southern England, 1850–1912*, Southampton: Foresters' Heritage Trust, 2006, p. 157.
38. Beito, *From mutual aid to the welfare state*, pp. 60–1.
39. Political and Economic Planning, *Report on the British health services: A survey of the existing health services in Great Britain with proposals for future development*, London: Political and Economic Planning, 1937, pp. 234–5.
40. Gorsky and Mohan, *Mutualism and health care*, p. 106.

41. See, e.g., Lawrence Friedman, "Philanthropy in America: Historicism and its discontents," in Lawrence Friedman and Mark McGarvie, eds., *Charity, philanthropy and civility in American history*, Cambridge: Cambridge University Press, 2003, pp. 1–21, at p. 18.
42. Harris, *Origins of the British welfare state*, p. 60; Finlayson, *Citizen, state and social welfare*, pp. 49–52.
43. Frank Prochaska, *Women and philanthropy in nineteenth-century England*, Oxford: Oxford University Press, 1980. See also Lindenmeyr, *Poverty is not a vice*, pp. 125–6; Kathleen D. McCarthy, "Women and political culture," in Lawrence Friedman and Mark McGarvie, eds., *Charity, philanthropy and civility in American history*, Cambridge: Cambridge University Press, 2003, pp. 179–98. The relationship between women and philanthropy is also discussed in Thomas Adam's contribution to this volume (see Ch. 7 below).
44. Harris, *Origins of the British welfare state*, p. 187.
45. Lindenmeyr, *Poverty is not a vice*, p. 132. For the expression of similar sentiments in a British context, see Harris, *Origins of the British welfare state*, p. 62.
46. See, e.g., Alan Kidd, "Civil society or the state: Recent approaches to the history of voluntary welfare," *Journal of Historical Sociology*, 15 (2002), 328–42, esp. pp. 337–8.
47. Stuart Woolf, *The poor in western Europe in the eighteenth and nineteenth centuries*, London: Methuen, pp. 158–97.
48. William B. Cohen, "Epilogue: The European comparison," in Lawrence Friedman and Mark McGarvie, eds., *Charity, philanthropy and civility in American history*, Cambridge: Cambridge University Press, 2003, pp. 385–412, at p. 399.
49. Christoph Sachße, "Public and private in German social welfare: The 1890s to the 1920s," in Michael Katz and Christoph Sachße, eds., *The mixed economy of social welfare: Public/private relations in England, Germany and the United States, the 1870s to the 1930s*, Baden-Baden: Nomos Verlagsgesellschaft, 1996, pp. 148–69, at p. 149.
50. Harris, *Origins of the British welfare state*, pp. 70–1, 189.
51. Robert Bremner, *American philanthropy*, Chicago: University of Chicago Press, 1960, pp. 144–51; David Hammack, "Failure and resilience: Pushing the limits in depression and wartime," in Lawrence Friedman and Mark McGarvie, eds., *Charity, philanthropy and civility in American history*, Cambridge: Cambridge University Press, 2003, pp. 263–80. See also Andrew Morris's contribution to this volume (Ch. 8 below).
52. Lindenmeyr, *Poverty is not a vice*, p. 221.
53. Bremner, *American philanthropy*, pp. 45, 50–3.
54. Harris, *Origins of the British welfare state*, pp. 133–4, 139, 146, 228.
55. Cohen, "Epilogue," p. 403.
56. Lindenmeyr, *Poverty is not a vice*, pp. 229–30.
57. Norman McCord, "The Poor Law and philanthropy," in Derek Fraser, ed., *The new poor law in the nineteenth century*, Basingstoke: Macmillan, 1976, pp. 870–110, at p. 97; Ellen Ross, "Hungry children: Housewives and London charity, 1870–1918," in Peter Mandler, ed., *The uses of charity: The poor on relief in the nineteenth century metropolis*, Philadelphia: University of Pennsylvania Press, 1990, pp. 161–96, at p. 164.
58. The figures compiled by Sampson Low suggest that more than 15 per cent of the money donated to charitable organisations in London in 1861 was used for domestic missionary work, whilst more than 26 per cent of the total sum was donated to organisations associated with missionary work overseas. See Harris, *Origins of the British welfare state*, p. 67.

59. Brian Harrison, "Philanthropy and the Victorians," *Victorian Studies*, 9 (1966), pp. 353–74, at pp. 363–4; Lindenmeyr, *Poverty is not a vice*, pp. 215–7.
60. Frank Prochaska, *The voluntary impulse: Philanthropy in modern Britain*, London: Faber and Faber, 1988, p. 86; ibid., "Philanthropy," in F. M. L. Thompson, ed., *The Cambridge social history of Britain, 1750–1950. Volume 3. Social agencies and institutions*, Cambridge: Cambridge University Press, 1990, pp. 357–94, at p. 357.
61. Peter Lindert, *Growing public: Social spending and economic growth since the eighteenth century*, Cambridge: Cambridge University Press, 2004, pp. 41–4.
62. Harris, *Origins of the British welfare state*, p. 68.
63. Lester Salamon and Helmut Anheier, "In search of the nonprofit sector II. The problem of classification," *Working Papers of the Johns Hopkins Comparative Nonprofit Sector Project*, no. 3, p. 1.
64. Susannah Morris, "Defining the nonprofit sector: Some lessons from history," *Voluntas*, 11 (2000), pp. 25–43, at p. 38; "Changing perceptions," p. 144. See also ibid., "Market solutions for social problems: Working-class housing in nineteenth-century London," *Economic History Review*, 54 (2001), 525–45.
65. Johnson, *Saving and spending*, pp. 16–19.
66. See, e.g., Johnson, *Mixed economies of welfare*, pp. 92–142.
67. Harris, *Origins of the British welfare state*, pp. 40–58, 202–4.
68. T. H. Marshall, "Citizenship and social class," in T. H. Marshall, *Class, citizenship and social development: Essays by T. H. Marshall*, New York: Doubleday, 1964, pp. 65–122, at pp. 72–3.
69. Ibid., pp. 80–1.
70. Harris, *Origins of the British welfare state*, pp. 34–5, 140–7, 157–65, 245–8, 294–7.
71. See, e.g., Lester Salomon and Helmut Anheier, eds., *Defining the nonprofit sector: A cross-national analysis*, Manchester: Manchester University Press, 1997.
72. See Organisation for Economic Cooperation and Development, *Social expenditure database* (www.oecd.org/els/social/expenditure), Paris: OECD, 2004.
73. For a recent survey, see Martin Powell, ed., *Understanding the mixed economy of welfare*, Bristol: Policy Press, 2007.
74. Marcel Mauss, *Essai sur le don. Forme et raison de l'échange dans les sociétés archaïques*, Paris: L'Année Sociologique, 1925. Republished as *The gift: Forms and functions of exchange in archaic societies*, London: Cohen and West, 1954.
75. See Chapter 4 below.
76. See Chapter 5, Table 14.
77. For an introduction to "policy transfer," see, e.g., D. Dolowitz and D. Marsh, "Who learns what from whom? A review of the policy transfer literature," *Political Studies*, 44 (1996), 343–57.
78. See Harris, *Origins of the British welfare state*, pp. 133–4.
79. See also Fairbairn, "Self-help and philanthropy."
80. See, e.g., Martin Gorsky, John Mohan, and Martin Powell, "British voluntary hospitals, 1871–1938: The geography of provision and utilisation," *Journal of Historical Geography*, 25 (1999), 463–82.

2 Charity and Poor Relief in England and Wales, Circa 1750–1914[*]

Bernard Harris

University of Southampton

The last twenty years have witnessed a significant change in the historiography of charity and philanthropy.[1] During the 1970s, Gareth Stedman Jones highlighted the way in which organisations like the Charity Organisation Society attempted to use charity to "remoralise" the London poor, but in the 1980s and 1900s writers such as Geoffrey Finlayson and Frank Prochaska offered a much more sympathetic account of the contribution that charity was able to make to meeting social needs.[2] As a result of this work, historians now have a much more nuanced view of the history of welfare provision. As Jane Lewis argued in 1995, "rather than seeing the story of the modern welfare state as a simple movement from individualism to collectivism . . . it is more accurate to see Britain as always having had a mixed economy of welfare, in which the state, the voluntary sector, the family and the market have played different parts at different points in time."[3]

However, as Lewis herself has recognised, it is not enough simply to describe the different components of this mixed economy; it is also necessary to explore the relationship between them. In her article on "the boundary between voluntary and statutory social service in the late-nineteenth and early-twentieth centuries," she explored the different ways in which supporters of the Charity Organisation Society and the Guilds of Help conceptualised the relationship between voluntary and statutory welfare in the late-Victorian and Edwardian periods.[4] This chapter seeks to extend Lewis's account by examining the relationship between charity and the Poor Law over the whole of the period between 1750 and 1914. It begins by examining the role played by charity in critiques of the Old Poor Law between 1750 and 1834. It then explores the contribution that charity made to the relief of poverty between 1834 and 1870. The final section shows how the relationship between charity and state welfare changed during the "Crusade against

---

[*]I should like to thank Paul Bridgen and Samantha Shave for some extremely helpful comments.

Outdoor Relief" and the subsequent expansion of state welfare provision between 1870 and 1914.

THE CAMPAIGN FOR POOR LAW REFORM

As Paul Slack has shown, both charity and the poor law played significant roles in the provision of social welfare in early-modern Britain. The amounts of money given by testators for the relief of the poor rose substantially between 1540 and 1660, and these bequests were augmented during the late-seventeenth and eighteenth centuries by the growth of subscriber charities, which played a key role in the development of schools and hospitals.[5] However, the provision of welfare by individuals and charities existed alongside an expanding system of public relief. The Poor Law Acts of 1597 and 1601 gave the churchwardens and overseers of each parish the right to levy a tax, or poor rate, on every inhabitant and occupier of land and made them responsible for "setting the poor on work," maintaining those who were unable to work, and securing apprenticeships for pauper children. The cost of this system grew rapidly during the second half of the eighteenth century, and this helped to fuel demands for its reform and, in some cases, abolition.[6]

One of the reformers' main complaints was that the existing system of poor relief meant that "men labour less and spend more, and the very system that provides for the poor, makes poor."[7] In 1786, the Rector of Pewsey, Joseph Townsend, argued that the Poor Laws weakened hope and destroyed fear—"the springs of industry"—because the poor knew that, if they worked hard, their efforts would be used to support others, whereas if they relied on others, "they shall be abundantly supplied, not only with food and raiment, but with their accustomed luxuries, at the expense of others."[8] Other writers shared these sentiments. John Davison argued that "the Poor Laws tell a man [that] he shall not be responsible for his want of exertion, forethought [or] sobriety,"[9] and James Geldart complained that "no encouragement is held out to industry, sobriety or good behaviour."[10] James Ridgway thought that the Poor Laws had fuelled the fires of unrest by taking away "the incitement to industry and good behaviour—the necessity of providing against occasional misfortune and old age, as well as the desire of making a provision for the support of a future family, has been removed."[11]

These critics were not simply concerned with the impact of the Poor Law on work incentives; they also felt that the provision of statutory relief undermined the proper relationship between poor relief and charity. In 1633, the poet and divine, George Herbert, argued that even though the wealthy should always be willing to give charity, the poor did not have an automatic right to receive it. This meant that charity should only be dispensed with discretion, which in turn would help to promote social order.[12] The expansion of poor relief threatened to undermine this position because it encouraged the poor to believe that their right to relief was no longer conditional on good behaviour. As Thomas Alcock complained in 1752: "The pauper thanks not me for anything he receives. He has a right to it, so he says, by law, and if I won't give, he'll go to the Justice and compel me. . . . This must of course create a good deal of ill-blood, hatred, murmuring and indignation on the side of the payer . . . and . . . still more disrespect, ingratitude and contempt on the part of the pauper."[13]

Alcock was not the only contemporary observer who believed that the creation of an "entitlement to welfare" weakened the natural bonds of society. Joseph Townsend argued that "a fixed, a certain, and a constant . . . provision for the poor . . . tends to destroy the harmony and beauty, the symmetry and order of that system, which God and nature have established in the world,"[14] and Frederic Morton Eden concluded that "the certainty of a legal provision weakens the principles of natural affection, and destroys one of the strongest ties of society, by rendering the exercise of domestic and social duties less necessary."[15] John Davison linked his concerns to the specific question of wage supplementation: "the labourer reckons half with his master and half with the overseer. Towards his master he has neither the zeal nor the attachment he ought to have to his natural patron and friend; and with his parish he keeps up a dependence which . . . [is] at once abject and insolent."[16]

Although these critics were particularly concerned with the impact of statutory relief on the morals of the recipient, they also thought that it was harmful to the giver. Thomas Alcock believed that the imposition of a compulsory levy tended to "crowd out" voluntary charity because "I'm obliged to pay so much to the poor by law, that I am not of ability to bestow in voluntary contributions," and he went on to express concern that "this checks and weakens the charitable principle within; and this principle, by not being exercised . . . grows weaker and weaker, and, in time, perhaps, is quite extinguished."[17] However, not all authors shared this pessimism. Frederic Eden, writing four decades later, thought that "the numerous appeals, even from impostors, which are made to the feelings of the humane and charitable, are a sufficient proof that voluntary charity flows in too copious a stream . . . if there is a defect in British benevolence, it is, that it is too unbounded and indiscriminate."[18]

Despite these differences, most commentators agreed that there was more virtue in voluntary charity than there was in a compulsory levy. Alcock argued that "all virtue must be free; if you force charity [*sic*], you destroy her," and that "as charity is said to cover a multitude of sins, a Christian by being forced to it, may think himself deprived of the blessing of it."[19] Eden quoted Edmund Burke's comments on the Church in support of his view that "it is better to cherish virtue and humanity, by leaving much to free will . . . than to attempt to make men mere machines and instruments of a political benevolence,"[20] and John Davison concluded that "the rich have been great losers, on their side, by the general substitution of a legal impost, for the natural cultivation of their own living, active and discriminating virtue."[21] The Scottish Evangelical Thomas Chalmers expressed a similar view when he claimed that the tenderness and delicacy of charity "have been put to flight by this metamorphosis of a matter of love" into one of "angry litigation."[22]

In view of these sentiments, it is not surprising that many contemporaries believed that charity could play an important role in helping to "lift" poor people off what might now be regarded as their "dependency" on poor relief. During the 1790s, Arthur Young published a series of accounts of charitable relief schemes in the *Annals of Agriculture*. John Critchley described a scheme which had been introduced in Rutland in 1785 to "promot[e] industry amongst the children of the labourers." The scheme was financed by a combination of parish payments and individual subscriptions and provided work opportunities to the children of poor families. The children who "produced the greatest quantity of work, of different kinds, and of the best quality" received small premiums, and premiums were also offered to young people who entered apprenticeships or went into service, and to day-labourers who had brought up four or more children ("born in wedlock") to the age of fourteen years without recourse to the parish.[23] A rather different scheme was introduced in the parish of Long Newton in 1800. This scheme offered 32 families the opportunity to become tenant farmers in return for an agreement to forego any future entitlement to poor relief. If a family was obliged to apply for relief (other than medical relief), the tenancy was forfeited.[24]

Although these schemes were designed, in part, to supplement the Poor Law, many writers argued that the scope of poor relief should either be restricted, or curtailed altogether, and replaced by voluntary provision. John Davison thought that the Poor Law should be gradually reduced, so that by the end of ten years "there would be a legal revenue for the support of the aged and infirm," and a voluntary fund for the relief of all other kinds of need, although he conceded that some form of statutory relief may still be necessary in "certain definite cases of severer distress."[25] Joseph Townsend went further. In 1786, he called for the poor law to be abolished altogether over a ten-year period and concluded that "to relieve the poor by voluntary donations is not only most wise, politic and just; is not only most agreeable both to reason and to revelation; but . . . is most effectual in preventing misery, and most excellent in itself, as cherishing . . . the most amiable affections of the human breast."[26]

As these extracts have demonstrated, there was substantial support for the view that there was a fundamental difference between the "forced" charity of the poor law and the voluntary charity of private philanthropy, and it is clear that many contemporaries believed that the balance between them needed to be readjusted, in favour of the latter. However, others believed that some form of public welfare provision was essential, partly because of the practical obstacles that stood in the way of complete abolition and partly because there was no guarantee that a purely voluntary system of social welfare would necessarily be fairer. In 1795, Capel Lofft argued that charity "is too precarious for the extent and importance of the object,"[27] and Jeremy Bentham observed that charity "is formed entirely at the expense of the most humane, of the most virtuous individuals in the society, often without proportion to their means."[28] The anonymous editor of the second edition of Joseph Townsend's *Dissertation on the Poor Laws* thought that nothing "could be more unwise . . . than to withdraw within so short a period as . . . *ten* years, the whole provision on which millions now depend for subsistence."[29] This was possibly one of the most important reasons why, when the Royal Commission on the Poor Law sat down to begin its investigations in February 1832, it focused its efforts on the reform of the poor law, rather than its abolition.[30]

CHARITY UNDER THE NEW POOR LAW

Although the Poor Law Amendment Act did not abolish poor relief, it was designed to restrict it, and this had significant implications for the role of charity, especially in urban areas where the introduction of the New Poor Law had faced initial resistance. The increased role played by charity in the relief of poverty has not always received the attention it deserves in debates about the introduction of the New Poor Law,[31] but its significance has emerged quite strongly in a number of local studies.

It would certainly be wrong to assume that the advent of the New Poor Law led automatically to an increase in charitable subventions. According to William Apfel and Peter Dunkley, the Assistant Poor Law Commissioner for Bedfordshire, D. G. Adey, "was unusually conscientious in scrutinising parish accounts, and by 1837 he felt able to assure Somerset House that the parochial use of 'private subscriptions' to circumvent the financial demands of the Boards of Guardians was no longer to be found in the county."[32] However, there is considerable evidence to suggest that the introduction of new restrictions on the distribution of poor relief did lead to the increased use of charitable resources in other parts of the country.

In Carlisle, the Poor Law Commission began the process of introducing the New Poor Law in the late 1830s, but the new regime faced its first real test when recession hit the town's textile industry in the spring of 1840. Four hundred and fifty weavers were placed on short-time work, and the Guardians saw little alternative but to revert to the traditional policy of subsidising the weavers' reduced wages from the poor rate. However, the Assistant Commissioner for Cumbria, Sir John Walsham, persuaded the Board to abandon this policy in favour of a stricter application of the "principles of 1834." Although the workhouse test was not applied formally, applicants for relief had to submit to an outdoor labour test, and relief was only granted to men who were wholly unemployed.

As R. N. Thompson has pointed out, this policy may have achieved the desired effect of reducing the poor rate, but only at the expense of increasing the hardship experienced by the weavers and their families. In the autumn of 1841, a detailed survey was carried out and this led to the establishment of a local mendicancy society "with the purpose of raising a subscription from the public, and distributing the proceeds to the needy." There was little common membership between the Board of Guardians and the mendicancy society but they were both drawn from the same local elite, and a joint committee was set up "to plan and coordinate their respective spheres of activity."[33]

Although Thompson argued that the establishment of the mendicancy society, and that of similar committees formed in Carlisle in the 1850s and 1860s, "represented a spontaneous but conscious effort by the local community to evade the restrictions of the official poor relief policy," it was not inconsistent with the aims of some of the early Poor Law reformers.[34] Although the Poor Law authorities were obliged to give relief to all those who met their "test of destitution," the mendicancy society was able to award relief to applicants on the basis that they were either "deserving" or "undeserving."[35] This was precisely the kind of discretionary approach to the relief of poverty that the critics of the Old Poor Law had been seeking to encourage when they advocated an enhanced role for charity before 1834.

Although the Poor Law Amendment Act was designed to lay the foundations for the development of a more uniform set of relief policies throughout England and Wales, it failed to give the Poor Law Commissioners a clear set of powers in relation to those areas that were already covered by local acts. One such area was Coventry, in the east Midlands, which received considerable amounts of advice and pressure from the central Commissioners but was not directly controlled by them. However, the city was brought under the authority of the Commission in 1842, and by 1844 "the united parishes had been brought as firmly under the control of the Poor Law Commission as any ordinary union."[36] The establishment of the new regime was accompanied by the virtual elimination of the payment of wage subsidies and a significant reduction in the number of families receiving poor relief.

The impact of the New Poor Law in Coventry meant that a greater burden was now placed on the provision of charitable relief. According to Peter Searby, "as the amount spent on statutory relief fell, the charities became relatively more important still. In no year between 1847 and 1860 did the cost of statutory outdoor relief reach £2000, and in 1853 it amounted to £800 only, while the most effective dole charities—the five controlled by the general charities trustees—alone disposed of £550 a year."[37] These sums were supplemented by special appeals during periods of particular need. More than £1000 was raised in the winter of 1847–8, and similar amounts were distributed in 1855 and the winter of 1857–8. However, when the city's weavers went on strike in protest against planned cuts in wages in the spring of 1860, only £390 was forthcoming.[38]

As Searby has pointed out, the much smaller amounts of money that were donated in the spring of 1860 illustrated the limits of mid-Victorian paternalism, but the relief funds were reopened in the autumn, after wages had been cut and the strike defeated. On this occasion, local funds proved quite inadequate and a national appeal was launched. This new appeal raised over £41,000, including donations from the Queen and from schools all over the country, but the funds were largely exhausted by the spring of 1862, and a second appeal had to be issued. This appeal raised a further £11,800, and the money was spent during the winter of 1862–3.[39]

Charity also played a critical role in the relief of distress in the Lancashire cotton districts. H. M. Boot found that "the average lag between becoming unemployed and receiving [poor] relief" in the late 1840s "was as long as six weeks" and that many individuals must have held out for much longer. He argued that their ability to do so "attests to the depth of private and communal resources they could resort to in times of distress, their hostility to the poor law, and the depth of poverty reached before they obtained relief from the poor law authorities."[40] Lynne Kiesling drew similar conclusions from her study of the relationship between unemployment and poor relief in the same areas during the cotton famine of the early 1860s: "The creation of local private relief committees . . . enabled many unemployed workers to avoid public relief entirely. . . . [Although] the private relief committees did not begin giving relief until mid-1862, [b]y early-1863 their expenditure . . . far outpaced public expenditure, reflecting both supply and demand constraints."[41]

In fact, Kiesling's account may be slightly misleading. On 12 May 1862, the Poor Law Board instructed H. B. Farnall to visit the cotton districts in order to ascertain "the manner and form in which the poor are either relieved out of the poor rates, or . . . by private subscriptions," and he compiled a series of reports over the next six weeks. Special relief funds had already been set up in Preston, Blackburn, and Ashton, and more than £10,000 had been distributed by the time of his visit; he also noted that a further £2888 had been distributed in the borough of Stockport (encompassing the townships of Stockport, Heaton Norris, Brinnington, Cheadle Bulkeley, and Cheadle Moseley) and that £45 had been distributed in the township of Hyde within the previous week.[42] In December 1862, when the total number of paupers throughout the cotton district reached its peak, 271,983 individuals (out of a combined population of 1,984,955) were dependent on statutory relief, and a further 236,310 people received assistance from local charity committees. The amount expended by the local Boards of Guardians on outdoor relief during the week ending 6 December 1862 was £18,728, whereas the amount expended by local charity committees in the week ending 27 December was £24,743.[43]

These accounts suggest that charity was likely to play a particularly important role in the relief of poverty during periods of exceptional hardship, but how significant was charity during "normal" periods? Derek Fraser argued that "the Poor Law was catering for only a minor part of the demonstrable need in Victorian England,"[44] and Ellen Ross has claimed that "in the 1870s, eleemosynary contributions were greater by far the whole national expenditure on poor relief."[45] Norman McCord also claimed that despite the problems involved in estimating the extent of charitable donations, "it is very clear that unofficial far outweighed official exertion."[46] However, these statements assume that even if the poor law authorities and charity organisations were not necessarily relieving the same people, they were directed towards the same ends. As Robert Humphreys argued in 1995, "If reference to the charitable generosity of the Victorians includes the vast amounts of capital used to build the public edifices that mushroomed in nineteenth-century Britain, this would have little bearing on the provision of direct financial relief to the poor in the sense of providing an alternative to poor law outdoor doles."[47]

One of the most intractable problems facing the historian who wishes to estimate the extent of charitable support in the nineteenth century is the fact that a great deal of charitable activity took place on an informal basis and was unlikely to be recorded. This is particularly true of what several authors have described as the "charity of the poor to the poor"[48] but may also have been true of other kinds of charity as well. During the 1890s and early 1900s, Jack Lanigan and his brother obtained a bowl of soup and a chunk of bread every day for lunch from the local police station, and Alice Foley recalled how the local priest, Canon Burke, "stuffed some food tickets" into her sister's hands "to help tide the family over a cruel Christmas."[49] It is very difficult to know the extent to which incidents of this kind are likely to have found their way into the tables of official charity statistics.

Instead of examining the records left by charity organisations and committees, some authors have attempted to use household budget surveys to assess the extent to which working-class families supplemented their incomes with charitable donations, but this evidence is also difficult to interpret. In 1887, the Paddington District Nursing Association examined the household budgets of 923 families in which a main earner was ill, but only a few were surviving on charitable donations, and the authors of a second survey, focusing on the families of unemployed men in the same year, found that only one household in eight was receiving assistance from the parish, benefit club, or charitable relief. However, as Ellen Ross has pointed out, such surveys are very likely to underestimate the extent to which poor families were receiving charitable assistance: "Investigators normally asked only about earnings in the form of wages, but charities . . . generally doled out goods in kind."[50]

One contemporary investigator who did attempt to estimate the extent of charitable provision was Charles Booth. In 1892 he published the results of an enquiry into the incomes of 9125 people over the age of sixty-five living in 262 rural parishes across the country. He found that 2008 individuals received some support from the Poor Law and that 2304 were either partly or wholly dependent on their relatives, but the extent of charitable support should not be underestimated. Even though only 112 individuals (1.3%) were wholly dependent on charity, a further 1552 (17%) used charity to supplement the income they obtained from other sources (see Table 2.1).[51]

In 1838, James Whishaw published a brief account of the characteristics of the endowed charities of Cornwall in the *Journal of the London Statistical Society*. The total number of such charities was 240, with a combined income (in 1836) of £3661 2s 9d. Whishaw calculated that just under half the total amount raised was given to charities for the benefit of "the poor." This included £510 for the "poor not receiving relief," £523 for the "poor generally," £435 for almshouses, and £352 as a contribution to the poor rate.

Table 2.1 Sources of Maintenance Among Elderly People in 262 Rural Parishes in 1892

	Number	*Percentage*
Parish only	458	5.02
Parish and charity	469	5.14
Parish and relations	462	5.06
Parish, charity, and relations	293	3.21
Parish and earnings	326	3.57
Charity only	112	1.23
Charity and relations	256	2.81
Charity and earnings	406	4.45
Charity, relations, and earnings	128	1.40
Relations only	486	5.33
Relations and earnings	369	4.04
Relations and means	211	2.31
Relations, earnings, and means	99	1.08
Earnings only	2224	24.37
Earnings and means	692	7.58
Means only	2134	23.39
Total	9125	100.00

Source: Charles Booth, *The aged poor in England and Wales*, London: Macmillan, 1894, p. 339.

Many of these charities failed to discriminate between the different categories of poor person and distributed relief in cash and in kind, but others specified that assistance should only be given to "poor labourers," the "deserving poor," "poor widows," the "poor of good character," and the "industrious poor," and offered assistance in the form of bread or clothing.[52]

Whishaw published a second paper, on the endowed charities of Herefordshire, in the following year. In 1836, there were 730 charities in Herefordshire, with a combined income of £13,153 3s 6d. The breakdown of expenditure was similar to that of Cornwall, but there were some differences. In Cornwall, 13.94 per cent of total income was used to support the "poor not receiving relief" and 14.29 per cent went to charities which supported the "poor generally," but in Herefordshire only 3.95 per cent of total income was used to support the "poor not receiving relief" and 33.18 per cent went to charities which supported the "poor generally," whilst only 0.37 per cent was used to subsidise the poor rates. However, the biggest differences were those between charities in the city of Hereford and those elsewhere in the county. In 1836, only 1.36 per cent of the money granted to charities in the city of Hereford was used to support the "poor not receiving relief" and a further 12.72 per cent was used to support the "poor generally," but more than 60 per cent of total income was used to support the city's eleven almshouses and hospitals (see Table 2.2).[53]

It is interesting to compare these figures with those obtained from other urban areas later in the century. Martin Gorsky's account of the history of the formation of Bristol's charities suggests that an increasing proportion of the charities formed from the 1830s onwards were concerned with moral and religious reform, but his figures also demonstrate the problems associated with any attempt to place individual charities within clearly defined boundaries. For example, Gorsky listed "Dorcas societies" under the general heading of "health," but they were also concerned with the relief of poverty and often had a strong religious purpose.[54] Similar arguments could be made about the large number of soup kitchens and similar activities provided by organisations such as the Salvation Army at the end of the nineteenth century. Although these organisations were primarily interested in saving people's souls, they also provided a wide range of social services, including visiting societies, provident funds, soup kitchens, mothers' meetings, coal and clothing clubs, blanket societies, infants' friends societies, penny banks, and maternity groups, which were directly concerned with people's material needs.[55]

Robin Dryburgh has recently examined the role played by charity in the relief of poverty in Bolton in the mid-nineteenth century. His account focuses on the town's endowed and associated (or subscription) charities, and he concludes that these organisations played a very minor role in the relief of poverty over the period as a whole, even though they made a much larger contribution during periods of particular distress. However, he also recognises that his estimates of charitable expenditure take little account of

Table 2.2 Incomes of the Endowed Charities of Cornwall and Herefordshire (Including the City of Hereford) in 1836

	Cornwall		Hereford (City)		Herefordshire (All)	
	£	Percentage	£	Percentage	£	Percentage
Schools and other purposes connected with education	982.61	26.84	140.59	6.82	3528.61	26.83
Poor not receiving relief	510.21	13.94	27.93	1.36	519.33	3.95
Poor generally	523.35	14.29	262.19	12.72	4364.87	33.18
Almshouses and hospitals[a]	434.94	11.88	1277.23	61.97	3771.35	28.67
Horwell's charity[b]	147.87	4.04	0.00	0.00	0.00	0.00
Apprenticing	52.00	1.42	83.03	4.03	310.97	2.36
Clergymen (for preaching sermons on particular days)	41.62	1.14	1.05	0.05	55.85	0.42
Repairs of churches (and otherwise in support of church rates)	608.20	16.61	15.80	0.77	117.04	0.89
Poor rates	352.13	9.62	0.00	0.00	49.20	0.37
Miscellaneous	8.21	0.22	253.21	12.29	435.96	3.31
Total	3661.14	100.00	2061.04	100.00	13,153.18	100.00

[a]In Cornwall, "the number of poor who are wholly or in part maintained in almshouses . . . is 63. They are generally selected from that class of indigent persons who contrive to support themselves without assistance from the parish rates." In Herefordshire, "170 poor persons are wholly or in part maintained and clothed in the endowed almshouses of this county." The total for Herefordshire included both almshouses and hospitals, but no bequests were made to endowed charities for hospitals in Cornwall.

[b]This charity received a total of £147 17s 4d "for maintaining and clothing . . . six poor boys." It also received £19 16s to pay for the cost of employing a schoolmaster to teach the boys reading, writing, and arithmetic and a further £25 as a contribution to their apprenticeship costs. The last two sums are shown under separate headings in the table.

Sources: James Whishaw, "Endowed charities in Cornwall," *Journal of the Statistical Society of London*, vol. 1, no. 3 (July, 1838), pp. 149–53, at pp. 151–2; ibid., "An account of the endowed charities in Herefordshire," *Journal of the Statistical Society of London*, vol. 2, no. 4 (July, 1839), pp. 234–50, at pp. 234–5, 240.

the "unknowable amount of private alms-giving," and that Bolton may not have been typical of other parts of the country. His conclusions on this point are similar to those reached by Keith Gregson in his study of charitable activity in the north-east of England later in the century.[56]

Some of the most detailed records on charitable income and expenditure come from London in the 1850s and 1860s. In 1862, Sampson Low Jr. published details of 640 metropolitan charities with a combined income from dividends and voluntary contributions of just over £2.4 million. His figures suggest that 15 per cent of total income was associated with charities that were primarily concerned with medical services, 10 per cent with benevolent pension funds and the relief of professional groups, and 11 per cent with education and children. However, the two largest categories were both associated with different forms of missionary work: 15.09 per cent of all funds belonged to charities that were engaged in domestic missionary work, and 26.06 per cent with charities engaged in missionary work overseas. Similar findings were also reported by George Hicks when he analysed the records of 364 London charities seven years later.[57]

These figures underline the importance of Humphreys's warnings about the need to avoid facile comparisons between the sums raised by voluntary charities and those distributed by the Poor Law, but it would also be wrong to underestimate the extent to which charity was being used to address genuine social needs. In 1869, Hicks commented that "it will not pass unobserved . . . that the names of some of our charities seem to speak for themselves of the inefficiency of the Poor Law. . . . Such, for instance, as those for homeless men, houseless men, refuges for the destitute, and others." Even though these organisations only accounted for a relatively small proportion of total charitable revenue, this did not prevent him from concluding that "there will always be large scope for individual charity [outside the Poor Law], but at present, the public, instead of supplementing . . . the Poor Law . . . is doing the work of the Poor Law itself."[58]

It is also important to recognise that neither Hicks nor Low believed that the analyses were exhaustive. When Low published the first edition of his survey in 1850, he explained that "this summary does not include local charities, or the charities in the gift of the corporate companies, etc.,"[59] and Hicks explained that "the prevailing absence of uniformity" and the "many highly-objectionable ways of preparing their balance sheets" meant that the records of many charitable organisations "[lacked] the value which would otherwise belong to them."[60] In 1869, Thomas Hawksley attempted to overcome these deficiencies by conducting his own analysis of the capital's charitable organisations. He estimated that the total income of the city's registered charities was £5.3 million, of which £4 million was spent in the capital itself. Approximately £630,000 was spent by charities concerned with the relief of disease, £1.7 million on "the ordinary necessaries of life," and a similar amount on "educational, moral and religious purposes." However, he also argued that these figures failed to take account of what he called "the benefactions of the charitable and the religious," the donations made by "the compassionate, the weak-minded and the thoughtless," the funds distributed by the Mendicity Society, those authorised by magistrates' courts, and those distributed by local and parochial funds. When these figures were added to the equation, he estimated that the total value of the funds distributed within the capital was at least £5.6 million.[61]

THE IDEOLOGY OF CHARITY IN
THE LATER-NINETEENTH CENTURY

Although George Hicks believed that charities were "doing the work of the Poor Law," this did not mean that mid-Victorian philanthropists wanted the state to relieve them of their responsibilities. As Sampson Low argued in 1862, those who "look upon charity merely as an economical resource, and who conceive that it ought to be dispensed with in favour of rates of shillings and pence in the pound" were "forgetting that this would destroy all opportunity for generous impulse and active faith, without ensuring the exercise of one whit more judgement."[62] Even the Charity Organisation Society believed that "no Christian society can exist unless there is a sphere for mutual sympathy, and mutual love, as well as justice."[63]

However, it was one thing to argue that charity should provide an opportunity for the exercise of judgement and discretion; another to believe that these qualities were being reflected in the way in which charity was currently being dispensed. During the 1860s, there was increasing disquiet about the "unsystematic and indiscriminate way" in which many charities operated, and a growing army of critics complained that the proliferation of charities was creating a new form of "welfare dependence."[64] In the first place, they complained that too many charities (and too many individuals) were dispensing charity without proper investigation or judgement; and, second, that their failure to coordinate their efforts with other charities led to unacceptable levels of what Lynn Lees has called "double- or even triple-dipping."[65]

These ideas were reflected in the development of a number of organisations designed to render charity more discriminating and more effective. These organisations included the Society for the Relief of Distress, founded in London in 1860; the Liverpool Central Relief Society (1863); and the Society for Improving the Condition of the Poor in Edinburgh, in 1867. However, the most important organisation was the Society for Organising Charity and Repressing Mendicity, or Charity Organisation Society, which was founded in London in 1869.[66]

As its full title suggests, the COS was concerned both to organise charity and to "repress mendicity." It established a network of District Committees, which, as David Owen has explained, were designed to be broadly coterminous with the capital's Poor Law Unions. Within each district, the Society aimed to coordinate the work of local charities and to ensure that no applicants received relief until their circumstances had been thoroughly investigated.[67] It also laid down strict conditions for the granting of relief. Applicants were only considered eligible if they were "doing all they can to help themselves" and if they were the kind of people for whom "temporary assistance is likely to prove a lasting benefit." Persons "who have thrown themselves out of employment through their own fault ought not to count upon being helped by charity," and those "of drunken, immoral or idle habits" should only expect to receive assistance if "they can satisfy the Committee that they are really trying to reform."[68]

The Society also aspired to play a key role in coordinating the relationship between charities and the Poor Law. In November 1869, the President of the Poor Law Board, George Goschen, issued a famous "Minute" in which he claimed that there had been a considerable increase in the number of outdoor paupers in London, and that this increase had been particularly marked in areas where charities were also known to operate. He argued that the "indiscriminate distribution of charitable funds" tended to increase, rather than decrease, the demand for public relief and that "it appears to be a matter of essential importance . . . to bring the authorities administering the Poor Laws and those who administer charitable funds to as clear an understanding as possible, so as to avoid the double distribution of relief to the same persons, and . . . secure . . . the most effective use . . . of the large sums habitually contributed by the public towards relieving such cases as the Poor Law can scarcely reach."[69]

Goschen believed that there ought to be a much stricter division of labour between the Poor Law and private charity. He argued that the Poor Law authorities should confine their attention to the relief of destitution, for which they had a legal responsibility, and that charities should confine their attention to the relief of those who were not already destitute. He also argued that there was no justification for charitable organisations to assist those who were already receiving poor relief, since the Poor Law authorities were obliged to ensure that the relief which they provided was itself "adequate." If charities did wish to "interpose" in such cases, "they should confine their assistance to donations of bedding and clothing, or any similar articles which the Guardians may not consider themselves bound to provide . . . and which can be easily distinguished from other relief."[70]

Although the responsibilities of the Poor Law Board were transferred to the Local Government Board in 1871, the Goschen Minute helped to lay the foundations for a more far-reaching change in Poor Law policy during the 1870s. In December 1871, the Local Government Board issued a circular (no. 20) prohibiting the distribution of outdoor relief to single able-bodied men and women, to women whose husbands had deserted them for less than twelve months, and to able-bodied widows with only a single dependent child. It said that outdoor relief should only be given to applicants after they had been visited by a relieving officer, and should be granted for no more than three months. The introduction of this "crusade" against outdoor relief led to a sharp reduction in the number of people receiving poor relief outside the workhouse. Between 1871 and 1880, the total number of "outdoor paupers" fell by more than 268,000, and the number of adult women and children (excluding "lunatics, insane persons and idiots") receiving outdoor relief fell by nearly 218,000.[71]

During the 1870s, branches of the Charity Organisation Society were set up in many parts of Britain, and in other cases local "charity organisation societies" were established that "corresponded" with the London society whilst remaining independent of it.[72] These organisations have often been cited as evidence of the popularity of COS thinking during this period. However, other writers have highlighted the tensions which existed between the London society and its provincial offshoots and the limited extent to which they were able to exercise a dominant influence on the development of both local charities and Poor Law policy.[73]

One of the main ways in which the COS sought to increase its influence was by campaigning actively to ensure that its supporters were elected as members of local Boards of Guardians. In 1875, a branch of the COS was set up in Southampton by a local Poor Law medical officer, Dr Richard Griffin, who claimed that the way in which the Poor Law was administered by the Southampton Board of Guardians meant that it was little more than a "system of pauper breeding."[74] During the next few years, a deputy president of the Southampton COS, George Lungley, was elected to chair the local Board of Guardians, and John Hill, a COS member, held the post of relieving officer from 1877 to 1890. These appointments helped the COS to become "the strongest force for strict Poor Law enforcement" in the city during this period.[75]

However, although the COS achieved some success in its efforts to change the broad direction of Poor Law policy in areas such as Southampton, it failed to achieve the closer working relationship that was an integral part of national COS policy. In Oxford, although the local Board of Guardians shared the Society's commitment to the crusade against outdoor relief, "it took about ten years to develop much liaison between the two agencies involving more than a semblance of coordinated action but even this was never 'formulated'."[76] In South Shields, there appears to have been "no vital cooperation between the Society and the Guardians and the numerous regional poor law sources . . . provide no evidence of such activity," and the Reverend Campion Mackgill of Croydon COS "did not see 'much chance of our Society working with the Board of Guardians'."[77] Although there were some examples of closer cooperation, they were comparatively rare. In West Hartlepool, the two organisations worked closely with each other during the 1890s, and in 1908 the Guardians agreed to make a contribution to the Society's funds, but there was little evidence to suggest that this degree of cooperation was replicated elsewhere in the north-east.[78]

The Society's efforts to forge closer links with Boards of Guardians were hampered by its failure to establish stronger ties with other charities.

Brighton's Charity Organisation Society regularly bemoaned its "failure to convert the town's charities," and in 1886 it was forced to admit that "the work of the Society is still only in its infancy." In 1890 an editorial in the local newspaper concluded that the Leamington Spa COS was "still decidedly unpopular and probably not even the Vigilance Association excites a more general sentiment of mistrust." In Oxford, members of the COS were confident that the "frightful condition of the population" could be improved if their principles "were more acted upon," but their meetings "failed to call forth much interest" and were "thinly attended." Reading's Charity Organisation Society faced persistent financial problems and complained of "some misunderstanding" with regard to the nature of its work.[79]

The Society's comparative isolation was particularly apparent during periods of economic crisis. In Manchester, "the willingness of a significant section of the middle class to give generously and unquestioningly at times of crisis seriously undermined the attempt of the poor law authorities and the charity organisers to restrict and contain relief-giving," and the Wood Street Mission attracted particular criticism when it opened its doors to homeless unemployed men in the winter of 1902–3.[80] These complaints echoed the criticisms that the secretary of the London Charity Organisation Society, Charles Stewart Loch, had aimed at the organisers of the Mansion House appeal in London in 1886: "Here, then, Society at large with a fund of £78,000 in its hand, became a panic-stricken pauperiser . . . able . . . to undo in a few weeks 'the quiet work of years'."[81]

One of the main reasons why the COS failed to achieve more prominence within the charitable sector was the contrast between its emphasis on the "scientific" nature of charity and the emphasis that others placed on its spontaneity. Charles Loch recognised that "the words Charity and Organisation" might appear to be "a contradiction in terms"[82] but the COS was unable to overcome the hostility that this contradiction often evoked. The "influential" Reverend Albert Wilberforce told a Poor Law conference in Southampton that even though he sympathised with the Society's aims, he "could hardly regard distress in the light in which it had been viewed by other speakers,"[83] and a Birkenhead clergyman doubted whether it would ever be possible for "heaven-born charity to pass through the rolling, pressing, squeezing, drying process of a vast piece of machinery and still preserve some of the aroma and flavour of its divine origin."[84] There are at least some similarities between these views and the sentiments expressed by the vice-chairman of the Newcastle Board of Guardians, William Todd, a few years earlier. Although he shared the COS's view that many charities were poorly managed and "a source of evil," he also recognised that "the moment you add organisation to [charity] . . . its lustre . . . light and life are gone." He therefore concluded that the only appropriate policy was to "leave it to its gladdening destiny, to cherish and comfort the deserving poor."[85]

COS traditionalists also found themselves increasingly isolated by changes in public welfare provision. Ironically, one of the first examples of this was triggered by legislation passed only a year after the Goschen Minute was issued and a year before the "Crusade against Outdoor Relief" was formally launched. When the Forster Education Act was passed in 1870, School Boards were given the power to make education compulsory for children between the ages of five and ten in the areas they served, but many parents were unable to afford the fees that the new schools charged. This meant that the school boards were forced to remit the fees charged to the children of parents on low incomes, but even though fee remission could be seen as a form of state benefit, it was provided outside the framework of the Poor Law and the parents were spared the disabilities that Poor Law provision would have implied.[86]

The arrangements for remitting school fees were not the only way in which changes in social policy affected the relationship between the state and the individual. When Parliament passed the Poor Law Amendment Act in 1834, it was primarily concerned with the payment of poor relief and the situation of the able-bodied male pauper, and had largely neglected the provision of medical relief, even though this had been an important part of the Old Poor Law.[87] However, in 1867 Parliament established a separate administrative authority—the Metropolitan Asylums Board—to oversee the development of Poor Law medical services in London, and in 1871 the board took an important step towards the creation of a public medical service when it agreed to admit nonpauper patients to the hospitals under its control. This provided an important precedent for the Medical Relief (Disqualifications Removal) Act of 1885, which meant that individuals who received medical assistance from the Poor Law's medical services were no longer subject to the same legal penalties that prevented the recipients of nonmedical poor relief from voting in parliamentary elections.[88]

These changes were primarily concerned with the funding of education and the provision of health care, but the period also witnessed changes in attitudes to the relief of poverty itself. The Charity Organisation Society had argued that individuals who were in need of assistance but outside the scope of the Poor Law should be supported by charity, but there was a growing demand for this assistance to be provided, or at least supported, by the state. In 1886, the president of the Local Government Board, Joseph Chamberlain, issued a circular inviting Boards of Guardians and other local authorities to investigate the use of public works to provide temporary relief to "artisans and others who have hitherto avoided Poor Law assistance," and in 1895 the Royal Commission on the Aged Poor highlighted the plight of poor elderly people who were too proud to apply for poor relief. During the early years of the twentieth century, the Liberals introduced a series of measures that have become known collectively as the "Liberal welfare reforms." In addition to the introduction of free school meals and school medical inspection, they also included old-age pensions, unemployment insurance, and health insurance.[89]

The slow expansion of state welfare had important implications for the development of the relationship between charity and the state. The founders of the Charity Organisation Society sought to distinguish between the "deserving poor," who were capable of being helped by charity, and the "undeserving poor," who should be left to the less tender mercies of the Poor Law. They wanted to be able to cooperate with Boards of Guardians in order to keep the two groups separate. However, the expansion of state welfare provision meant that a growing number of the "deserving" poor were likely to receive assistance from public agencies, and this led to a very different view of the role that voluntary organisations might play in the development of welfare provision.[90]

These new ideas affected the development of social thought inside and outside the Charity Organisation Society. As José Harris and others have shown, the COS was prepared to cooperate with other agencies in the provision of statutory benefits and services, but it often did so with a certain amount of ill grace. During the 1880s and 1890s the COS supported the establishment of public-works schemes for unemployed workers but only when the schemes were administered under its control.[91] After 1906, the London COS also played a key role in the development of the Children's Care Committees, which were set up by the London County Council to supervise the provision of free school meals under the Education (Provision of Meals) Act.[92] However, this did not prevent leading members of the society from condemning the introduction of free school meals as a gross assault on the principle of parental responsibility, and when the Care Committees were established, COS members used their position to ensure that the food provided "was of such a character as to constitute in itself a definite test of need."[93]

Although the COS felt that it had little option other than to cooperate with state agencies in circumstances where they had already taken the decision to expand the benefits of state provision, other agencies, such as the Guilds of Help and the Councils of Social Welfare, were much more positive.[94] These organisations often used methods similar to the COS— they also emphasised the importance of individual casework and the links between middle-class "helpers" and their working-class "clients"—but they showed a much greater understanding of the economic causes of poverty and were more sympathetic to the expansion of state-sponsored solutions to it.[95] As a result, they not only represented a significant departure from the "old" philanthropy of the Charity Organisation Society but also anticipated the development of the "new philanthropy," which achieved its full flowering during the interwar years.[96]

CONCLUSION

As José Harris observed in 1983, "writers on social questions often refer to 'social policy' as though it were a peculiarity of modern or advanced societies, but this view is misplaced. All political regimes have social policies of some kind, even if such policies consist simply in leaving the pursuit of welfare to the family or the local community or the corporation or the market."[97] One important dimension of this is the question of how far needs should be met by state provision, and how far they should be met by private charity. This chapter has tried to examine how the boundary between statutory and voluntary provision changed, in the specific context of the relief of poverty and destitution, between circa 1750 and 1914. At the beginning of this period, a growing number of commentators began to argue that more emphasis should be placed on the importance of voluntary provision and that the provision of welfare by public agencies should be sharply curtailed. This led to a significant increase in the relative importance of the role played by charity in the relief of poverty in many parts of the country after 1834. However, by the early years of the twentieth century, it was widely accepted that the state would have to play a greater role in welfare provision, and voluntary organisations became increasingly concerned with the question of how far they could find a role for themselves in the new world which was beginning to emerge.

These issues became increasingly important after 1914. The First World War generated a new sense of entitlement on the part of those in need of state welfare, and the rise of mass unemployment after 1918 forced the state to accept a much greater responsibility for welfare provision. The voluntary sector was also forced to reconsider its position. Although voluntary organisations continued to play an important part in meeting general relief needs, especially during the 1920s, they also began to argue that their most important role was not to provide an alternative to state welfare but to complement it by offering services for which the state had not yet taken responsibility. As G. D. H. Cole explained in 1945, after 1918 "the old Charity Organisation Society case against outdoor relief simply went by default; and all the voluntary charities had to accommodate themselves . . . to the changed situation."[98] Elizabeth Macadam tried to reflect this in her book *The New Philanthropy*. She argued that the voluntary sector should use its ability to provide a "more flexible, closely-individualised and highly-specialised" service to develop schemes "which are experimental and of insufficiently-recognised value to have yet acquired a claim on the state" and to bring "pressure to bear on the state to amend existing and introduce fresh provision for social needs."[99]

Many of these issues have resurfaced in more recent debates about the role of the state and the relationship between the statutory and voluntary sectors. During the 1970s and 1980s, there was renewed argument about the threat of "welfare dependency" and the need to reinvigorate "civil society" by placing greater reliance on the voluntary sector, and many of these arguments have continued under "New Labour."[100] However, whereas earlier debates focused on what Beveridge called the "moving frontier" between charity and state welfare,[101] this frontier has become increasingly blurred as governments have explored new ways of delivering public services through voluntary agencies.[102]

NOTES

1. In 1980, Olive Checkland argued that the terms "charity" and "philanthropy" ought to be interpreted rather differently, but Frank Prochaska has argued that they can be used interchangeably. See Bernard Harris, *The origins of the British welfare state: Social welfare in England and Wales 1800–1945*, Basingstoke: Palgrave Macmillan, 2004, pp. 59–60.

2. See Gareth Stedman Jones, *Outcast London: A study in the relationship between classes in Victorian society*, Harmondsworth: Penguin, 2nd ed., 1984, pp. 262–80 (1st ed. published 1971); Frank Prochaska, *Women and philanthropy in nineteenth-century England*, Oxford: Oxford University Press, 1980; ibid., *The voluntary impulse: Philanthropy in modern Britain*, London: Faber, 1988; "Philanthropy," in F. M. L. Thompson, ed., *The Cambridge social history of Britain, 1750–1950. Vol. 3, Social agencies and institutions*, Cambridge: Cambridge University Press, 1990, pp. 357–94; Geoffrey Finlayson, *Citizen, state and social welfare in Britain 1830–1990*, Oxford: Oxford University Press, 1994.

3. Jane Lewis, *The voluntary sector, the state and social work in Britain: The Charity Organisation Society/Family Welfare Association since 1869*, Aldershot: Edward Elgar, 1995, p. 3; see also ibid., "Voluntary and informal welfare," in Robert Page and Richard Silburn, eds., *British social welfare in the twentieth century*, Basingstoke: Palgrave Macmillan, 1999, pp. 249–70, at p. 249.

4. Jane Lewis, "The boundary between voluntary and statutory social services in the late-nineteenth and early-twentieth centuries," *Historical Journal*, 39 (1996), 155–77.

5. Paul Slack, *The English poor law, 1531–1782*, Cambridge: Cambridge University Press, 1995, pp. 42–3; see also Joanna Innes, "The 'mixed economy of welfare' in early-modern England: Assessments of the options from Hale to Malthus (c. 1683–1803)," in Martin Daunton, ed., *Charity, self-interest and welfare in the English past*, London: UCL Press, 1996, 139–80, at pp. 147–9; ibid., "State, church and voluntarism in European welfare, 1690–1850," in Hugh Cunningham and Joanna Innes, eds., *Charity, philanthropy and reform from the 1690s to 1850*, Basingstoke: Macmillan, 1998, pp. 15–65, at pp. 37–8; Steve Hindle, *On the parish? The micropolitics of poor relief in rural England, 1550–1750*, Oxford: Clarendon Press, 2004; Paul Fideler, *Social welfare in preindustrial England*, Basingstoke: Palgrave Macmillan, 2006.

6. Harris, *Origins of the British welfare state*, pp. 40–5.

7. Thomas Alcock, *Observations on the defects of the poor laws and on the causes and consequences of the great increase and burden of the poor, with a proposal for redressing these grievances, in a letter to a Member of Parliament*, London: R. Baldwin and R. Clements, 1752, p. 11.

8. Joseph Townsend, *A dissertation on the poor laws*, London: Ridgway, 1817 (2nd ed.; 1st ed., 1786), pp. 14–15.

9. John Davison, *Considerations on the poor laws*, Oxford: University Press, 1818 (2nd ed.; 1st ed., 1817), p. 69.

10. James Geldart, *A short dissertation on the poor laws, with remedies suggested for their evils and defects, and a plan for improving the condition of the poor*, Cambridge: J. Smith, 1819, p. 11.

11. James Ridgway, *General remarks on the state of the poor and poor laws, and the circumstances affecting their condition*, London: James Ridgway, 1832, pp. 12–13.

12. See Hindle, *On the parish*, pp. 129–31.

13. Alcock, *Observations*, pp. 13–14.

14. Townsend, *Dissertation on the poor laws*, pp. 40–1.

15. Frederic Morton Eden, *The state of the poor*, London: J. Davis, 3 volumes, 1797, vol. 1, p. 467.
16. Davison, *Considerations*, p. 58.
17. Alcock, *Observations*, pp. 11–12.
18. Eden, *State of the poor*, vol. 1, p. 458.
19. Alcock, *Observations*, p. 11.
20. Eden, *State of the poor*, p. 467.
21. Davison, *Considerations on the poor laws*, p. 118.
22. Boyd Hilton, *The age of atonement: The influence of Evangelicalism on social and economic thought, 1795–1865*, Oxford: Clarendon Press, 1988, p. 101.
23. John Critchley, "Management of the poor in Rutlandshire," *Annals of Agriculture*, vol. 22 (1794), pp. 416–26.
24. Thomas Estcourt, "An account of the result of an effort to better the condition of the poor in a country village," *Annals of Agriculture*, vol. 43 (1804), pp. 1–8.
25. Davison, *Considerations on the poor laws*, p. 121.
26. Townsend, *Dissertation on the poor laws*, p. 107.
27. Capel Lofft, "Relief of the poor," *Annals of Agriculture*, vol. 24 (1795), pp. 559–62, at p. 561.
28. John Bowring, ed., *The works of Jeremy Bentham*, Edinburgh: William Tait, 1843, vol. 1, p. 315.
29. Townsend, *Dissertation on the poor laws*, p. viii.
30. See Harris, *Origins of the British welfare state*, p. 46.
31. See also the comments by Peter Searby in Peter Searby, "The relief of the poor in Coventry, 1830–63," *Historical Journal*, 20 (1977), pp. 345–61, at p. 346.
32. William Apfel and Peter Dunkley, "English rural society and the New Poor Law: Bedfordshire, 1834–47," *Social History*, 10 (1985), 37–68, at p. 43. "Somerset House" was the physical location of the headquarters of the Poor Law Commission.
33. R. N. Thompson, "The working of the Poor Law Amendment Act in Cumbria, 1836–71," *Northern History*, 15 (1979), 117–37, at p. 122.
34. Ibid.
35. Ibid., p. 123.
36. Searby, "The relief of the poor in Coventry," p. 354.
37. Ibid., p. 358.
38. Ibid., p. 359.
39. Ibid., pp. 359–60.
40. H. M. Boot, "Unemployment and poor relief in Manchester, 1845–50," *Social History*, 15 (1990), 217–28, at p. 22.
41. L. Lynne Kiesling, "Institutional choice matters: The poor law and implicit labor contracts in Victorian Lancashire," *Explorations in Economic History*, 33 (1996), 65–85, at p. 74.
42. PP 1862 (389) xlix, Part 1, 89, Copy of Mr Farnall's reports to the Poor Law Commissioners on the distress in the cotton manufacturing district. See especially pp. 3 (Preston), 7 (Blackburn), 10 (Wigan), 13 (Ashton), 18 (Stockport borough and Hyde).
43. PP 1864 (60) lii, 9. Copy of report of H. B. Farnall, Esq., of the 28th day of June, on distress in the cotton manufacturing districts, pp. 1–2, 6.
44. Derek Fraser, "Introduction," in D. Fraser, ed., *The new poor law in the nineteenth century*, Basingstoke: Macmillan, 1976, pp. 1–24, at p. 11.
45. Ellen Ross, "Hungry children: Housewives and London charity, 1870–1918," in Peter Mandler, ed., *The uses of charity: The poor on relief in the nineteenth century Metropolis*, Philadelphia: University of Pennsylvania Press, 1990, pp. 161–96, at p. 164.

46. Norman McCord, "The Poor Law and philanthropy," in Derek Fraser, ed., *The new poor law in the nineteenth century*, Basingstoke: Macmillan, 1976, pp. 87–110, at p. 97.
47. Robert Humphreys, *Sin, organised charity and the poor law in Victorian England*, Basingstoke: Macmillan, 1995, p. 170.
48. See, e.g., Prochaska, "Philanthropy," p. 362.
49. John Burnett, ed., *Destiny obscure: Autobiographies of childhood, education and family from the 1820s to the 1920s*, London: Allen Lane, 1982, pp. 88, 92.
50. Ross, "Hungry children," p. 170.
51. Charles Booth, *The aged poor in England and Wales*, London: Macmillan, 1894, pp. 339–40; see also David Thomson, "Public, private and the English elderly," in Michael Katz and Christoph Sachße, eds., *The mixed economy of social welfare: Public/private relations in England, Germany and the United States, the 1870s to the 1930s*, Baden-Baden: Nomos Verlagsgesellschaft, 1996, pp. 319–39.
52. James Whishaw, "Endowed charities in Cornwall," *Journal of the Statistical Society of London*, vol. 1, no. 3 (July, 1838), pp. 149–53, at pp. 151–2.
53. Ibid., "An account of the endowed charities in Herefordshire," *Journal of the Statistical Society of London*, vol. 2, no. 4 (July, 1839), pp. 234–50, at pp. 234–5, 240
54. Martin Gorsky, *Patterns of philanthropy: Charity and society in nineteenth-century Bristol*, Woodbridge: Royal Historical Society/Boydell Press, 1999, p. 138; Harris, *Origins of the British welfare state*, pp. 64–6.
55. David Bebbington, *Evangelicalism in modern Britain: A history from the 1730s to the 1980s*, London: Unwin Hyman, 1989, pp. 122–3.
56. Robin Dryburgh, "'The mixed economy of welfare':. The New Poor Law and charity in mid-nineteenth century England," University of Oxford D.Phil. thesis, 2004, pp. 291–2. Gregson's conclusion was that the north-east "experienced all shades of activity from an almost total lack of charitable effort and cooperation with the Poor Law, through a cooperation with the Poor Law, to a cooperation almost verging on integration." See Keith Gregson, "Poor law and organised charity: The relief of exceptional distress in north-east England, 1879–1910," in Michael Rose, ed., *The poor and the city: The English poor law in its urban context, 1834–1914*, Leicester: Leicester University Press, 1985, pp. 94–131, at p. 122.
57. See Harris, *Origins of the British welfare state*, pp. 65–8.
58. George Hicks, "A synopsis of reports of some of the Metropolitan charities," *Times*, 11 February 1869, pp. 3–5; ibid., "The metropolitan charities," *Times*, 11 February 1869, p. 5.
59. Sampson Low, Jr., *The charities of London, comprehending the benevolent, educational and religious institutions, their origin, design, progress and present position*, London: Sampson Low, 1850, pp. 451–2.
60. Hicks, "The Metropolitan charities."
61. Thomas Hawksley, *The charities of London and some errors of their administration, with suggestions for an improved system of private and official charitable relief*, London: John Churchill and Sons, pp. 3–7; see also Harris, *Origins of the British welfare state*, p. 68.
62. Sampson Low, Jr., *The charities of London in 1861, comprising an account of the operations, resources and general condition of the charitable, educational and religious institutions of London*, London: Sampson Low, Son & Co., 1862, p. xiii.
63. Quoted in Michael J. D. Roberts, "Charity disestablished? The origins of the Charity Organisation Society revisited, 1868–71," *Journal of Ecclesiastical History*, 54 (2003), 40–61, at p. 47.

64. David Owen, *English philanthropy, 1660–1960*, Cambridge, MA.: Belknap Press, pp. 215–8.
65. Lynn Hollen Lees, *The solidarities of strangers: The English poor laws and the people, 1700–1948*, Cambridge: Cambridge University Press, 1998, pp. 268–9.
66. Kathleen Woodroofe, *From charity to social work in England and the United States*, London: Routledge and Kegan Paul, 1962, pp. 25–8; Owen, *English philanthropy*, pp. 218–21. See also Roberts, "Charity disestablished?."
67. Owen, *English philanthropy*, pp. 222–3.
68. Woodroofe, *From charity to social work*, p. 41.
69. "Relief to the Poor in the Metropolis—Minute of the Poor Law Board," *Twenty-second Annual Report of the Poor Law Board, 1869–70* (PP 1870 C. 123 xxxv, 1), p. 9.
70. Ibid., p. 10.
71. PP 1872 C. 516 xxviii, 1. *First Report of the Local Government Board 1871–2*, pp. 63–8. See also Harris, *Origins of the British welfare state*, pp. 54–5.
72. Charles Loch Mowat, *The Charity Organisation Society 1869–1913:Iits ideas and work*, London: Methuen & Co., 1961, p. 92.
73. Finlayson, *Citizen, state and social welfare*, pp. 149–50; Robert Humphreys, *Sin, organised charity and the poor law in Victorian England*, Basingstoke: Macmillan, 1995, p. 7.
74. Ruth Hutchinson Crocker, "The Victorian Poor Law in crisis and change: Southampton, 1870–1895," *Albion*, 19 (1), Spring 1987, 19–44, at p. 23.
75. Ibid., p. 36.
76. Humphreys, *Sin, organised charity and the poor law*, p. 83.
77. Gregson, "Poor law and organised charity," p. 103; Humphreys, *Sin, organised charity and the poor law*, p. 86.
78. Gregson, "Poor law and organised charity," p. 118.
79. Humphreys, *Sin, organised charity and the poor law*, pp. 64–83.
80. Alan Kidd, "Outcast Manchester, voluntary charity, poor relief and the casual poor, 1860–1905," in Alan Kidd and Kenneth Roberts, eds., *City, class and culture: Studies of cultural production and social policy in Victorian Manchester*, Manchester: Manchester University Press, 1985, pp. 48–73, at pp. 60–3.
81. Jones, *Outcast London*, p. 300.
82. Charles Stewart Loch, "Charity organisation," *Charity Organisation Society Occasional Papers*, 1st series, no. 36 (1894), p. 153; quoted in Judith Fido, "The Charity Organisation Society and social casework in London, 1869–1900," in Anthony Donajgrodski, ed., *Social control in nineteenth–century Britain*, London: Croom Helm, 1977, pp. 207–30, at pp. 211–2.
83. Crocker, "The Victorian poor law," pp. 39–40.
84. Humphreys, *Sin, organised charity and the poor law*, p. 92.
85. Gregson, "Poor law and organised charity," p. 121.
86. Alan Gillie, "The origin of the poverty line," *Economic History Review*, 49 (1996), 715–30.
87. Michael Flinn, "Medical services under the New Poor Law," in Derek Fraser, ed., *The New Poor Law in the nineteenth century*, Basingstoke: Macmillan, 1976, 45–66; see especially pp. 45–8.
88. See Harris, *Origins of the British welfare state*, pp. 56, 97.
89. Ibid., pp. 56–8, 157–65.
90. As the organiser of the Bradford Guild of Help, Walter Milledge, explained in 1908, "The state is assuming responsibilities which have hitherto been . . . very partially undertaken by philanthropic agencies. The result, however, will be to broaden the outlook for the philanthropist and to enlarge his [*sic*] opportunities for constructive work." Quoted in Keith Laybourn, "The Guild of Help

and the changing face of Edwardian philanthropy," *Urban History*, 20 (1993), pp. 43–60, at p. 49.

91. José Harris, *Unemployment and politics: A study in English social policy 1886–1914*, Oxford: Oxford University Press, 1972, pp. 109–10.

92. Lewis, *The voluntary sector*, pp. 62–5. See also Ross, "Hungry children," pp. 178–9.

93. Helen Bosanquet, *Social work in London, 1869–1912: A history of the Charity Organisation Society*, London: John Murray, 1914, pp. 249–59; Jane Lewis, "The boundary between voluntary and statutory social services in the late-nineteenth and early-twentieth centuries," *Historical Journal*, 39 (1996), 155–77, at p. 167.

94. For more information about these organisations, see Michael Moore, "Social work and social welfare: The organisation of philanthropic resources in Britain, 1900–14," *Journal of British Studies*, 16 (1977), pp. 85–104; Michael Cahill and Tony Jowitt, "The new philanthropy: The emergence of the Bradford City Guild of Help," *Journal of Social Policy*, 9 (1980), pp. 359–82; Laybourn, "The Guild of Help and the changing face of Edwardian philanthropy"; ibid., *The Guild of Help and the changing face of Edwardian philanthropy: The Guild of Help, voluntary work and the state, 1904–19*, Lampeter: Edward Mellen Press, 1994; Lewis, "The boundary between voluntary and statutory social service."

95. Laybourn, "The Guild of Help," p. 49.

96. See Harris, *Origins of the British welfare state*, pp. 186–90.

97. José Harris, "The transition to high politics in English social policy, 1880–1914," in Michael Bentley and John Stevenson, eds., *High and low politics in modern Britain: Ten studies*, Oxford: Clarendon Press, 1983, pp. 58–79, at p. 58.

98. G. D. H. Cole, "A retrospect of the history of voluntary social service," in A. F. C. Bourdillon, ed., *Voluntary social services: Their place in the modern state*, London: Methuen and Co., 1945, pp. 11–30, at p. 24.

99. Elizabeth Macadam, *The new philanthropy: A study of the relations between the statutory and voluntary social services*, London: George Allen and Unwin, 1934, pp. 18, 287.

100. Some of the arguments about the "crisis" of the welfare state during the 1970s and 1980s and the rise of "welfare pluralism" were reviewed in Norman Johnson, *The welfare state in transition: The theory and practice of welfare pluralism*, Brighton: Wheatsheaf, 1987. On New Labour and the voluntary sector, see Edward Brundson and Margaret May, "Evaluating New Labour's approach to independent welfare provision," in Martin Powell, ed., *Evaluating New Labour's welfare reforms*, Bristol: Policy Press, 2002, pp. 61–84, at pp. 61–71.

101. Geoffrey Finlayson, "A moving frontier: Voluntarism and the state in British social welfare, 1911–49," *Twentieth Century British History*, 1 (1990), pp. 183–206.

102. See, e.g., Jane Lewis, "What is New Labour? Can it deliver on social policy?," in Jane Lewis and Rebecca Surender, eds., *Welfare state change: Towards a third way*, Oxford: Oxford University Press, 2004, pp. 207–38.

3 The Mixed Moral Economy of Welfare

European Perspectives[*]

Thomas M. Adams

National Endowment for the Humanities

The concept of a "mixed economy of welfare" is well established. It came to the fore as historians of welfare recognized that their work had too often focused exclusively on official provision of assistance through public sources. Christoph Sachße and Michael Katz edited a volume in 1996 that highlighted the coexistence of private and public sources of social provision in the European and American contexts from the 1870s to the 1930s. The interest in the relationship between voluntary and state assistance on the part of British historians echoed twentieth-century policy debates over the balance between these components of social provision.[1] Investigation of the various forms, public and private, of welfare provision has received a further impetus from modern social historians seeking to write the history of welfare from the perspective of the recipient. Thus, the contributors to a collection of perspectives on poor relief in the nineteenth-century metropolis focused on the survival strategies of the poor themselves, highlighting the "agency" of the poor and their resourcefulness in contriving a patchwork quilt of social protection. Olwen Hufton had earlier coined the phrase "an economy of makeshifts," in describing how the poor of eighteenth-century France combined meagre sources of public and private relief with other precarious sources of income.[2]

Underlying the provision of welfare is a "moral economy," a complex amalgam of justifications and motives that inspires the behaviour of providers and recipients and gives legitimacy to their transactions. The concept

*The views expressed by the author are his own and do not necessarily reflect those of his employer, the National Endowment for the Humanities. He wishes to acknowledge the support of the NEH in the form of released time for independent reading. An earlier version of this paper was presented at the European Social Science History Conference in Berlin in March 2004. The author wishes to thank the editors of this volume, Bernard Harris and Paul Bridgen, and all the others who have contributed to enlightening discussions of European social welfare history at ESSHC conferences, with the support of the Social Inequality Network and the International Institute for Social History in Amsterdam.

of a "moral economy" was formulated most dramatically perhaps by E. P. Thompson in his interpretation of the "moral economy" underlying crowd behaviour in the early modern period. He focused particularly on the widely held popular assumption that in times of dearth, the local authorities and the agents of higher authority held a responsibility to ensure the availability of subsistence and to control the marketplace so that those who traded in foodstuffs would not have free rein to exploit the opportunity for gain at the expense of a famished population. The notion was applied in various studies on provisioning and crowd behavior in the early modern period. One point that emerged from such studies in France was that even in the midst of conflicts between poor consumers and well-to-do traders in commodities, authorities acknowledged the validity of such expectations, at least insofar as a *bonne police* required that the authorities take all necessary precautions to allay the fears of the hungry and to intervene actively in provisioning the marketplace.[3]

The concept of a "moral economy" can perhaps be applied more broadly to any action that is based on the moral underpinnings of the social order. Here, it will be considered applicable to the broad domain of welfare provision. While the term is not always invoked so broadly, students of welfare have explored very extensively the underlying assumptions and expectations held in different sectors of society regarding public and private obligation to those in need.[4]

It should be noted that the "moral economy" of welfare in a given milieu is "mixed" in ways that cut across public and private provision. That is to say, a common set of assumptions about the social order may govern both public and private provision of welfare measures and accompanying measures of control or repression, or these assumptions may diverge in certain respects. For example, in eighteenth-century France, the obligation of the able-bodied poor to provide for their subsistence through work was recognized by public authorities and by private donors. There were many locally organized projects to provide work through the beneficence of local philanthropists in addition to the royally financed *ateliers de charité*. However, the belief that all begging, even by the poor living close to home (the "domiciled" beggars), should be sanctioned by confinement was not universally shared when it was carried into practice by royal (public) authorities. To cite but one example, private individuals in Rennes (seat of Brittany's *parlement*) continued a customary practice of giving to familiar beggars who came to their doors on Mondays. Prohibitions on begging, confinement of the poor, and sanctions against the giving of manual alms all met a greater or lesser degree of public resistance at various times and places, in forms ranging from the discourse of learned treatises to the scuffles of lackeys and artisans with the municipal *archers des pauvres* or the royal *cavaliers de la maréchaussée* responsible for carrying out arrests in public places. Such resistance was rooted in certain notions of a moral economy, reflecting in many cases a belief that the receiving and giving of alms were privileged acts and that the civil authority had no business judging the wisdom or discernment of the spiritually motivated donor.[5]

The complementarity and interpenetration of the private and public "spheres" or domains may thus be as important as their distinctiveness. In order to examine how this is so, I will seek to identify certain continuing strands in the history of charity and welfare that are intertwined: the perennial relationship between the historiography of welfare provision and the advocacy of policy, the social psychology of stewardship as an amalgam of altruism and self-interest, the conundrum of discipline and autonomy, and the coexistence of social inequality and citizenship. The notion of subsidiarity, now formally recognized as a guiding principle of the European Union, will be examined as a framework for reconciling such antinomies and tensions. A notion with a complex pedigree, subsidiarity may prove useful as a conceptual tool, among others, for adapting the multiform heritage of European welfare states to a host of challenges.

To begin with historiography. Dorothy Porter recently commented on efforts to correct a "linear" historiography of welfare as "the growth of government," concurring in the view that historians of welfare have been, in large part, "as much advocates of social democracy as analysts of it." While conceding that a "Whig history" of welfare shortchanges the historical importance of private initiatives, Porter calls on historians to strike a balance in their revision of prevailing welfare-state historiography. Crediting Finlayson and others with focusing renewed attention on the role of voluntarism and private association, Porter nonetheless argues for the continued importance of "the history of political collectivism" in any further study of "the complex history of ideologies of citizenship in civil society."

Two supporting arguments in Porter's article point to important continuities in the history of social welfare. One is her point that historians of the medieval and early modern period have shown the distinction between public and private to be in many respects quite fluid. A second point concerns the ideological underpinnings of the welfare state. Porter observes that while the architects of the modern welfare state saw the principle of universal state entitlement as an antidote to the structural inequality generated by an industrial capitalist society, they "did not lose sight of an equally long tradition in which entitlements were earned through the fulfillment of social obligations."[6] Both of these points illustrate continuities in the mixed moral economy of welfare over the very long term.

Pursuing the first of these points, I would like to suggest that the modern practice of social citizenship overlies a deep substratum of long-held European ways of thinking about an individual's public responsibility. This continuity tends to be obscured by the fact that the motivation for the public good was often mixed with motives that appear to the modern eye to be "impure" or defective and therefore unrelated to the ideals of social citizenship. In particular, those who aided the poor or the sick in the past were often inspired by the hope of securing spiritual salvation, social or economic aggrandizement, status, power, or influence.

Although scholars of late-medieval and early-modern charity and social provision are well inoculated against any romanticized view of a society in which the bountiful rich cared for all the needs of "their" poor in a selfless outpouring of charity and human compassion, their work demonstrates that the practice of charity was widely institutionalized in European urban society and internalized in its cultural values. Admittedly, it is easy to be misled by a few famous examples, and organized charities were always skilled at promoting themselves and their works. But it is well established that those towns that could afford to be more generous on account of their relative commercial prosperity commonly took pride in preserving a well-ordered and prosperous community through attending to specific wants among their populations. Scholars now recognize that preserving the social order entailed substantial provision for those who had suffered a decline in their social status through a relative "impoverishment." If charity was thus expended to protect against downward mobility of the upper tiers of society and to spare "the shamefaced poor" among the better artisan class from the necessity of begging, it also served intermittently to provide the bare essentials for the common labourer in times of dearth or an interruption in trade. For the purpose of this essay, I leave aside rural charity, which appears to have been far less organized, but about which, by the same token, far less is known. There were, to be sure, important connections between urban and rural charity. For one thing, the notion of parish responsibility is widely invoked throughout Europe, providing a link between rural and urban provision that is often invoked in theory, in some cases in law, and to some degree in practice. For example, the Elizabethan Poor Law took effect in rural as well as urban parishes. A second point to be noted is that the obligation of the feudal lord to provide protection to his tenants often bore a concomitant expectation of charitable provision, an important element in the ideology and practice of charity that complemented urban ideals of civic solidarity.[7]

J. S. Henderson's study of Florence in the fourteenth and fifteenth centuries reveals with special clarity the cultural ideal of a well-governed city in which the public good—conceived both in religious and secular terms—includes providing for the security and subsistence of its members. Members of the governing elite of the city were also leaders in the civic-religious associations that provided for large-scale distributions of grain in times of food shortage, and funds were allocated for this purpose from public funds as well as from private contributions. Brian Pullan's study of Venice, primarily in the fifteenth and sixteenth centuries, portrays the guilds' involvement in charity for various categories of workers. This is not to suggest that all needs were provided for, since such aid was "residual" and selective in nature. Monica Chojnacka's study of women's networks in early-modern Venice serves as a reminder that newcomers especially had to rely on informal networks of information and support at best.[8]

Marco van Leeuwen has proposed some generalizations about the workings and motivations for welfare in major urban centers of preindustrial modern Europe based on his study of Amsterdam in the early nineteenth century and some comparisons with work on other cities throughout the early-modern period. From this he concludes that both the resources for social provision and the motivations of its organizers were characteristically "mixed." His schema of motives for the elites includes: regulating the labour market, stabilizing social order, averting turmoil, reducing risk of infection, civilizing the poor, status, career and patronage, and salvation. The poor, in turn, were adept at piecing together aid that would offer at least some partial relief in times of their distress. Some were more adept than others, and some were favoured while others were turned away or punished as miscreants.[9]

Because the modern conception of social citizenship has been forged in the cauldron of modern democratic revolutions, such mixed motives as these can easily be categorized as the values of a predemocratic society—values definitively superseded and rejected. But for more than one reason, the continuities are significant. Social arrangements in modern Western states are still, to a greater degree than we would like to admit, solidly hierarchical. While Western states profess to promote social mobility through public education and to cushion insecurity through provision of social services, the avenues to social and economic "success" continue to be heavily conditioned by family status, resources, and lifestyle. In terms of "moral economy," the belief that civilization could not survive without substantial inequality is by no means confined to the United States.

If the promise of democracy has been limited in ways that preserve social inequality, the need to "civilize the poor" and the concern to provide safeguards against attacks on the social order also continue in new guises. Such social imperatives need not be seen as purely negative and undemocratic, either in the past or in the present. Disruption and conflict in a society have almost invariably caused greater harm to the lowly than to the high and mighty. Thus, the enlightened self-interest of elites, and, in our day, of a prosperous middle class, in maintaining social "order" (in early modern parlance *une bonne police* or *gute Polizei*) is not an entirely selfish goal. Elite strivings for social integration should not be seen solely as "social control" but also as an expression, in however limited a form, of social solidarity.[10] Of course, it would be absurd to argue that traditional paternalistic charity is no different from a modern conception of social citizenship, especially one based on universalist principles. Nonetheless, solidarity draws on old forms and old habits and performs some of the same functions as in past centuries even as it comes to serve new principles of citizenship.

Here I would like to identify two key aspects of the solidaristic dimensions of a mixed moral economy of welfare—with continuities linking contemporary social citizenship to earlier historical experience. One is the social psychology of stewardship; the other is the relationship between discipline and autonomy.

"Blessed is he that considereth the poor," the psalmist sang, and the care of the poor has been defined in Christian tradition as a function that brings blessings upon the entire community as well as upon the steward.[11] It is too easily assumed that public functions can only be performed through completely disinterested motives, or, to put it another way, if those concerned have their own self-interest in view they cannot be effective stewards of the poor. Rather, it is possible for selfish motives to mix with disinterested ones. It is a delicate balancing act for the historian to be neither too cynical nor too trusting in such matters, but bias and distortion have not always favoured the empowered donor. Europeans have a long tradition of debunking charitable motives, calling people to account for the results of their stewardship, and skewering the hypocrisy of a mere show of charity. The humanist scholar Juan Luis Vives, author of an early sixteenth-century treatise on poor relief, waxed indignant at the aristocratic coxcomb who wished to be excused his sins for a few pennies of charity tossed to a street beggar. The nineteenth-century novelist Juan Galdos sharpened his satirical pen on the lavish social display of charitable ladies in Spain. Jean-Pierre Gutton cites the sources of a "black legend" of abuse and incompetence by those professing to serve the poor in eighteenth-century French hospitals. Such instances of the unmasking of hypocrisy in charitable practice abound and represent an integral element in the moral economy of welfare.[12]

The various studies of eighteenth-century hospital administrators collected by Gutton paint a picture of a group selected from an urban elite, varying in composition from place to place, more often than not including men successful in trade or manufacture, as well as professional men of the law, with an influential role played by a local aristocrat, high cleric, or representative of royal authority. In practically all cases, serving the poor enhanced the social status of those involved. Holders of municipal offices had generally served at some point on the boards of charitable institutions, and in some cases a place of honour on these boards was reserved for those who had retired from the highest municipal offices. Usually board members were expected to make substantial financial contributions to their institutions as well as attending regular meetings, performing services depending on their expertise, and intervening as advocates or sponsors. Contributions of time and effort might involve oversight of personnel and of their adherence to regulations, inspection of provisions, auditing of accounts, and handling of legal matters. Studies of individual institutions reveal great differences from one institution to another, even within France in the eighteenth century. Nevertheless, it may be generally stated that in preindustrial Europe charitable oversight and a significant portion of the day-to-day administration of charities were conducted in large part through volunteer service that involved substantial contributions of time, effort, and personal resources. Women drawn from the elites of society also had a large role in administering certain classes of religious institutions consecrated to charitable missions. In seventeenth-century France, women of lower social standing were also recruited through the establishment of the Sisters of Charity by Vincent de Paul and Louise de Marillac.[13]

It goes without saying that administrators were not always successful in their efforts. In France and elsewhere, the management of land or buildings bequeathed to charitable institutions proved to be a particularly time-consuming process that rarely realized the hoped-for financial benefits. Relatives of the deceased frequently contested the terms of charitable bequests, and the terms of those bequests that were sustained often imposed obligations that proved onerous.[14] Regardless of such shortcomings, the desire to be seen as devoted, sober stewards of a community's charitable institutions prevailed widely. Dutch paintings of governing boards capture a corporate spirit of municipal pride in charitable activity. Many trustees never had their service so immortalized but contributed their time and effort from various motives secular and religious, base and noble, including a recognition that social status came with civic obligations. Daniel Hickey invokes the notion of "social capital" and Bourdieu's concept of *habitus* to account for such expectations, which were implicitly acknowledged in the behavior of hospital administrators in early modern France.[15]

The psychology of stewardship undoubtedly partook of a strong dose of enlightened self-interest. Maintaining social integration through social provision that allowed the less well off to sustain themselves through difficult economic times expressed a solidaristic acknowledgment of a shared self-interest. Charity during economic downswings or food shortage not only protected property against the desperate but served to maintain a skilled labour force that would be needed at the first sign of an upturn. Lyon's reputation for charity was buttressed by such reasoning. Likewise, the administrators of the *mont-de-piété*, or pawnshop, in Avignon, who were drawn from the city's merchant class, readily made loans to silk workers lest they relocate upstream to Lyon in bad times.[16] In the historiography of "social control" in France, the fact that local hospital boards were not particularly enthusiastic about enforcing royal orders of 1724 to confine beggars and vagabonds was taken to be a sign of their sluggishness and devotion to routine. Jean-Pierre Gutton alerted us, however, to the fact that some of these hospital administrators actively chose to give priority to providing support to local citizens in need, rather than expending limited resources on the less-productive mission of locking up and "correcting" beggars who happened to be wandering far from home.[17]

The matter of maintaining a workforce relates to the broader theme of social discipline and autonomy and to the somewhat vaguer notion identified by Marco van Leeuwen as "civilizing the poor." While the provision of aid could be a positive incentive to a worker to continue contributing to his employer's enterprise, urban elites also took measures to discourage behaviour that deviated from an industrious norm, notably the practice of begging and wandering from place to place. The social control of the poor by their more prosperous brethren presents the most problematic element in the moral economy of welfare. How is it possible to view such elements of social policy as anything but exploitation designed to maintain the subservience of the poor to the rich?

The answer to that question lies in part in the observation by Dorothy Porter cited earlier, namely, that the rationale for social provision has generally carried an assumption of mutual obligation. Surely, the poor through the ages have not rebelled against the obligation to work as such? What must always have been most galling was having to take work that was too ill paid to provide subsistence for a family and to have little if any control over their conditions of work.[18] The poor may also have found it hard to explain how those who lived from the work of others would be entitled to demand punishment for "idleness" that was often the result of an involuntary cessation of a wage earner's employment. The harshness of measures to instill "regular" work habits among the lower orders has been a sinister thread in social history, and that thread has not disappeared in spite of claims that Europeans are today cosseted with generous guarantees of security that enervate their willingness to work. The avowed principle of "less eligibility" that was enshrined in English public policy with the promulgation of the "new" Poor Law of 1834 had ample precedents in preceding centuries. The work of grinding brazilwood to make sawdust for dye in the Amsterdam "Rasphuis" and similar projects of obligatory toil in other seventeenth-century cities were predicated on the belief that an inmate who had been subjugated to such arduous and strenuous labor would willingly take up the tasks offered to him for a wage upon his release.[19]

That said, there was frequently in centuries past a solidaristic impulse to foster social integration in measures taken to instill discipline and self-sufficiency among the poor. This is most evident in those workshops or public-works sites that were set up to provide work for the unemployed poor. Some of the best known instances are the various *ateliers de charité* established in the eighteenth century in France as a kind of countercyclical employment, leading to larger scale experiments that failed eventually for a variety of reasons in the French Revolution and again in 1848. A relatively unexplored subject, however, is the degree to which public works in cities throughout Europe were managed with an eye to providing wages for the unemployed poor. This theme has drawn attention in scattered instances from medieval historians as well as from social and economic historians of the modern period. Studies of measures of welfare and police directed at beggars and vagrants have pointed to many instances of "free" charity workshops coexisting with those in which arrested beggars were put to work under physical compulsion.[20]

Much thought has been given ever since the Middle Ages as to how work projects could be designed so as to provide those employed in them a marketable skill. These efforts generally encountered a host of obstacles not unfamiliar to social planners today. One of the most common fallacies was to expect a training workshop to pay its own way or to make a profit. The costs were generally higher than anticipated, the challenges of organization and marketing more complex, and the problems of maintaining quality with a ragtag and reluctant workforce greater. A successful workshop encountered resistance among those artisans with whose production it competed. This was the central complaint of Daniel Defoe in his pamphlet of 1704, *Giving Alms No Charity*, which took aim at publicly financed work projects for the poor. Work may be, as an eighteenth-century writer proclaimed, the true philosopher's stone, but it is a remedy not cheaply or easily administered. Be that as it may, it is a constant feature of a mixed moral economy in the past and today to attempt to make the unemployed productive either by training and discipline that are designed to qualify them for the open labor market or by creating a parallel market through various forms of public employment.[21]

Perhaps the most illuminating continuities with the present in this regard are to be found in the various institutionalized efforts to train young orphans and foundlings for trades that would make them self-sufficient. The Aumône-Générale of Lyon, established in 1534, is a well known example that implemented the suggestion that the seed for a local silk industry could be planted by teaching silk manufacture to the youths who would otherwise be without a means to earn a living. Not surprisingly, such schools of industry reflected hierarchical assumptions that prevailed among ruling elites and the options of those being trained were often severely limited. In the care of orphans in Amsterdam from the sixteenth to the nineteenth century, it is interesting to observe that the orphans of established citizens were trained for artisanal trades, whereas those of migrants from without were trained only for general labour. Ironically, a charitable institution that was particularly successful in training its charges might find that members of the elite jostled for the opportunity to place their own clients in them, as, for example, the San Telmo orphanage in Seville, which trained boys for seamanship and navigation through the eighteenth and early-nineteenth centuries.[22]

One case drawn from Thomas Safly's account of seventeenth-century Augsburg can perhaps serve to make the point that charitable authorities responsible for the apprenticing of orphans recognized the need to find an occupation suitable to their young charges in order to provide them an autonomous livelihood. He documents the persistence of the directors in the case of a youth who ran away from successive masters and tangled with the law, noting their repeated efforts on his behalf.[23] Such persistence may be explained in part by a desire to convey symbolically the directors' fatherly concern for errant youths, a theme that Philip S. Gorski remarks upon in his treatment of the Calvinist regimen applied both to orphanages and workhouses in the Netherlands. Gorski in turn expands upon a theme developed by the German scholar Gerhard Oestreich, namely, the importance of "discipline from below" and the maintenance of a disciplined community in the development of state authority in the early modern period.[24]

The question of discipline and autonomy is especially problematic where the provision of welfare to women and the "police" of their behavior were concerned. The study of gender in the history of social protection in recent decades has squarely addressed questions of moral economy as they impinged on the economic roles that women played and as they determined women's access to resources of all kinds. While women were often the special objects of charity and welfare, they were also subject to an especially coercive regimen. Institutions serving women have tended to reflect an ideology based on the subordination of women and a sexual double standard. Those that provided for the rehabilitation of repentant prostitutes may be seen as particularly coercive, projecting a view of the moral "weakness" of women.[25]

Here again, perhaps a single case may be adduced to suggest that the motivations for instilling discipline and "virtue" in poor women were not exclusively inspired by misogyny and a desire to subject women to patriarchal domination. The published regulations for a house that confined repentant prostitutes in seventeenth-century Dijon began by stating that men were to blame for the fact that women became prostitutes, contrary to the frequent charge that some inherent vice in women was the cause of men's waywardness. A regulation of the same hospital a century later stated that the regime of the house was to train these women to be domestic servants. The work they were asked to do was hard, the author of the brochure admitted, but only as needed in order to prepare the women for what would be expected of them if they were to be retained successfully as household servants. Such a statement may not strike the contemporary ear as a particularly impressive affirmation of respect for women's autonomy, but given the context of seventeenth-century society, the rationale for the discipline of the institution was indeed to train women to be able to choose honest work as an alternative to prostituting themselves.[26]

In exploring the theme of "the mixed moral economy of welfare," I have sought to establish that the continuity of certain important themes in welfare history tends to be obscured by the assumption that the democratic foundations of modern social citizenship entail a total break with the undemocratic "prehistory" of the modern welfare state. To round out this argument for continuity, a few further remarks may serve to suggest how the mixed moral economy of welfare carries over into the development of the modern welfare state. For this purpose, I will focus on France, with sidelong glances toward its English and German neighbors.

In France, debates over proposed social welfare legislation in the two decades before the First World War stimulated a debate among historians over the legacy of the French Revolution in this domain. Léon Lallemand spoke for a Catholic tradition of institutional charity, vandalized by the Jacobins in the Revolution of 1789 and once again threatened a century later by anticlerical politicians of the Third Republic. Taking up cudgels for the lay republican cause, Camille Bloch edited the reports of the Committee on Mendicity of the Constituent Assembly and combed the archives to argue for the emergence of the concept of "assistance as a public service" that began with the systematic review of charitable legislation by Turgot when this iconic minister-*philosophe* was in charge of French finance from 1774 to 1776.[27]

The conception that Bloch and the early twentieth-century advocates of welfare legislation found in the eighteenth century was indeed the corner-stone of social citizenship under the aegis of the nation state. Provision for need became a mutual obligation of citizenship. In Dorothy Porter's terms, it embodied, on the one hand, a notion that entitlement was accompanied by obligation, and, on the other hand, a notion that the multiform task of securing welfare for those in need was to be accomplished by coordinating efforts at various levels of government and society. Philanthropy would not be banished but would take new civic forms. In his oft-cited article for the *Encyclopédie* on "endowments," Turgot encouraged his fellow citizens not to let the English outshine them in displaying "the spirit of the citizen" through civic engagement and philanthropic association. The revolutionary assemblies solemnly received "patriotic gifts" from private citizens.[28]

Current historiography has brought to light the various forms of philanthropic activity that developed in France from the Revolution through the nineteenth century and has also focused on the evolution of a municipally focused approach to promoting a mix of private and public initiatives. Timothy Smith has argued persuasively that the emergence of the welfare state in twentieth-century France may be seen as an evolution of a municipally based practice of welfare provision. The municipal impulse was intensely localistic throughout the nineteenth century, but after World War I its spokesmen sought to integrate local institutions into a national framework of support and coordination. Even in Lyon, self-styled "capital of charity" in centuries past, municipal and professional elites came around to the conclusion that their stewardship of the needy could only be effective in conjunction with national stewardship and support. Turgot would certainly have approved of this development, but, having attacked the corporate influence of craft guilds, he would no doubt have been chagrined to see the strong converging influence of mutualism and other working-class movements in bringing legislative form to the concepts of social citizenship that unfolded over the following decades. Indeed, the principle of consultation with "social partners," meaning primarily confederations of unions and other professional organizations, has become thoroughly institutionalized not only in France but throughout the European Union. Workers and owners of the means of production were not the only influences on the social policies of the Third Republic: A veritable constellation of social reform toward the end of the nineteenth century took shape through networks of professional organizations such as criminologists and psychologists.[29]

Although Turgot praised the civic-mindedness of the English in their approach to social provision, many of his compatriots over the next two centuries saw England as a negative example. From Malesherbes in the 1770s to the critics of proposed French welfare legislation in the 1890s, England's Poor Law, old, new, or reformed, was viewed as an object lesson in heavy-handed direction by the central state. "Moral economy" was in fact at the heart of French critics' contention that social provision through national legislation would entail a disastrous cooling of civic commitment to local institutions and charitable largesse.[30] In England, debates over the Poor Laws and the respective spheres of public law and private charity went through several phases, but in each phase the "moral economy" of the recipient was under scrutiny. The reciprocity of entitlement and obligation was at issue, as was the proper locus of stewardship. The New Poor Law of 1834 aimed to nullify the recipient's presumed repugnance for work by providing relief only in exchange for work "less eligible" than the choices offered by employers. The subsequent rise of the Charity Organization Society (COS) in the private sphere was intended to regulate and supplement this scheme of moral economy by "scientific" investigation of claims of need, case by case, that would result in a clear identification of the "deserving poor." The volunteers of the COS would organize the resources of private philanthropy to serve the needs, strictly defined, of those who deserved support. The "undeserving" remainder were free to seek employment or apply to the Poor Law authorities, who would implement "the workhouse test." The COS itself came to recognize the need for certain forms of state intervention in the alleviation of mass poverty and lent support to experimentation in the private sector, such as the movement for University Settlements.[31]

Other contributions to this volume examine in depth the relationship between public and private provision in England. They lend support to Dorothy Porter's assertion that a concern to link entitlement with obligation remains a constant theme in English social-welfare history. If voluntarist traditions of social provision appear to be overborne to an increasing degree by a collectivist impulse, the benefits of maintaining a mix of motivations and bases for action, on the local, associational, and personal level, continue to be debated.[32]

The French looked to Germany as well as to England for comparison in the second half of the nineteenth century. They were at once appalled and fascinated by the example of compulsory state action in fields as diverse as public health and pension plans.[33] If Germany under Bismarck appeared to be an extreme model of state centralization, its social services reflected long traditions of civic, municipal, and voluntary engagements. Some of these traditions were defined by long-established sectarian religious affiliation and by a statist tradition of cameralism; some were newly defined in terms of political parties, unions, and associations of professional experts. War and industrial transformation overwhelmed Hamburg's exemplary municipal welfare reforms of the 1780s, characterized by Enlightenment principles of civic oversight and a rational assessment of need, but the Elberfeld system established in the Rhineland in the 1850s inherited many of its features, recruiting a cadre of voluntary citizen inspectors of the poor to serve neigh-borhoods inhabited by industrial workers.[34] The question of defining the locus of stewardship proved especially controversial in the area of child welfare, the battleground of religious and political organizations through-out the nineteenth century, and throughout the troubled life of the Weimar Republic. The claim of professionals and scientific experts to provide the most authoritative stewardship of the public welfare manifested itself in this domain and in others, notably public health and hygiene, housing and urban design, criminology, psychiatry, and social work. Universities and new professional organizations served as platforms for asserting the claim of stewardship on behalf of the community at large.[35]

World War I opened new discussions over the moral economy of social provision, as the claims of veterans and their widows raised questions about the entitlements and obligations of all citizens. While the Weimar constitu-tion gave sweeping guarantees of state responsibility for the social protection of all citizens, the most troublesome challenge came from the large class of middle-class citizens who were dispossessed when their savings evaporated in the inflation of the 1920s.[36] The Nazi regime appealed to some as a means of resolving deadlock over social policy, but any such hopes faded rapidly as the new regime ran roughshod over the weak and the unfit. The welfare state as it evolved in West Germany after World War II rested on the stewardship of government officials committed to maintaining free market competition exercised jointly with representatives of labor and management.[37]

The growth of the welfare state in its various European forms had a predictable impact on private charity and profoundly affected the "moral economy" of social provision. Advocates of the welfare states generally assumed that the function of private initiative would be largely superseded by a new moral economy of public "social citizenship," but by and large even the most ardent advocates of the new regime did not argue that pri-vate initiatives had no place at all. Indeed, the failure of the welfare state to provide certain pressing needs revived interest in private initiatives. In France, for example, the abbé Pierre's discovery of seventeen homeless Pari-sians frozen to death in the winter of 1954 launched a movement and served as a call to action in both public and private spheres.[38] To describe how a place for a "third sector" of traditional charity and philanthropy evolved in each country would be to tell a long tale. A few observations on the debates surrounding this process may serve here to support the argument that the historical legacies of a "mixed moral economy" of welfare retain a practical pertinence to contemporary policy.

In the early decades of European reconstruction and widening prosperity after World War II, it was assumed that relatively full employment would place social provision on a firm foundation of workers' earnings and com-plementary contributions, with a small residual population in need of assis-tance over and above those too young or too old to work. By the late 1970s, it became clear that the welfare state was carrying a larger burden of social protection than such a model would have predicted, and global economic circumstances gave practical urgency to lightening any burden on the economy that would slow down the growth of productivity and competitiveness. Moreover, there was an ominous echo of Disraeli's "Two Nations"—rich and poor—in analysts' conclusions that the welfare state was creating new forms of socially entrenched inequality. The moral economy of the welfare state was coming into question. Such critiques were particularly vocal in France and Germany.[39] When Amartya Sen surveyed strategies for promoting social justice and combating poverty in the developed as well as the undeveloped countries, he cited Europe's tolerance of high levels of unemployment as a critical source of injustice, characterized by "capability deprivation" of a an entire class of citizens.[40]

Critics argued that the welfare state became the victim of its own success. The "utopian" impulse behind the creation of the welfare state had spent itself, Jürgen Habermas argued in a speech before the Cortes of Spain in 1984. Depending on the rules of a free market to generate wealth and jobs, the welfare state could deploy its authority to provide compensation for adverse contingencies, but it could not realize the vision of a universally productive and autonomous citizenry. The bureaucratic mode of operation of the welfare state, he argued, was experienced as a detriment to individual autonomy rather than as a tool of self-realization; new technologies of communication did not give voice to the individual citizen in the policy arena.[41] After three decades of an "economic miracle," corresponding to the "*trente glorieuses*" of the French welfare state, the German model ran into increasing difficulties, giving rise to talk of a breakdown of moral cohesion, the rise of welfare cheats and a new generation of the "workshy."[42] The abuse of social provision by those working and middle-class citizens who might be termed the "proprietors" and "rulers" of the welfare state gave scandal to its supporters and detractors alike. Abuse of disability provisions and what in earlier periods would have been decried moralistically as "malingering" or "shirking" seemed to be a spreading social disease, along with tax evasion, especially through unreported employment.[43]

Debates over the moral economy of social citizenship led to a variety of political and administrative responses in the 1980s, some of them successful. In the Netherlands, for example, disability policies were reviewed and abuses were brought under control, while productivity became the object of a shared corporatist policy engaging the labour unions as well as state actors. Sweden tamed the costs of its universalist provision.[44] In Germany, Christian Democrats called for a revitalization of the private and voluntary sector in the domain of social services and for a greater devolution of social policy within the German federal system. Inaugurating a sixteen-year ascendancy of his party in 1982, Helmut Kohl declared,

> We want citizens to help themselves and each other more. The political principle that provides the structure for this is subsidiarity. This calls

for giving priority to the ever smaller social unit. What the smaller is capable of providing should not be taken over by the larger. Family, neighbourhood, independent providers, self-help and support groups and social service organizations can engender a greater sense of citizenship and citizen responsibility than any big and anonymous institution could ever do.[45]

In this speech, Helmut Kohl invoked a term that Christian Democrats had only recently adopted as a watchword. "Subsidiarity" referred to a concept that had achieved prominence through its use in a papal encyclical of the 1930s, a declaration aimed particularly at defending the autonomy of the family against the power of the state. Christian Democrats called for a "new subsidiarity" that would galvanize individuals and groups to take responsibility for themselves and their communities in a myriad of new ways. Although critics were quick to point out the conflicting assumptions that could accompany the use of the term, Social Democrats promoted their own positive interpretation of the term. While Christian Democrats touted new forms of "self-help" in Berlin's depressed neighborhoods, Social Democrats organized workers' enterprises in Cologne. While Christian Democrats revived to some extent the role of denominational charities, the Social Democrats called for an expanded role for unions in organizing social action.[46]

The term "subsidiarity" has since taken on a broader European significance. It was in conversation with German union leaders and political leaders active in the various Länder that the French Social Democrat Jacques Delors was persuaded of the utility of the concept in the emerging discussions among European states about a closer European Union.[47] As commissioner of the European Community, leading the drive to ratify the Maastricht Treaty, Delors argued that the formula of subsidiarity incorporated in the treaty should put to rest fears that a common currency, and its attendant coordination of policies in areas ranging from labour mobility to environmental regulation, would undermine national sovereignty and impose top-down legislation. It stated that

> in areas which do not fall within its exclusive competence, the Community shall take action, in accordance with the principle of subsidiarity, only if and in so far as the objectives of the proposed action cannot be sufficiently achieved by the Member States and can therefore, by reason of the scale or effect of the proposed action, be better achieved by the community.[48]

Delors was particularly aware of concerns that a stronger European Union would either impose new welfare burdens across the board or dilute strong provisions already established at the national level. His broader vision of Maastricht was that it represented a wager that a "European social model" was not incompatible with global competitiveness. Delors emphasized the point that the concept of subsidiarity laid an obligation on the "higher" authority, not only to respect "lower" initiatives, but to exercise its legitimate power in ways that would foster the vitality of other levels of government and administration. He spoke of the concept as "the pedagogy of the federalist approach," and even "as the keystone, on the political plane, of the organization of a common life and, on the institutional plane, of the shared exercise of sovereignty in those domains—and only in those domains— where such a sharing has been determined."[49]

By invoking a concept that had particular resonance among Christian Democrats, Jacques Delors no doubt aimed to build on the common ground that they and the Social Democrats had found since World War II in advancing the measures of social protection that defined the welfare state.[50] In Germany, in particular, the term has been invoked in recent discussions of the fiscal crisis of the German welfare state by the Christian Democrat Kurt Biedenkopf, who articulated the principle of subsidiarity a quarter century ago, as well as by Green foreign minister Joschka Fischer in connection with the elaboration of a "constitution" of an expanded European Union.[51] Critics initially viewed the formula as little more than an agreement to disagree. Some argued thereafter that the formula was being used in practice in an exclusively negative sense, as a means to veto any effective EU initiatives in the domain of social policy.[52] On the other hand, the formula of subsidiarity has allowed some degree of consensus to emerge on the minimal elements of states' responsibility for social provision, accompanied by a gradualist advance of procedures for monitoring policies and their effectiveness.[53]

For a history of a "mixed moral economy of welfare," the significance of the concept of subsidiarity lies in the continuities it evokes—in its reworking of a complex array of old traditions into a search for effective ways to coordinate levels of governance and enable citizen participation. Discussion of the concept has contributed to a reexamination of Europe's historical inventory of jurisprudence and institutional practice, encouraging the quest for alternative frameworks of social action, whether they be municipal, corporatist, or more generally associative in form.[54] In arguing for forms of social services that are administered more closely to the recipient, French sociologist Robert Castel suggests that the remedy for the ills of the modern *état providence* may entail to some degree a reinvention of the localistic and personal relationships of medieval and early modern charity.[55] While the concept of subsidiarity seems to have found little echo in the UK, Paul Slack remarked, in a series of historical lectures on reform and improvement in England, that recent discussions of the role of "civil society" in the provision of social services indicate a desire to resurrect certain features of institutions and social arrangements that prevailed on the eve of the modern era.[56]

From the foregoing it would appear that a "mixed moral economy" is not merely a recognizable feature of social provision in centuries past but remains as a legacy to be drawn upon in a form appropriate to present circumstances. Perhaps, as economist Joseph Schumpeter speculated, the very survival of a new model of society may depend for its existence on values that arose from the daily practice of an earlier society, serving as "flying buttresses" to hold up the walls of a towering edifice.[57] Although Schumpeter was arguing that the edifice of capitalism was shored up by principles other than those of the free market, the edifice of the welfare state may likewise require for its support forms of action other than those initiated through the machinery of the centralized nation-state. The prospect for a positive coordination of economic and social policies in an expanding Europe may depend as much on the success of institutional and associational life at all the "lower" levels as it does on the codifying ingenuity of bureaucrats, who can engineer an appropriate schema for "*subsidium*" and harmonization only if the moral economy of social provision is flourishing in a variety of institutional forms within and across the nations of the union.

NOTES

1. Gunter Frankenberg, "Shifting boundaries: The private, the public, and the welfare state," in Michael B. Katz and Christoph Sachße, eds., *The mixed economy of social welfare: Public/private relations in England, Germany, and the United States, the 1870s to the 1930s* (Baden-Baden: Nomos, 1996), pp. 72–94; Joanna Innes, "The 'mixed economy of welfare' in early modern England: Assessments of the options from Hale to Malthus (c.1683–1803)," in *Charity, self-interest and welfare in the English past*, ed. Martin Daunton (London: University College London Press, 1996), pp. 139–80; the "mixed economy of welfare" emerges as a perduring theme in European welfare history in the collection edited by Peregrine Horden and Richard Smith, *The locus of care: Families, communities, institutions and the provision of welfare since antiquity* (New York: Routledge, 1998), especially pp. 9 (editors' introduction) and 22 (Peregrine Horden, "Household care and informal networks: Comparisons and continuities from antiquity to the present. ")
2. Peter Mandler, ed., *The uses of charity: The poor on relief in the nineteenth-century metropolis* (Philadelphia: University of Pennsylvania Press, 1990); Olwen Hufton, *The poor of eighteenth-century France, 1750–1789* (New York: Oxford University Press, 1974), pp. 69–127. For England, see Anne Crowther, "Health care and poor relief in provincial England," in *Health care and poor relief in 18th and 19th century Northern Europe*, ed. Ole Peter Grell, Andrew Cunningham, and Robert Jütte (Aldershot, UK: Ashgate, 2002), pp. 203–19, especially p. 206. On the importance of "subsidiary bodies," see Paul Slack, *From Reformation to improvement: Public welfare in early modern England* (Oxford: Clarendon Press, 1999), p. 132.
3. E. P. Thompson, "The moral economy of the English crowd in the eighteenth century," *Past and Present* 50 (1971), 76–136. George Rudé, *The crowd in history: A study of popular disturbances in France and England, 1730–1848* (New York: Wiley, 1964); Cynthia A. Bouton, *The flour war: Gender, class, and community in late ancien régime French society.* (Pennsylvania State University Press, 1993). Among the pertinent works of Steven L. Kaplan, see especially his *Bread, politics and political economy in the reign of Louis XV*, 2 vols. (The Hague: Martinus Nijhoff, 1976) and *The famine plot persuasion in eighteenth-century France; Transactions of the American Philosophical Society*, 22:3 (Philadelphia, 1982).

4. See the more general discussion of the prescriptive customary rights of the poor in Lynn Hollen Lees, *The solidarities of strangers: the English Poor Laws and the people, 1700–1948* (Cambridge: CUP 1998), p. 74, and Paul Slack, *From Reformation to improvement*, p. 65, on the impact of Stuart prerogative on the entitlements of the poor.

5. Thomas McStay Adams, *Bureaucrats and beggars: French social policy in the Age of the Enlightenment* (New York: Oxford University Press, 1990), pp. 15–16 and 119.

6. Dorothy Porter, "Health care and the construction of citizenship in civil societies in the era of the Enlightenment and industrialization," in Grell, Cunningham, and Jütte, *Health Care and Poor Relief*, 15–31, especially p. 18; David Thomson, "Welfare and the historians," in L. Bonfield and R. M. Smith, eds., *The world we have gained: Historians of population and social structure* (Oxford: Basil Blackwell, 1980), pp. 355–76. Thompson argues that "Whig historians" of welfare tend to exaggerate the shortcomings of older arrangements and to create false expectations of the new.

7. Richard C. Trexler, "Charity and the defense of urban elites in the Italian communes," in Frederic Cople Jaher, ed., *The rich, the well born, and the powerful: Elites and upper classes in history* (Urbana: University of Illinois Press, 1973), pp. 64–109. Local studies of rural charity include Patrice Berger, "Rural charity in late seventeenth-century France: The Pontchartrain case," *French Historical Studies*, 10:3 (Spring 1978), 393–415. On the rural poor and the extension of the Poor Law in seventeenth-century England, see Paul Slack, *Poverty and policy in Tudor and Stuart England* (New York: Longman, 1988), pp. 62–7; 170.

8. J. S. Henderson, *Piety and charity in late medieval Florence* (Oxford: Clarendon, 1994); Brian Pullan, *Rich and poor in Renaissance Venice: The social institutions of a Catholic state* (Cambridge, MA: Harvard University Press, 1971); Monica Chojnacka, *Working women of early modern Venice* (Baltimore: Johns Hopkins University Press, 2001).

9. Marco van Leeuwen, "Histories of risk and welfare in Europe during the 18th and 19th centuries," in Grell, Cunningham, and Jütte, eds., *Health Care and Poor Relief*, pp. 32–66. See also Van Leeuwen, *The logic of charity: Amsterdam, 1800–1850* (New York: Saint Martin's Press, 2000), pp. 182–4.; and Herman Diedericks, "La politique économique et sociale à Amsterdam et Leyde," in Jacques-Guy Petit and Yannick Marec, eds., *Le social dans la ville en France et en Europe, 1750–1914* (Paris: Les Éditions de l'atelier/Éditions ouvrières, 1996), pp. 254–69, esp. p. 260.

10. The solidaristic dimension of charity has been examined systematically in terms of the concepts and roles of family and community in Katherine A Lynch, *Individuals, families, and communities in Europe, 1200–1800* (New York: Cambridge University Press, 2003), pp. 21 (announcing the theme of "family") and 213 (underscoring "the very fine line that existed between the world of voluntary associations and the world of local urban officials.")

11. The phrase "Beatus qui intellegit super egenem et pauperum" is frequently cited in writings devoted to charitable concerns. It appears among other biblical injunctions to serve the poor in J. L. Vives, *De subventione pauperum sive de humanis necessitatibus Libri II* (Introduction, critical edition, translation, and notes), ed. C. Matheeussen and C. Fantazzi, with the assistance of J. de Landtsheer (Leiden and Boston: Brill, 2002), 64–5. It is the opening verse of Psalm 41 in the King James version.

12. Jean-Pierre Gutton, "Pour l'histoire d'un élite," in *Les administrateurs d'hôpitaux dans la France d'ancien régime*, ed. Jean-Pierre Gutton (Lyon: Presses Universitaires de Lyon, 1999), pp. 7–18, especially p. 13; Benito Pérez Galdos,

Marianela, ed. Francisco Caudit (Madrid: Cátedra, 2003), the story of a blind waif who becomes the object of charity; Vives's comments are in an annotation to his Latin edition of Augustine's *Civitas Dei*; I have consulted the English translation of this edition in the Library of Congress: *St. Avgvstine, of the Citie of God: With the learned comment of Io. Lod. Vives, englished by John Healey* ([London]: Printed by G. Eld, 1610), Book 21, Chapter 7, "Against those who think those sinnes shall not be laid to their charge, where-in they mixed some work of mercy." In a note, Vives castigates those who think it is "a great man's part" to let "Ducats by the thousands" be lost at the gambling table, "but ask a penny for Christ's sake, and they are either as mute as stones, or grieve at the sight of the guift they part from."

13. Daniel Hickey, *Local hospitals in ancien régime France: Rationalization, resistance, renewal, 1530–1789* (Montreal: McGill Queens Press, 1997), pp, 134–74, especially p. 148; Henry Légier Desgranges, *Hospitaliers d'autrefois: Hôpital general de Paris, 1656–1790* (Paris: Hachette, 1952), p. 29 ("les supérieures), and 83 ("les officières"); on the work of new associations, especially those involving women, in seventeenth-century Lyon, see Jean-Pierre Gutton, *La société et les pauvres: L'exemple de la généralité de Lyon, 1534–1789* (Paris: Société d'édition "les belles lettres," 1971), 373; on the evolution of charitable motives among aristocratic Parisian women, see Barbara B. Diefendorf, *From penitence to charity: Pious women and the Catholic Reformation in Paris* (New York: Oxford University Press, 2002).

14. Jean-Pierre Gutton, "Pour l'histoire d'un elite," *Les administrateurs d'hôpitaux dans la France d'ancien régime*, ed. Jean-Pierre Gutton (Lyon: Presses Universitaires de Lyon, 1999), pp.7–18. Among the essays in the same volume that point to the level of effort contributed by administrators, note especially Philippe Loupès, "Les administrateurs des hôpitaux du Sud-Ouest sous l'Ancien Régime: Etude comparée de quatre établissements," in Ibid., pp. 97–109, and Philippe Maret, "Les recteurs et le patrimoine rural: Bonne ou mauvaise gestion," Ibid., pp. 137–46.

15. Daniel Hickey, "Les mécanismes de la stratégie sociale. Bienfaiteurs et administrateurs des hôpitaux locaux en France au XVIIe et XVIIIe siècles in *Les administrateurs d'hôpitaux dans la France d'ancien régime*, ed, Jean-Pierre Gutton (Lyon: Presses Universitaires de Lyon, 1999), 19–41.

16. Madeleine Ferrières, "Les administrateurs du Mont-de-Piété d'Avignon," in Ibid., pp. 11–122 (especially p. 116).

17. Jean-Pierre Gutton, *L'état et la mendicité dans la première moitié du xviiie siècle: Auvergne, Beaujolais, Forez, Lyonnais* (Lyon: Centre d'Études Foréziennes, 1973), pp. 108, 118–26, 222;

18. "Working men preferred independence to pauperism and not simply because pauperism had been stigmatized," observes Derek Fraser in the context of nineteenth-century England, in "The English Poor Law and the origins of the British welfare state," in W. J. Mommsen, ed., *The emergence of the welfare state in Britain and Germany, 1850–1950* (London: Croom Helm; German Historical Institute, 1981), pp. 9–31, esp. p. 27.

19. C. Lis and H. Soly, *Poverty and capitalism in pre-industrial Europe* (Atlantic Highlands, NJ: Humanities Press, 1979), p. 119; Pieter Spierenburg, *The prison experience: Disciplinary institutions and their inmates in early modern Europe* (New Brunswick, NJ: Rutgers University Press, 1991), p. 127. Spierenberg argues, however (p. 129), that houses of correction functioned more as symbols of repression than as actual "training schools" producing disciplined laborers.

20. Hufton, *The poor of eighteenth century France*, pp. 182–93; Robert Castel, *Les metamorphoses de la question sociale: Une chronique du salariat* (Paris:

Fayard, 1995), pp. 139–40; Michael Stolberg, "Health care provision and poor relief in the electorate and kingdom of Bavaria," in Grell et al., eds., *Health care and poor relief*, pp. 112–35, especially p. 118. For a medieval instance, see the discussion following the article by Philippe-Jean Hesse, "Artistes, artisans et sécurité sociale au moyen âge," in Xavier Barral i Altet, ed., *Artistes, artisans et production artistique au moyen âge: Colloque international*, Vol. 1, *Les hommes* (Paris: Picard, 1986), pp. 85–92.

21. Abram de Swaan, *In care of the state: Health care, education and welfare in Europe and the USA in the modern era* (New York: Oxford University Press, 1988), p. 46; Pierre Rosanvallon, *La nouvelle question sociale: Repenser l'état providence* (Paris: Seuil, 1995), p. 139; Claude Seibel, "Le chômage de longue durée et les politiques d'emploi," Tony Atkinson et al., *Pauvreté et exclusion*. La documentation française. Conseil d'Analyse Economique (Paris: La documentation française, 1998), pp. 93–112, especially p. 111.

22. Natalie Zemon Davis, "Poor relief, humanism, and heresy," in Davis, *Society and culture in early modern France: Eight essays by Natalie Zemon Davis* (Stanford: Stanford University Press, 1975), pp. 17–64; Thomas M. Adams, "The provision of work as correction and assistance in France, 1534–1848," in Donald T. Critchlow and Charles H. Parker, eds., *With us always: A History of private charity and public welfare* (Lanham, MD: Rowman and Littlefield, 1998), pp. 55–76; Anne E. C. McCants, *Civic charity in a golden age: Orphan care in early modern Amsterdam* (Urbana: University of Illinois Press, 1997), pp. 63–83, especially p. 76. Valentina K. Tikoff gave a paper on "Orphans as agents of empire: The naval orphanage of San Telmo in Seville, 1681–1847" at the annual meeting of the American Historical Association held in Chicago, January 2000.

23. Thomas Max Safley, *Charity and economy in the orphanages of early modern Augsburg* (Atlantic Highlands, NJ: Humanities Press, 1997), pp. 266–73.

24. Philip S. Gorski, *The disciplinary revolution: Calvinism and the rise of the state in early modern Europe* (Chicago: University of Chicago Press, 2003), pp. 29–30 and 63–7; see also the essays in Christoph Sachsse and Florian Tennstedt, eds., *Soziale sicherheit und sozial disziplinierung: Beiträge zu einer historischen theorie des sozialpolitik* (Frankfort-am-Main, Germany: 1996), and a skeptical view of the concept in Martin Dinges, "Frühneuzeitliche armenfürsorge als sozialdisziplinierung? Probleme mit einem konzept," *Geschichte und Gesellschaft*, 17 (1991), 5–29.

25. Sandra Cavallo, "Charity as boundary making: Social stratification, gender and the family in the Italian states" in Hugh Cunningham and Joanna Innes, eds., *Charity, philanthropy and reform: From the 1690s to 1850s* (New York: St. Martin's Press, 1998), pp. 108–29; also Cavallo, *Charity and power in early modern Italy: Benefactors and their motives in Turin, 1541–1789* (Cambridge: Cambridge University Press, 1995), and Sherrill Cohen, *The evolution of women's asylums since 1500: From refuges for ex-prostitutes to shelters for battered women* (New York: Oxford University Press), pp. 14, 42–43, 127, 171.

26. Bibliothèque de l'assistance publique de Paris (BAAP), Dijon B-45, *Fondations ... hospital St. Esprit et de Notre Dame de la Charité, N.D. de la Charité, 1649*, p.55, "Du devoir des maistresses qui ont charge de monstrer les ouvrages aux filles"; the author states that whatever truth there may be to the charge that women are the cause of evil in the world, it only applies to the vicious, "et ne touche point les bonnes et vertueuses, qui peuvent faire du bien, qui en ont fait en tout temps, et qui en font encore journellement. Que si à leur occasion il s'en fait par des hommes perdus, qui sont sans crainte de Dieu et sans respect de leur semblables, ce n'est plus aux femmes qu'il s'en faut prendre, mais aux

hommes." The statement on work comes from a later regulation, *Règlement du 11 juin 1752, concernant la nourriture et le travail des pauvres à l'hôpital de Notre-Dame de la Charité, etabli en la ville de Dijon*. Dijon, Antoine de Fay, 1752 (BAAP, A-971). On the perceived need to prepare women for working roles, see Lynch, *Individuals, families, and communities*, pp. 154–5.

27. Léon Lallemand, *Histoire de la charité*, 4 vols. (Paris, 1902–1912); Camille Bloch, *L'assistance et l'état en France à la veille de la Révolution: Généralités de Paris, Rouen, Alençon, Orléans, Soissons, Amiens (1764–1790)* (Paris, 1908); Alan Forrest, *The French Revolution and the poor* (New York: St. Martin's Press, 1981), pp. 76–7.

28. Adams, *Bureaucrats and beggars*, pp. 34–35, with further discussion of Turgot's views on "mendicité" as *intendant* and controller-general; on "patriotic gifts," see Lynch, *Individuals, families, and communities*, pp. 181–3.

29. Catherine Duprat, *Le temps des philanthropes: La philanthropie parisienne des lumières a la monarchie de juillet*, Vol 1. (Paris, 1993); Steven M. Baudouin, "Without belonging to public service: Charities, the state, and civil society in Third Republic Bordeaux, 1870–1914," *Journal of Social History*, 31,3 (Spring 1998), 671–99; Timothy Smith, *Creating the welfare state in France, 1880–1940* (Montreal: McGill-Queens University Press, 2003); Paul V. Dutton, *Origins of the French welfare state: The struggle for social reform in France 1914–1947* (Cambridge: Cambridge University Press, 2002); Christian Topalov, ed., *Laboratoires du nouveau siècle: La nébuleuse réformatrice et ses réseaux en France, 1880–1914* (Paris: EHESS, 1999); Janet Horne, *A social laboratory for modern France: The musée social and the rise of the welfare state* (Durham, NC: Duke University Press, 2002).

30. Timothy B. Smith, "The ideology of charity, the image of the English Poor Law, and debates over the right to assistance in France, 1830–1903," *The Historical Journal*, 40, 4 (December, 1997), 997–1032; for Malesherbes's remarks, see Pierre Grosclaude, *Malesherbes: Témoin et interprète de son temps* (Paris, 1961), pp. 348–49; and Adams, *Bureaucrats and beggars*, p. 154.

31. Bernard Harris, *The origins of the British welfare state: Society, state, and social welfare in England and Wales, 1800–1945* (New York: Palgrave Macmillan, 2004), pp. 72–75; Derek Fraser, *The evolution of the British welfare state*, 3rd ed. (New York: Palgrave Macmillan, 2003), p. 157; Robert Humphreys, *Sin, organized charity and the Poor Law in Victorian England* (New York: St. Martin's Press, 1995), pp. 151, 157.

32. Geoffrey B. A. M. Finlayson, *Citizen, state, and social welfare in Britain, 1830–1990* (New York: Oxford University Press, 1994), pp. 297, 400; see the caveats against simplistic historical assumptions in Peregrine Horden and Richard Smith, ed., *The locus of care: Families, communities, institutions, and the provision of welfare since antiquity* (London: Routledge, 1998), pp. 1–18 (editors' introduction), especially pp. 4–6.

33. Allan Mitchell, *The divided path: The German influence on social reform in France after 1870* (Chapel Hill: University of North Carolina Press, 1991).

34. Christoph Sachße and Florian Tennstedt, *Geschichte der armenfúrsorge in Deutschland, Vo.l 1, Vom Spätmittelalter bis zum 1. Weltkrieg*, 2nd ed. (Stuttgart, Germany: Kohlhammer, 1998), p. 215; Mary Lindemann, *Patriots and paupers: Hamburg, 1712–1830* (New York: Oxford University Press, 1990), p. 12; Gerhard A. Ritter, *Der sozialstaat: Entstehung und entwicklung im internationaler vergleich* (Munich: Oldenbourg, 1991), p. 85; George Steinmetz, *Regulating the social: The welfare state and local politics in imperial Germany* (Princeton, NJ: Princeton University Press, 1993), p. 216.

35. Edward Ross Dickenson, *The politics of German child welfare from the Empire to the Federal Republic* (Cambridge, MA: Harvard University Press,

1996); Constantin Goschler, *Rudolf Virchow: Medizin, politiker, anthropologe* (Cologne, Germany: Boehlau, 2002); David F. Crew, *Germans on welfare from Weimar to Hitler* (New York: Oxford University Press, 1998), p. 137; for two transatlantic perspectives, see Kathryn Kish Sklar, Anja Schüler, and Susan Strasser, eds., *Social justice feminists in the United States and Germany: A dialogue in documents, 1885–1933* (Ithaca, NY: Cornell University Press, 1998); and Daniel T. Rodgers, *Atlantic crossings: Social politics in a progressive age* (Cambridge, MA: Harvard University Press, 1998), pp. 82–111.

36. Crew, *Germans on welfare*, p. 89; Young-Sun Hong, *Welfare, modernity, and the Weimar state, 1919–1933* (Princeton, NJ: Princeton University Press, 1998), p. 111.

37. Gerhard Ritter, *Sozialstaat*, 163; A. J. Nicholls, *Freedom with responsibility: The social market economy in Germany, 1918–1963* (Oxford: Clarendon, 1994), p. 396.

38. Boris Simon, *Abbé Pierre and the ragpickers of Emmaus* (New York: J. P. Kennedy and Sons, 1955).

39. See the introductory essay by the editors in *Politik der armut und die spaltung des sozialstaats*, eds. Stephan Leibfried and Florian Tennstedt (Frankfurt-am-Main, Germany: Suhrkampf, 1985), p. 17, and their explicit references to the undermined "moral economy" of the welfare state in "Armenpolitik und arbeiterpolitik: Zur entwicklung und krise der traditionellen sozialpolitik der verteilungsformen," in ibid., pp. 64–93, esp. pp. 65 and 92; Eckart Pankoke and Christoph Sachsse, "Armutsdiskurs und wohlfahrtforschung am deutschen weg in die industrielle moderne," in Stephan Liebfried and Wolfgang Voges, *Armut im modernen wohlfahrtstaat*, published by the *Kólner Zeitschrift für Soziologie und Sozialpsychologie*, Sonderheft 32 (1992), pp. 149–178, esp. pp. 168–9; for a similar diagnosis for France, see Colette Bec, *L'assistance en démocratie* (Paris: Belin, 1998), pp. 146 and 191 in particular.

40. Amartya Sen, *Development as freedom* (New York: Alfred A. Knopf, 1999), pp. 94–6; *The Frankfurter Allgemeine Zeitung* reported March 2, 2005, that unemployment had reached a record high of 5.2 million, or 12.6 percent. For an indictment of French "solidarity" in practice, see Timothy B. Smith, *France in crisis: Welfare, inequality and globalization since 1980* (New York: Cambridge University Press, 2004).

41. Jürgen Habermas, "Die krise des wohlfahrtsstaates und die erschöpfung utopischer energien," in Habermas, *Zeitdiagnosen: Zwölf Essays, 1980–2001* (Frankfurt-am-Main, Gernany: Suhrkampf, 2003), pp. 27–49 (text first published 1985, based on a speech of 24 November 1984); see the typology of various diagnoses of the ills of the welfare state by Jens Alber, "Der deutsche sozialstaat in der Ära Kohl: Diagnosen und daten," in Stephan Leibfried and Uwe Wagschal, eds., *Der deutsche sozialstaat: Bilanzen—reformen—perspectiven* (Frankfurt/New York: Campus Verlag, 2000), pp. 235–275.

42. Siegfried Lamnek, *Tatort sozialstaat: Schwarzarbeit, leistungsmissbrauch, steuerhinterziehung und ihre (hinter) grunder* (Opladen, Germany: Leske and Budrick, 2000), p. 18; the central importance of an ethic of self-help is developed in a historical context by Peter Gross, "Selbsthilfe und selbstverantwortung als normativen leitideen der sozialpolitik," in Christoph Sachsse and H. Tristam Engelhardt, eds., *Sicherheit und freiheit: zur ethik des wohlfahrtsstaates* (Frankfurt-am-Main, Germany: Suhrkampf, 1990), pp. 85–105.

43. For critical perspectives on these issues, see Siegfried Lamnek and Jens Luedtke, eds., *Der sozialstaat zwischen "markt" und "hedonismus"?* (Opladen, Germany: Leske and Budrich, 1999), esp. the concluding chapter summarizing the analysis of social deviance, pp. 368–85; Lutz Leiserung and Stephan Leibfried, *Time and poverty in Western welfare state: United Germany in perspective*

(New York: Cambridge University Press, 1999), examines longitudinal case studies of recipients of public assistance.

44. Jelle Visser and Anton Hemerijk, *"A Dutch miracle": Job growth, welfare reform, and corporatism in the Netherlands* (Amsterdam: Amsterdam University Press, 1997); Urban Lundberg and Klas Amark, "Social rights and social security: The Swedish welfare state, 1900–2000," *Scandinavian Journal of History*, 26:3 (2001), 157–176.

45. Rolf G. Heinze, Thomas Olk, and Josef Hilbert, *Der neue Sozialstaat: Analyse und reformperspektiven* (Freiburg-im-Breisgau, Germany: Lambertus Verlag, 1988), p. 101; my translation of Kohl's words (the term *gemeinschaft* carries the resonances of "community" in contradistinction to "society"): "Wir wollen mehr selbst- und nächstenhilfe der bürger füreinander. Das politische strukturprinzip dafür ist die subsidiarität. Es verlangt die vorfahrt für die jeweils kleinere gemeinschaft. Was diese zu leisten vermag, soll ihr die grösser nicht abnehmen. Familie, nachbarschaft, freie träger, initiativ- und selbsthilfegruppen und sociale dienste können mehr bürgersinn und bürgerverantwortung erzeugen, als es grossen und anonymen institutionen je möglich sein wird."

46. Ibid., p. 106; Eric Jakob, *Europa und der sozialphilosophische hintergrund der subsidiaritätsprinzips* (Bern: Stämpfli; Zurich: Schultheis, 2000), p. 47; see the nuanced critique of self-help arguments in Ernst von Kardorff and Elmar Koenen, "Armenpolitik und selbstorganisation," in Leibfried and Tennstedt, *Politik der armut*, pp. 357–79; .

47. Ken Endo, "The principle of subsidiarity: From Johannes Althusius to Jacques Delors," *The Hokkaido Law Review*, 44:6 (1994), 652–553 (pagination in descending order); for an unsympathetic view of Delors and his conception of subsidiarity, see John Gillingham, *European integration, 1950–2003: Superstate or new market economy* (New York: Cambridge University Press, 2003), pp. 157–163

48. Bernard Rudden and Derrick Wyatt, eds., *Basic community laws*, 5th ed. (Oxford: Clarendon Press, 1994), p. 29.

49. Jacques Delors, "Le principe de subsidiarité" (au Colloque de l'institut Européen d'Administration Publique à Maastricht, le 21 mars 1991), in Delors, *Le nouveau concert européen* (Paris, 1992), pp. 163–76. As president of the European Commission, Jacques Delors framed the argument for a policy that ensured social rights in a global marketplace in the EU document, *Pour entrer dans le XXIe siècle: Emploi, croissance, compétitivité: Le livre blanc de la Commission Européenne* (Paris: Michel Lafon, 1994); original report published 1993, pp. ii and 33).

50. See Paul Misner, "Christian democratic social policy: Precedents for third-way thinking," in Thomas Kselman and Joseph A. Buttigieg, eds., *European Christian democracy: Historical legacies and comparative perspectives* (Notre Dame, IN: University of Notre Dame Press, 2003), pp. 68–92, especially pp. 85–8; Harold L. Wilensky, "Leftism, Catholicism, and democratic corporatism: The role of political parties in recent welfare state development," in Peter Flora and Arnold J. Heidenheimer, *The development of welfare state in Europe and America* (New Brunswick, NJ.: Transaction, 1990), pp. 345–82, esp. pp. 351–53; Ignazio Massulli, *Welfare state e patte sociale in Europa: Gran Bretagna, Germania, Francia, Italia, 1954–1985* (Bologna: CLUEB, 2003), p. 261 (on the center-left political alliance); Jacques Delors evokes the Italian contribution in citing A. Spinelli's recourse to the term "subsidiarity" in a report of 1975 on the Commission of the European Union and the ensuing treaty of 1984 (*Nouveau concert*, p. 164).

51. Hertie Roundtable: "The welfare state: Past present, and future in transatlantic perspective: A discussion with Kurt Biedenkopf," Monday, February 2,

2004, at the German Historical Institute, Washington, DC; "From confederacy to federation–Thoughts on the finality of European integration," speech by Joschka Fischer at the Humboldt University in Berlin, 12 May 2000, obtained on line in 2000 from: http:www.german-embassy.org.uk/speech_of_foreign_minister_fis.html; Jacques Delors, *Le nouveau concert européen* (Paris, 1992), p. 124 (speech of 14 July 1985).

52. For critical commentary, see Yves Chassard, "La construction européenne et la protection sociale à la veille de l'élargissement de l'union," *Droit Social,* March 1999, pp. 268–78; Wolfgang Merkel, "Die Europäische integration und das elend der theorie," *Geschichte und Gesellschaft,* 25 (1999), 302–338, Bernhard Ebbinghaus and Jelle Visser, "European labor and transnational solidarity: Challenges, pathways, and barriers," in Jytte Klausen and Louise Tilly, eds., *European integration in social and historical perspective: 1850 to the present* (Lanham, sMD: Rowman and Littlefield, 1997), pp. 51–70; and Wolfgang Streeck, "European social policy after Maastricht: The 'social dialogue' and 'subsidiarity,'" *Economic and industrial democracy* (London: Sage), Vol. 15 (1994), pp. 151–77, esp. p. 171.

53. For a judicious assessment of the degree of progress achieved by consultation, goal setting, and benchmarking, see Robert Geyer, *Exploring European social policy* (Oxford, UK: Blackwell, 2000), pp. 163, 208–12.

54. A number of conferences and symposia have focused on the concept of subsidiarity, its intellectual genealogy, and its applications, including, for example, Alois Riklin and Gerard Batliner, eds., *Subsidiarität: Ein interdiziplinäres Symposium des Liechtenstien-Instituts 23–25 September 1993* (Vaduz: Verlag der Liechtensteinischen Akademischen Gesellschaft, 1994).

55. Castel, *Metamorphoses de la question sociale,* pp. 55–58 and 471; Jean-Paul Fitoussi and Pierre Rosanvallon, *Le nouvel âge des inégalités* (Paris: Seuil, 1996), pp. 191–99. For a treatment of subsidiarity that explicitly accentuates its positive potential for France and Europe, see Claude de Granrut, *La citoyenneté européenne: Une application du principe de subsidiarité* (Paris: Librairie Générale de Droit et de Jurisprudence, 1997).

56. Paul Slack, *From Reformation to improvement,* p. 151; Richard Smith focuses on the historical importance of "a view of welfare that serves to promote self-sufficiency and self-interest" in his essay, "Charity, self-interest, and welfare: Reflections from demographic and family history," in Martin Daunton, ed., *Charity, self-interest and welfare in the English past* (London: University College of London Press, 1996), pp. 23–49, esp. p. 45; see also the discussion of the concept of "community care" in Mathew Thomson, "Community care and the control of mental defectives in inter-war Britain," in Horden and Smith, eds., *Locus of care,* pp. 198–216.

57. J. A Schumpeter, *Capitalism, socialism, and democracy* (New York: Harper, 1950; 1st ed., 1944), p. 139; cited by Gøsta Esping-Anderson, *Three worlds of welfare capitalism* (Princeton, NJ: Princeton University Press, 1990), p. 27.

4 Supporting Self-Help
Charity, Mutuality, and Reciprocity in Nineteenth-Century Britain

Daniel Weinbren

Open University

Since at least 1697, when Daniel Defoe contrasted friendly societies and charitable institutions, friendly societies have been regarded as separate from charities. Many scholars have maintained the distinction. There is little on friendly societies in Roberts's book on charities, nor is there much material about charities in Hopkins's work on working-class self-help.[1] Winter stressed that "mutual aid is not paternalism, neither is it charity nor is it philanthropy," and O'Neill argued that "friendly societies were not charities."[2] Others too have not categorised friendly societies with charities, instead presenting them as linked to either trade unions or insurance companies.[3] However, such a taxonomy, which obscures the overlapping range of activities, functions, members, and structures of friendly societies and charities, has not always been adopted.[4] Gorsky has shown how in eighteenth-century Britain many charities were "coloured by mutualist sentiment," and Prochaska argued that in the nineteenth century "the boundaries between religion, philanthropy and mutual aid were less marked than in the past."[5] Harris too has suggested a porous boundary in the nineteenth century, noting that because it was viewed with ambivalence by recipients, some charitable activity was presented in terms of mutual aid.[6] In this chapter, the importance of networks of obligation for both friendly societies and charities are highlighted in order to illuminate the circulation of power within and between these bodies.

In the *Common Origins* section, the importance of the guild traditions to both friendly societies and charities will be demonstrated by reference to the guilds, charities, and friendly societies of Lynn, west Norfolk.[7] This recognition of the historical precedents is followed by the employment, in *The Gift Relationship* section, of Marcel Mauss's conceptualisation of a cycle of giving, receiving, and returning "gifts." The importance of building networks rather than engaging in single transactions was widely recognised. Reciprocity was pervasive within working class communities. In the early 1870s, a report on Poor Law administration commented on the practice of collections to help widows:

What amounts to interchange of charitable assistance among the poor in London is not uncommon ... they assist each other to an extent which is little understood. ... It is scarcely possible to conceive a form of charity which combines so completely its highest reciprocal benefits with the absence of mischief so frequently incident to almsgiving.[8]

The implications of this widespread acceptance of reciprocation are assessed in *The Familiarity of Reciprocity* section. Over the course of the nineteenth century, many of the symbiotic ties between the friendly society and charitable patrons, on the one hand, and working class members and recipients, on the other hand, remained. Overt control of friendly societies diminished, but ties of trust with charities were created and renewed. Through reference to the work of Mark Granovetter, who has provided a useful framework for understanding such relationships with his categorisation of ties as being either "weak" or "strong," these shifts are explored in the *Independence and Patronage* section. Through this emphasis on the significance of cycles of exchange and networks, the promotion by charities and friendly societies of self-help, independence, loyalty, and a sense of community can be understood as evidence of the extent to which these bodies bolstered and reflected widely held values.

COMMON ORIGINS

In that they promoted collective self-help, Christian morality, elections, costumes, feasting, ceremonies, and visits to the homes of the recipients of largesse, medieval and early-modern religious and craft guilds can be seen as the parents of both friendly societies and charities. Guilds took a variety of forms, but among their most frequently expressed aims were fellowship, charity, commerce, conviviality, and a commitment to endow members with trading privileges. For most, the central function was to enable men to assemble in order to ensure the welfare of both members and others. Although not the only source for the tradition of such charitable feasting as fund-raising dinners and "charity ales," the annual banquets of medieval parish guilds, which were held in honour of patron saints, involved sharing with paupers and "celebrated, in the view of guests, a spirit of solidarity, friendship, and peace." As such, they were a significant precedent for charities and friendly societies.[9]

In fourteenth-century Lynn, probably half the men of the town were members of guilds, associations that were organised to provide for members who were unable to work due to fire, theft, or old age. There was also a long-standing tradition of these guilds honouring their dead and of members dressing in regalia on parades and providing for widows and orphans. Although assisting the needy was seen as a means of improving an individual's prospects of reaching heaven, Lynn's guilds were discriminating. They favoured members over others and the deserving over the undeserving. Even after the Reformation, guilds played an important role within the corporation, an élite body that held feasts and processions, had regalia and rituals, and elected the mayor of what has been called a "city state."[10] Lynn's Trinity Gild had ceremonial and civic activities, was wealthy, exclusive, and its officers visited those in receipt of payments.[11] Guild traditions continued to resonate within popular memory throughout the nineteenth century. In 1880, to mark the annual conference of the Manchester Unity Oddfellows being held in Lynn, there was a reception of the Guildhall, a procession through the town, a fête, a gala, and a banquet presided over by the mayor.[12] In 1906, a leading member of the Ancient Order of Foresters Friendly Society (AoF), Charles Ward, related the popularity of the AoF in Lynn to the large number of social and benevolent guilds, thirty-one in 1744, whose "work appears to have been on very similar lines to the modern friendly society."[13] Highlighting their understanding of their roots, the term *guild* was employed by a variety of later bodies. In late nineteenth-century Bristol, there was a friendly society called the Guild of St Mary and St Joseph and Guilds of Help were formed to "minister to the needs of the honest poor" and promote thrift and self-help in Bradford (1904), Wimbledon (1907), and a number of other towns.[14]

The late nineteenth-century registrar of friendly societies, Edward Brabrook, remarked that the small, simple village society resembled the benefit system of the guilds, Toulmin Smith referred to the guilds' spirit of "mutual self-help" and "manly independence," and Walford argued that the roots of modern insurance lay in the guilds.[15] In the 1920s, Clapham rhetorically argued that friendly societies' graveside duties and drinking were "an old inheritance. Did not Anglo-Saxon gilds pay a subscription in malt"?[16] More recently, Walker has demonstrated that seventeenth-century friendly societies had "the weight of guild heritage behind them," and Gorsky concluded that "gild mutualism was to be the template for the practices of later benefit clubs."[17]

Charities also drew on guild traditions seeking to help the poor and bind together recipients and donors. In eighteenth-century Bristol, the annual meetings of charities typically included a Christian service, a procession, and a feast in one of the old guild halls. The founders of the late eighteenth-century charity, the Strangers Friend Society, made visiting a regular part of its work with a system of checks similar to those developed by many friendly societies. Members subscribed money and placed suggestions as to suitable recipients in a box. A committee assessed the proposals and dispatched visitors to check on the recommended individuals. If appropriate, a second visitor would check again and then hand over the charity.[18] Subscriber democracy spread to other charities. Funding was collected from the members, who elected a committee of higher status members and constructed an elaborate hierarchy of grades of membership. "Voting charities" drew up a list of candidates eligible for relief and provided subscribers with a number of votes proportionate to their subscriptions.

Like the guilds in the earlier period, many charities and friendly societies in the nineteenth century sought to promote solidarity by reinforcing
the sense of mutual obligation among members. Relief was seen as meeting institutional as well as individual needs. For both guilds and friendly
societies, a member's inability to carry on his trade or profession was the
principal criterion for deciding who deserved assistance. Members who met
this criterion would have been classed with the deserving poor, a group
that included orphans, widows, the aged, the sick, the maimed, and otherwise self-supporting men and women who had fallen on hard times due
to events beyond their control.[19] Like some of the guilds, friendly societies
developed systems for paying "travelling brothers," that is, members who
were supported in their search for work in towns other than their own.[20]
Many developed secret rituals, partly to ensure that new arrivals were genuine "travelling brothers." In a similar fashion, the Society of Friends had a
national, organized, charitable system to support travelling Friends, apprentices, and paupers with medical and funeral costs, while the organisers of
the Anglican-run charitable mothers' meetings ensured that recipients were
deserving by sifting through their membership to reduce the number of
"travellers" who abused the system. Many guilds and friendly societies had
explicit behavioural regulations, forbidding gambling, for example. Some
charities, and many friendly societies, had costumes and ceremonies, such as
the Warwick Bread Dole or the buttons decorated with shears on the clothing provided by a tailor's charity in Atherstone, Warwickshire.[21] To ensure
institutional survival, members, whether of guilds or friendly societies, had
to be bound together into a cohesive whole. This could be accomplished
through the shared experiences of fraternal life and the mutual obligation to
be respectful and to pray for members. Similarly, charities sought to develop
a sense of obligation and commitment to the public good.

THE GIFT RELATIONSHIP

Marcel Mauss's theory about the gift relationship can be used to illuminate
the similarities between friendly societies and charities. He argued that a
cycle of giving, receiving, and returning *prestations* (gifts that could include
religious offices, rank, possessions, and labour) lay at "the heart of normal
social life." Attending funerals, comforting the bereaved, visiting the sick,
holding office, or deference could be manifestations of gift giving, as could
supporting an MP who was indebted to his electorate and moral behaviour,
which implied a need for a response. Linking charity and fair dealing, Mauss
suggested that alms were the "gift morality raised to the position of a principle of justice" but that "friendly societies are better than mere personal
security guaranteed by the nobleman to his tenant, better than the mean life
afforded by the daily wages handed out by the managements and better even
than the uncertainty of capitalist savings." By accepting a "gift," the recipient

also accepted the obligation to reciprocate. If gifts were a mixture of altruism and selfishness based on the principle of *do ut des* (I give so that you may return), then "generosity and self-interest are linked in giving." People employed the tangible in a fashion which bound them through unspoken contracts: "Sentiments and personas are mingled. This confusion of personalities and things is precisely the mark of exchange contracts." Relationships within the cycle of exchange were not necessarily equal. A generous donor could maintain social divisions because, as there was no such thing as a free gift, a refusal to reciprocate was "a declaration of war." Until the debt was requited, the recipient had to act deferentially towards that donor. Mauss pointed out that

> The great acts of generosity are not free from self-interest . . . between vassals and chiefs, between vassals and their henchmen, the hierarchy is established by means of these gifts. To give is to show one's superiority, to show that one is something more and higher. . . . To accept without returning or repaying is to face subordination, to become a client . . . if one hoards it is only to spend later on, to put people under obligation and to win followers.[22]

Even though the poor preferred mutual aid to overt charity and the friendly societies stressed their independence, in terms of the Maussian gift economy, friendly society membership was akin to being a recipient of or donor to charity, in that it was a means by which strategic, financial, and social gifts were exchanged for social or other capital. Both charities and friendly societies sought to increase trust between members, or clients and patrons, by placing upon them that which Mauss saw as the triple obligation to give, receive, and return "gifts." In the 1860s, considerable emphasis was placed on the importance of personal relationships between charitable donors and recipients, although "ideally the gift was an organic relationship . . . in a large urban area where the rich and poor had been separated, the social powers supposedly inherent in the gift had disappeared." The Charity Organisation Society (COS) was established in 1869 to force the malingering poor to "relearn the virtues of thrift and self help" while encouraging the poor to help themselves. Such an approach was also a prominent feature of the settlements such as Toynbee Hall, which was established in 1883.[23] Reciprocity was more than an economic survival strategy; it helped to create communities based on obligation.

THE FAMILIARITY OF RECIPROCITY

Much of Mauss's focus was on "archaic" non-European societies. He examined the cycle of exchange in the Trobriand Islands and concluded that, in a gift economy, what mattered when objects, even those of great value, changed hands was the relations between people. He argued that gift exchange merged people and objects, interest and disinterest, and that by the nineteenth century in Europe these had become disaggregated with the "victory of rationalism and mercantilism."[24] However, there is evidence that, although often associated with the premodern marketplace (where exchanges were dependent on credit and typically were solidified only after hours of negotiation in a local tavern, over drinks and in front of witnesses), personal credit and attendant ideas of a moral economy persisted well into Victorian times.[25] For the middle class, it continued to be safest to extend credit only to those of good character.[26] For working men and women, there are examples of reciprocity being the basis of relationships in many areas of the United Kingdom. In the nineteenth century, reciprocity and trust within economic relations were familiar and stabilizing notions. Employing the language of reciprocity made sense to many people.[27] It was argued that malingering or moral hazard would be reduced if friendly society members or charitable donors or recipients felt that they would be adversely affected if they lost the regard of others.

Engels was one of many observers who commented upon the extent of working-class mutual help.[28] According to the satirical magazine *Porcupine* in 1880, the poor "have a system of mutual assistance, a habit of helping each other, which prevents many of them ever becoming rich in anything but nobleness of character."[29] Reports of the 1832 pay negotiations between the Durham and Northumberland-based Coal Miners' Friendly Society and the employers indicate that "the language of fairness and reciprocity was central to this culture of bargaining and negotiation."[30] On other coalfields, friendly societies promoted cooperation between employers and workers.[31] County court judges refused to enforce credit contracts that had not been mediated by personal contact between traders and poor consumers.[32] By the mid-nineteenth century, high-volume, low-markup, multiple shops were selling at single publicly posted fixed prices for cash. However, small shops continued to offer items "on tick" in return for loyalty. Customers only settled their accounts and purchased goods elsewhere if the cycle of reciprocity broke down.

In London, Lees described how "Irish neighbours contributed money for funeral expenses, if the dead person's kin could not raise enough. Neighbours loaned money."[33] In the East End, "the bulk of women's day-to-day sharing was exchange: In theory, at least, reciprocity was the rule."[34] White provides examples of mutual aid among the poor of Islington, including "pudding bowl collections for bereavements . . . neighbourhood-based 'diddlum' clubs for savings and credit . . . and the Vernon 'Help-One-Another Society'," formed in 1899.[35] Walsworth vicar Arthur Jephson wrote of the Waterloo area of the 1880s that "as long as one person has anything to share, they are willing to share it. . . . The starving can always secure help from neighbours in distress, for the poorest never know when their turn to starve may not come."[36] In Preston, it was "well-nigh essential to make every effort to keep in contact with, or enter into reciprocal assistance with, kins-men, if life chances were not to be seriously imperilled" and in the Potter-ies there is evidence of "reciprocity negotiated between family members"[37] Archie Cameron described the "mutual aid" between the poor of the island of Rhum, which, between 1843 and 1957, was a privately owned estate.[38] In rural Perthshire, *lovedargs* were both a system of neighbourly reciproc-ity and one used by the wealthy to embed their social superiority.[39] In early nineteenth-century Wales, community not conjugality was highlighted at weddings when the entire neighbourhood was invited to give presents. Each practical gift would be noted and an appropriate gift returned, if not to the individuals then to their descendants.[40] In Ireland, farmers did not pay off their debts to suppliers in order to maintain a state of mutual indebted-ness to neighbours engaging in reciprocal support.[41] In rural England, one of the most popular forms of supported self-help, familiar from the 1840s and provided for one in three male agricultural labourers by 1873, was allotments. These were a means by which clerics and landowners provided assistance in order to improve morality, reduce the rates, local taxes, and increase social stability.[42] Provided for the deserving and taken from rule breakers, allotments were "about moral issues and moral improvements" and often linked to other landlord-inspired improvements such as medical and clothing clubs.[43] They too can be seen as evidence of the continuing importance of a notion of reciprocity.

Perhaps because, as Mauss pointed out, "charity wounds him who receives, and our whole moral effort is directed towards suppressing the unconscious harmful patronage of the almoner," some charities stressed the importance of reciprocity.[44] John Money has suggested that the Freemasons conceived of charity in terms of mutual aid, that they saw "charity primar-ily in terms of their own self-realisation. To 'make' a mason, archetypically formed and regularly tested to the 'working' of his lodge was itself the best form of charity because it conferred those attributes of 'character' without which charity was wasted on the recipient."[45]

Durr argued that the Freemasons had a concept of "fraternal charity," that is, "an ideology of interdependence, its practical manifestation being giving and receiving."[46] Other bodies also blurred the distinctions between charitable and mutual-aid activities. Ellen Ranyard founded a mission which sold Bibles. It also offered advice to poor women and created schemes to pay for clothing, coal, food, and furniture. In 1857, that is, within a decade of the foundation of this mission, £44,000 had been collected through its provident funds.[47] Despite its name, the Girls' Friendly Society was not legally a friendly society. However, this popular Anglican-dominated body, which had gained over 150,000 members within 25 years of its foundation in 1875, provided benefits for the virtuous and sought to create a sense of fictive kinship for young unmarried women away from home. Its object was "to create a bond of union between ladies and working girls . . . forming a Society, a kind of Freemasonry among women, of which the sign manual shall be Purity and the hand held out shall be Fellowship."[48] In Scotland, with its different legal system from England and Wales, the poor had limited rights to poor relief, which was distributed by ministers and elders of the kirk and landowners before the passage of the Scottish Poor Law of 1845. Relief was sometimes dependent on voluntary assessments from parish inhabitants because landowners, often absentee, evaded assessments for poor relief. It was also sometimes presented as mutual aid. An Edinburgh cabinetmaker said that workmates raised seven pounds to pay for a colleague's funeral and enable his widow to be free, as they put it, from "charity." Such acts were common and Winter argued that "poor people would perceive this as mutual aid, not charity." He called this "begging . . . disguised as a form of mutual aid," which marginalizes that the two were sometimes indistinguishable, indeed, as he concludes, "relief from friends could be thought of as a reciprocal arrangement."[49] These charitable practices and formulations enabled people to retain their dignity and social standing because they were understood to be part of a cycle of reciprocity. Even after the 1845 legislation, applicants for relief did not present themselves as victims but active agents, and in both England and Scotland "the relationship between people and parish was one of negotiation."[50] In rural England, too, advocates of allotments argued that, although it was the wealthy who provide the land, it was important to "avoid any appearance of charity."[51]

Some friendly societies provided charity. A number of lifeboats donated by friendly societies carried the name of the donors, and when, in 1884, four men were rescued by the Cleethorpes-based *Manchester Unity* lifeboat, the story was publicized through the *Oddfellows' Magazine*.[52] In 1800 in Manchester, a Union of Friendly Societies collected donations and distributed food cheaply to the poor. In 1877, the Free Gardeners of Redcar provided a lifeboat house with reading room and accommodation for the coxswain and a lifeboat, named the *United Free Gardener*.[53] In 1906, the Henry Flowers Manchester Unity Odd Fellows lodge, Salthouse Norfolk, the treasurers of which had been vicars between 1894 and 1900, started a distress fund to which all members contributed and from which those in need of additional help received payments.[54] There was also charitable help for individuals. The Druids held a concert at which the opportunity was taken to present "an injured brother a sum of £40 and on another occasion £25 was given to a disabled member." The Crewe Co-operative Industrial and Friendly Society ran a dentist and sick-benefit club for employees, donated to local people, famine relief in India, locked-out engineers in 1897, and the local hospital, to which it also recommended patients.[55] Members of the larger, affiliated, friendly societies could appeal to their lodges for help beyond that which was expected, and then their region and finally the national organizers. For example, at its annual delegate meetings the Foresters decided on which members were worthy of additional charitable help from its funds.

Some donors to charity expected reciprocity. Being treated in many hospitals often required the support of a patron, that is, a letter from a subscriber or governor.[56] These patrons included friendly societies. For example, between 1765 and 1814, sixteen friendly societies donated to Northampton General Hospital and thus secured places for their members.[57] The 1831 opening ceremony of Huddersfield Infirmary was attended by the Manchester Unity Odd Fellows, Royal Foresters, Ancient Order of Shepherds, and various local societies. By the 1870s, the annual Friendly Societies Demonstration made several hundred pounds each year for the hospital. The rules of the hospital made provision for the treatment of subscribing friendly societies. In its inaugural year, six friendly societies paid an annual subscription, twenty-four years later it was thirteen, and by 1865, sixteen societies. Many also made donations. In return, the infirmary provided for a number of patients. A similar system operated at Wakefield Infirmary.[58] In Crewe, the friendly societies were generous donors to the Crewe and District Hospital Sunday Fund. They held a fête for the fund and a fund-raising annual gala from 1865. Other friendly societies sought reciprocity in different forms. In 1846, members of the Birmingham Catholic Friendly Society subscribed to the Queen's Hospital, "for the benefit of charity and also to convince our fellow townsmen that Catholics are at least as ready and willing to forward good works as any others."[59] The Saturday Fund, founded in 1874, raised money for hospitals through "monster demonstrations" and the collection of a penny a week from numerous people. It campaigned for more working-class governors and the right to determine which patients were admitted to hospital. Although it may have been a contributory insurance scheme, it was presented by hospital authorities as a form of self-help philanthropy.[60] In its aims, "it partly reflected the mutual aid societies by offering its supporters the possibility of a return on their contribution in time of sickness," and indeed it was criticised as being an attempt at working people's self-help.[61]

Some charities established friendly societies. In 1800 in Warrington, the Masonic Lodge of Lights had both a Masonic Benefit Society and links to the White Hart Benefit Society. In Bristol, the Colston collecting societies, named after a local philanthropist, combined mutuality, charity, and guild traditions, and the Temple Lodge Benefit Society was both a Masonic Lodge and a friendly society.[62] In general, "the friendly society values of Freemasonry are evident throughout in the late eighteenth and early nineteenth centuries." The Masonic Lodge of Friendship, Oldham, gave a grant to a brother whose wife was ill, purchased a coffin for a deceased brother, and made payments to imprisoned brothers. It started a benevolent society in 1828 and a sick fund in 1829. The local Unitarian church, run in the 1860s by a Freemason, had long been involved in welfare work and had its own sick and clothing clubs.[63] In the 1880s, the Oxford COS was central to the creation and subsequent development of the Oxford Working Women's Benefit Society.[64] The COS "argued that even the very poor could join friendly societies, sick clubs, or even keep savings accounts and therefore should not need poor relief."[65] In 1908, Freemason Lord Baden Powell established a charity, the Scout Association, and in 1914 became president of an associated fraternal body whose first trustees were all peers, the Scouts Friendly Society. Many nonconformist bodies, which were charities, including the Salvation Army and numerous Sunday schools, ran their own friendly societies.[66] The near-ubiquitous philanthropic mothers' meetings often had savings banks and friendly sick-benefit clubs attached and "saturated the poor with a mix of benevolence and self-help."[67] Operating within separate, but comparable, spheres, wives and husbands could support their families through single-sex gatherings outside the home, with the former sewing at charitable mothers meetings and the latter drinking in the friendly society lodge.

In his 1948 report on voluntary activity, William Beveridge distinguished between the motives associated with mutual aid and those associated with charity.[68] However, many of the motives assigned to those involved in friendly societies could be applied to charitable donors. Harrison has argued that there were shared values of decency, independence, and animosity towards the undeserving poor.[69] Doran noted of the early friendly societies that "they intentionally organised themselves around notions of friendship, brotherly love, charity."[70] Many friendly society rule books indicate the importance attached to helping members develop their self-control, moderation, and manners. Some suggest that friendly societies could be used to build solidarity and fraternity across class lines or within a specific locality, to gain a sense of personal, Christian virtue or to ensure that the poor spent their money wisely. The original rules of the Independent Order of Rechabites Friendly Society, which was founded in 1835, indicate that its objectives were similar to those of many charities: "Our objects are to improve the morals of our brethren, and to promote brotherly love, to relieve the distressed, to administer to the wants and necessities of the afflicted and to smooth the dying pillow."[71]

The Manchester Unity Odd Fellows Lecture of the White Degree begins: "The first point which our Order ordains to admonish you is no less than that of the first friendly duty to mankind—Charity."[72] Whether supporting mutual aid or charities, employers may have sought to demonstrate their interest in their workforce. Other donors or patrons may have felt a sense of civic pride or an interest in improving national efficiency, a sense of humanitarian sympathy or religious obligation, possibly derived from relevant personal experiences, or guilt about how they acquired their money. Friendly societies sought to create a sense of brotherhood and promoted a sense of obligation and reward for acts of kindness towards kin, however broadly defined, while for many, such as F. D. Mocatta, "charity took the place of a family."[73]

Cycles of exchange, whether balanced and asymmetrical, may have encouraged docility and deference in recipients while enhancing the status of donors, be they fellow friendly society members or wealthy patrons.[74] A widespread acceptance of a notion of reciprocity may have helped the élite retain differentiation from their social inferiors, so that people knew their place within the hierarchy, and also nurtured social interaction across that hierarchy.[75] Charities drew on such traditions when they sought to bring donors and recipients closer together in a continuing relationship.[76] For members of friendly societies, the importance of familial and charitable networks was clear because, even at the time when the societies had millions of members, those members often had to rely on kinship ties during periods when the household income was reduced.[77]

INDEPENDENCE AND PATRONAGE

There are many examples of patronage within friendly societies in the early nineteenth century. The labourers of Ashdon invited their new vicar to contribute to their club in 1820. The vicar made a donation, enlisted seven honorary members, and by 1824 had sufficient authority within the club to summon members to meetings and to produce plans to abolish the biannual feasts.[78] This was a period in which in South Lindsey friendly society lodges were named after the local gentry and contributions begged from local farmers.[79] Reverend Becher, who was active within the friendly society movement, argued that independence required support and that friendly society patrons could help "the industrious members of the community to attain a state of independence which is intimately connected with moral rectitude."[80] It was common for local gentry to draft the rules of village friendly societies and to attend their feasts while local clergy served as officers.[81]

The extent of this overt domination by middle-class patrons diminished during the course of the century, as Cordery and Gorsky have demonstrated.[82] This was in some measure due to the association of the societies with the strengthening of trade unionism in, for example, the northeast coalfields, Yorkshire and Lancashire.[83] There was also legislation in 1871 that enabled unions to secure legal recognition of their funds if the union registered under the Friendly Societies Act. The consensus is that, as Cordery put it: "Trade unions after 1850 looked and sounded like friendly societies."[84] By the 1870s, of the two million registered friendly society members in England and Wales, fewer than 43,500 were in societies controlled by honorary members. In 1896, only two of the 3551 English Ancient Order of Foresters' Courts (that is, branches) had secretaries who were clergymen, and only fifteen had clerical treasurers. Garrard called British friendly societies the "most democratically impressive" of working-class voluntary organisations, which were "likely to enhance the independence of their members," unlike charities that were "instruments of class-formation"; and Tholfsen concluded that the societies took "a conscious and responsible decision not to surrender to middle-class values."[85] Savage has also stressed the importance of independence. He characterised the collective efforts of Victorian artisans to protect against exploitation and uncertainty as "mutualistic" and contrasted such activity with taxation-funded state welfare, controlled by the middle class.[86]

Nevertheless, there were examples of gentry-financed friendly societies existing throughout the nineteenth century in Gloucestershire, Essex, Yorkshire, and rural Shropshire.[87] In Frimley, Surrey, "Rectors and Curates were prominent amongst the Courts's secretaries and treasurers . . . until well after the Second World War."[88] There are also examples of employer-dominated friendly societies at many collieries and large firms such as Marshalls of Leeds, which owned several flax mills. Across the country, by 1870, there were about 80 railway company-sponsored friendly societies.[89] Many female friendly societies were dominated by patrons. There are examples of such societies in York, Sheffield, Bishops Castle and Lydbury (Powys), Southill (Bedfordshire), Wakefield, Huddersfield, Leeds, and elsewhere.[90] Within such societies there was reciprocity, but it was uneven and in many cases the structures were similar to those of charities. Some female friendly societies also shared another form of internal hierarchy with many charities. By the 1890s, there were 20,000 paid female officials in philanthropic societies. These agents encouraged the establishment of branches, often with elaborate constitutional arrangements but also with sufficient autonomy to encourage local initiative. There were parallels with the structures of friendly societies that relied on the frequent collection of small sums from working people. Some paid commission to collectors and the Bristol-based Female Friendly Clothing Society employed visitors.[91]

Kidd, after comparing charities and friendly societies, concluded that it was only charities that were "fundamentally unequal."[92] However, even within the more independent friendly societies there was often a continuing leadership role for members of the highest social class in the locality. These leaders were often clergy, gentry or employers, but in some cases they were artisans. Some friendly societies developed internal hierarchies which echoed those of charities. Gosden found that business-owners constituted a majority of over 100 principal leaders of the Manchester Unity, Independent Order of Odd Fellows, and the Ancient Order of Foresters in the nineteenth century.[93] In Cambridge, "although the majority of ordinary friendly society members were from the working class, the leadership of the movement was dominated by members from the lower middle class."[94] The Foresters' Courts in Stokenchurch, Buckinghamshire, and Tadley, Hampshire, were probably initiated in 1874 and 1884, respectively, by relieving officers and gentry.[95] The Compton Pilgrims Benefit Society was founded by a Primitive Methodist in 1835. By 1888, the annual meeting was chaired by the mayor of Newbury, and in 1907, an Anglican cleric took the chair.[96] Between 1867 and 1915 there were 60 men who held the posts of provincial grand master, deputy provincial grand master, corresponding secretary, or trustees in the King's Lynn and West Norfolk District of the Independent Order of Oddfellows, Manchester Unity. The occupations of twenty-nine of them in 1881 can be identified. These include a ship owner, a brewer, a timber merchant, a rector, a solicitor, several tradesmen, and only one agricultural labourer. The Manchester Unity Oddfellows provincial grand master in 1871, a butcher, owned land from which he derived an annual income of £6.10s. Only twelve of 106 of the secretaries and treasurers of the ninety-five Ancient Order of Foresters Courts in Norfolk in 1885 were agricultural labourers. The others identified themselves as craftsmen, tradesmen, or farmers in the 1881 census. Other local studies have revealed that those who were the most literate, and had fewer ties to local employers, tended to have positions of authority. One Norfolk friendly society noted: "We are a plain lot of uncultivated agricultural labourers [who need] 10 or 20 percent of middle class to keep [us] straight."[97] In a farming hamlet in southwest Norfolk in the 1880s and 1890s, the Manchester Unity Oddfellows were dominated by a local tailor, later coal merchant, and chair of the Rural District Council.[98] Skilled workers were more likely to be society officials, and in rural areas it was the village artisans who generally ran the lodges. It was a woollen weaver and employer who became the first secretary of a Philanthropic Order of True Ivorites Lodge in Glamorganshire, holding the post for sixteen years until his death.[99] While the rhetoric of friendly societies emphasized brotherhood, there were still overt hierarchies, between officials and members, and covert ones as to who became officials. From 1856, the Foresters published the names of the nobility and MPs who became honorary members. Analysis indicates that following the extension of the franchise there was "an unseemly rush" by MPs to become Foresters. In 1889, twenty of the sixty diners at the Court Brownlow, Chesham, annual dinner were honorary members.[100] Although a growth in membership brought greater financial independence, as friendly societies and charities grew, so they became more like vast companies. "Friendly societies have been praised as agencies of self-help . . . with the growing size of societies, their centralisation and increasing complication of their administrative machinery, the ideal of democratic control proved to be another fallacy."[101] While independence grew in importance for working men, the influence of patrons and employers continued throughout the century.[102]

From the time of the first legislation aimed at them, the Statute of Charitable Uses (passed in the same year as the Poor Law, 1601, and for similar reasons) and the 1793 Act for the Encouragement and Relief of Friendly Societies (which aimed at "diminishing the Publick Burdens"), a desire to reduce the rates, drove much of the regulation and quantification of the activities of charities and friendly societies. The poor, and particularly the ill poor, were perceived as a burden on the rates, and in the nineteenth century, the emphasis was on selective, coordinated, effective, efficient, and educative relief. The 1819 legislation on friendly societies was influenced by parliamentary committee discussions on the Poor Law.[103] At that time, ratepayers could receive rates-funded assistance with pensions or funeral expenses, and friendly society arrears could be paid from the rates in order to stop people becoming more of a burden on the rates.[104] John Tidd Pratt, the registrar of friendly societies for four decades from the post's creation in 1834, was one of those who drafted the 1834 Poor Law (Amendment) Act. It was in part based on the 1829 Friendly Societies Act and was in turn a model for the 1875 Friendly Societies Act.[105] Both friendly societies and Poor Law administrators were regulated in regions by district auditors, and both sought to measure lives in similar ways.[106] The regulation of those in receipt of friendly society pensions and those in receipt of state pensions, former military, postal, and naval personnel, reflected the similarities in the ways that these bodies rewarded those who were loyal and moral.[107] One commentator argued in 1867 that charitable hospitals were, as a means of reducing reliance on relief, "an important agent against pauperism."[108] There was an attempt to use a charity to support ratepayers in another way in the early twentieth century. In 1900, William Sutton left his fortune to provide housing for the poor. By 1913, the Local Government Board and several councils had become dominant trustees of the charity. They sought to use it to maintain the income of ratepaying local landlords.[109] Throughout the nineteenth century, charities and friendly societies were part of a broad concern, expressed in part through the considerable growth in the collation of government data with occupational ill-health, morbidity, and morality, which were conceptualized as the main causes of working-class poverty.[110] Indeed, "if there is a single thread running through early English population statistics it is insurance."[111] The widespread importance attached to "self-help" and the discourse of the "deserving poor," a discourse that was articulated through legislation, framed much charitable and friendly society activity.

Although, the role of working-class men within the friendly societies movement grew in the later part of the nineteenth century, so too did the importance of the weak ties that societies had to charities. Within the friendly society lodge, what Granovetter has called "strong ties" could be developed.[112] These could lead to the creation of cliques that supported weaker members and helped establish a sense of security. At a time when the legal framework for contract enforcement (against embezzlement of friendly society funds, for example) was weak, internal sanctions had to be strong and strong ties provided collective insurance against debt and an inability to work.[113] However, weaker, more impersonal, bonds that connected, for example, friendly society lodges to one another or to a charity were also of value. Such weaker ties, in effect low-cost screening devices, required less time or contact to maintain but increased the number of possible transactions, facilitated the flow of information, and reduced uncertainty. Through only a few brokers of loose ties, connections could be made that enabled members of a number of organizations to improve their decision making in a variety of fields. Mark Sykes, Unionist MP and heir to the largest landed estate in East Riding, was not strongly tied to any one friendly society. However, when he accepted invitations to 22 friendly society feasts in 1909 and attended 17 of them, he linked friendly societies members to a cycle of exchange that stretched well beyond the individual clubs and lodges.[114]

The importance of weak ties can be gauged through analysis of their development in Norfolk. On the one hand, there were a number of ties between Primitive Methodism, friendly societies, and trade unions in the county. A union for agricultural labourers thrived between 1872 and 1896, was revived in 1906, and in 1911, under the National Health Insurance legislation, was "approved" to act as a friendly society. From the 1870s and in parallel with the union, Farmers' Defence Associations, an echo of the earlier Hundred Associations of employers' who rewarded loyalty and service within the Hundreds, arose. These defence associations rewarded compliance and loyalty and sought to punish trade unionists. Some landowners and vicars sought to maintain loyalty to Anglicanism, through providing charity only to those who attended church. Perhaps in order to promote trust and ameliorate potential social division, there were other attempts to create weak ties between employers and working men. In the 1880s, a number of squires attended the Aylsham Oddfellows' Lodge anniversary dinners and most of Lynn's Town Council joined the Oddfellows, who also received support from the Prince of Wales, who lived nearby in Sandringham. Lynn's only Masonic lodge between 1851 and 1906, the Philanthropic Lodge No. 107, was dominated by the wealthy of the area and included the Prince of Wales among its members. However, it initiated John Rust (later a grand master of the Manchester Unity Oddfellows), William Hyner (later an Ancient Order of Foresters high chief ranger, that is, national president), and a number of other leading friendly society officials. Moreover, landowner and Freemason Hamon Le Strange initiated an Oddfellows lodge in Hunstanton, where he lived, and in the 1890s, Lord Winchilsea established the National Agricultural Union, which stressed loyalty to the parish, estate, and workplace and independence from outsiders. He encouraged landowners to support friendly societies. By the late nineteenth-century, friendly societies, unions and Freemasons all presented themselves as independent. Friendly societies ceased to have as many overt patrons but weak ties, which were often significant links, continued to connect charitable and mutual aid bodies to one another.[115]

CONCLUSION

Charities and friendly societies were linked to one another by virtue of both enjoying rapid growth during a period of industrialisation and urbanisation when there was much interest in organisations that could increase social stability and reduce social divisions through the promotion of self-help, reciprocity, and patronage. Many charities and friendly societies had similar internal structures and hierarchies. Those involved in both could hope to gain respect, self-confidence, self-discipline, and new skills (notably bookkeeping, secretarial work, decision making, and publicity). Some of those involved in both charities and friendly societies may have sought affection or a desire to promote closer links between religious and social welfare. There are a number of examples of individuals who were simultaneously influential in both charities and friendly societies. Employing the notions of reciprocity and the strength of weak ties for analysis does not diminish the differences between many charities and friendly societies. Rather, it recognizes that both forms were, through the interactions of gift exchange, capable of generating varying degrees of solidarity. It highlights their common roots in the guilds, their continuing common interest in institutionalizing benevolence through creating social relationships and mutual ties based on loyalty, and their interest in transcending economic transfers between recipients and donors, or members, by extending them to involve emotional and social relationships.

NOTES

1. D. Roberts, *Paternalism in early Victorian England*, London: Croom Helm, 1979; E. Hopkins, *Working-class self-help in nineteenth-century England: Responses to industrialisation*, London: UCL Press, 1995.
2. J. Winter, "Widowed mothers and mutual aid in early Victorian Britain," *Journal of Social History*, 17, 1 1983, p. 115; J. O'Neill, *In the club, Female Friendly Societies in Nottinghamshire 1792–1913*, Nottingham: Trent Valley History Group, 2001, p. 3.
3. Hobsbawm closely linked friendly societies to trade unions. See, for example, E. J. Hobsbawm, *Primitive rebels*, Manchester: Manchester University Press, 1959, pp. 152–54, and E. J. Hobsbawm, "Artisan or labour aristocrat?," *Economic History Review*, 37, 3 1984, p. 361. Supple presented friendly societies in terms of insurance. See B. Supple, *The Royal Exchange Assurance: A history of british insurance 1720–1970*, Cambridge: Cambridge University Press, 1970, p. 310.
4. For the breadth of the activities of philanthropists and friendly societies, see D. Owen, *English philanthropy*, Cambridge, MA: Harvard University Press, 1965, p. 472, and D. Weinbren, "'Imagined families': Research on friendly societies," *Mitteilungsblatt des Instituts für die Geschichte der sozialen Bewegungen*, 27, 2002.
5. M. Gorsky, *Patterns of philanthropy: Charity and society in nineteenth-century Bristol*, Woodbridge, UK: Boydell, 1999, pp. 18, 117; F. Prochaska, *Christianity and social service in modern Britain: The disinherited spirit*, Oxford: Oxford University Press, 2006, pp. 11, 10.
6. B. Harris, *The origins of the British welfare state: Social welfare in England and Wales, 1800–1945*, Basingstoke: Palgrave, 2004, pp. 72, 77.
7. The town has been called a number of names, including Bishop's Lynn, King's Lynn, and King's Regis. To clarify matters, and in keeping with current local usage, it is here referred to as Lynn.
8. *Local Government Board, Report, 1873–74* (Appendix B, report 14, Henry Longley on Poor Law Administration in London), p. 186.
9. J. M. Bennett, "Conviviality and charity in medieval and early modern England," *Past and Present*, 134, 1992, pp. 33–35. Mauss stressed the importance of feasts within the gift economy; see M. Mauss, *The gift. Forms and functions of exchange in archaic societies*, London: Cohen & West, 1954, translated by I. Cunnison, first published 1925, p. 19. On other sources for such traditions, see E. Clark, "Social welfare and mutual aid in the medieval countryside," *Journal of British Studies*, 33 1994, p. 404.
10. P. Richards, *Kings Lynn*, Chichester: Phillimore, 1990, pp. 61–63, 103, 116, 120–22.

11. On the importance of mutual obligation to fraternal culture, see A. Black, *Guilds and civil society in European political thought from the 12th century to the present*, Ithaca, NY: Cornel University Press, 1984, pp. 508, 26–27, and M. Clawson, *Constructing brotherhood: Class, gender and fraternalism*, Princeton, NJ: Princeton University Press, 1989, pp. 41–42.

12. *Oddfellows' Magazine*, April 1880, pp. 455, 457.

13. C. E. Ward, "Forestry in King's Lynn and District," was published both in *Foresters' directory* and the *Guide to King's Lynn*, 1906, which was produced by the AoF to mark their holding of their High Court in the town in that year. Ward was the high chief ranger.

14. Gorsky, *Patterns*, p. 181; K. Laybourn, *The Guild of Help and the changing face of Edwardian Philanthropy: The Guild of Help, voluntary work and the state, 1904–1919*, Mellen: Ceredigion, 1994.

15. E. W. Brabook, *Provident societies and industrial welfare*, London: Blackie & Son, 1898, p. 57; T. Smith, ed., *English Gilds 1870*, reprint Oxford: Oxford University Press, 1963l; C. Walford, *Gilds: Their origin, constitution, objects and later history*, London: George Redway, 1888, p. 5.

16. J. H. Clapham, *An economic history of modern Britain*, Vol. 1, Cambridge: Cambridge University Press, 1926, pp. 296–298.

17. M. J. Walker, "The extent of guild control of trades in England, c. 1660–1820," PhD Cambridge 1986, p. 345; Gorsky, *Patterns*, p. 115.

18. J. M. Gardiner, *History of the Leeds Benevolent or Strangers Friend Society, 1789–1889*, Leeds, 1890, cited in R. J. Morris, "Voluntary societies and British urban élites, 1780–1850: An analysis," *Historical Journal*, 26, 1, 1983, p. 107.

19. B. R. McRee, "Charity and gild solidarity in late medieval England," *Journal of British Studies*, 32, 1993, pp. 198, 204, 209–10.

20. R. A. Leeson, *Travelling brothers*, London: George Allen & Unwin, 1979.

21. S. M. Pinches, "Objects of charity: Fads and fashions in founding charities over 400 years in Warwickshire," paper read to the Family and Community Historical Research Society conference, 13 May 2005.

22. Mauss, *The gift*, pp. 11, 12, 15, 18, 67, 72, 73.

23. G. Stedman Jones, *Outcast London: A study in the relationship between classes in Victorian society*, Harmondsworth, UK: Penguin, 1984, pp. 256, 257, 259.

24. Mauss, *The gift*, p. 76.

25. C. Muldrew, *The economy of obligation: The culture of credit and social relations in early modern England*, New York: St. Martin's Press, 1998.

26. M. C. Finn, *The character of credit: Personal debt in English culture, 1740–1914*, Cambridge: Cambridge University Press, 2003.

27. G. Stedman Jones, "Rethinking Chartism," in G. Stedman Jones, *Languages of class: Studies in English working class history 1832–1982*, Cambridge: Cambridge University Press, 1983, pp. 112–44.

28. F. Engels, *The condition of the working class in England*, Oxford: Oxford University Press, 1958, pp. 100, 102, 140.

29. *Porcupine*, 29 May 1880, p. 138.

30. J. A. Jaffe, *Striking a bargain: Work and industrial relations in England 1815–1865*, Manchester, UK: Manchester University Press, 2000, pp. 67, 136–37.

31. J. Benson, "Coalminers, coalowners and collaboration: The miners' permanent relief fund movement in England, 1860–1895," *Labour History Review*, 68, 2, 2003, pp. 184, 191.

32. M. Finn, "Working-class women and the contest for consumer control in Victorian county courts," *Past and Present*, 161, 1998.

33. L. H. Lees, *Exiles of Erin: Irish immigrants in Victorian London*, Manchester, UK: Manchester University Press, 1979, p. 83.

34. E. Ross, "Survival networks: Women's neighbourhood sharing in London before World War I," *History Workshop Journal*, 15, 1983, p. 11.

35. J. White, *The worst street in north London: Campbell Bunk, Islington, between the wars*, London: Routledge & Kegan Paul, 1986, pp. 73–74, 274.

36. Quoted in A. Davin, *Growing up poor: Home, school and street in London 1870–1914*, London: Rivers Oram, 1996, p. 59.

37. M. Anderson, *Family structure in nineteenth-century Lancashire*, Cambridge: Cambridge University Press, 1971, p. 137; M. Dupree, *Family structure in the Staffordshire potteries, 1840–1880*, Oxford: Oxford University Press, 1995, p. 350.

38. A. Cameron, *Bare feet and tackety boots. A boyhood on Rhum*, Barr, UK: Luath Press, 1988, p. 3.

39. G. J. West, "Charity labour gatherings in rural Perthshire 1850–1950," *Scottish Studies*, 33, 1999, p. 134.

40. T. Owen, *Welsh Folk Customs*, Cardiff, UK: National Museum of Wales, 1978, pp. 161–162.

41. C. M. Arensberg, *The Irish countryman: An anthropological study*, Gloucester, UK: Peter Smith, 1937; A. O'Dowd, *Meitheal: A Study of Co-Operative Labour in Rural Ireland (Aspects of Ireland)*, Dublin: Comhairle Bhealoideas Eireann, 1981.

42. J. Burchardt, *The allotment movement in England, 1793–1873*, Woodbridge, UK: Boydell, p. 181.

43. J. E. Archer, "The nineteenth-century allotment: Half an acre and a row," *Economic History Review*, 1997, Volume 50, pp. 25, 27, 35.

44. Mauss, *The gift*, p. 63.

45. J. Money, "The masonic moment: Or, ritual, replica, and credit: John Wilkes, the Macaroni Parson, and the making of the middle class mind," *Journal of British Studies*, 32, 1993, p. 384.

46. A. Durr, "Chicken and egg—the Emblem Book and Freemasonry: The visual and material culture of associated life," *Transactions of Quatour Coronati Lodge*, February 2005, pp. 8–10.

47. Prochaska, *Christianity*, p. 113.

48. Anon., *The Girls' Friendly Society*, London: Hatchards, 1877, p. 2.

49. Winter, "Widowed mothers," pp. 121–23.

50. A. Blaikie, "Nuclear hardship or variant dependency? Households and the Scottish Poor Law, *Continuity and Change*, 17, 2, 2002, p. 275.

51. Burchardt, *The allotment*, p. 80.

52. *Oddfellows' Magazine*, January 1884, p. 32.

53. D. Philipson, *Redcar's forgotten lifeboat*, privately printed, 1977, pp. 3, 12.

54. B. Stibbins, "'A highly beneficial influence': Friendly societies in Norfolk in the nineteenth century, with particular reference to north Norfolk," *MA*, University of East Anglia, 2001, pp. 20, 43.

55. F. Edwards, "The treatment of poverty in Nantwich and Crewe 1730–1914," *MA*, 1990, Keele University, pp. 487, 491, 501–506, 523.

56. K. Waddington, *Charity and the London Hospitals 1850–1898*, Woodbridge, UK: Boydell, 2000, p. 33.

57. A. Berry, "Patronage, funding and the hospital patient c1750–1815: Three English regional case studies," *PhD*, Oxford, 1995, pp. 109–10.

58. H. Marland, *Medicine and society in Wakefield and Huddersfield 1780–1870*, Cambridge: Cambridge University Press, 1987, pp. 186, 196.

59. Minutes quoted in S. M. Pinches, "Philanthropy and locality: An examination of the ways in which charity reflected and reinforced local identity in the eighteenth and nineteenth centuries," paper read at the European Social Science History Conference, The Hague, March 2002.

60. M. Gorsky and J. Mohan, *Medicine and mutual aid: British hospital contributory schemes in the twentieth century*, Manchester, UK: Manchester University Press, 2006.
61. Waddington, *Charity*, pp. 70–71, 152; Gorsky, *Patterns*, pp. 161, 184.
62. Gorsky, *Patterns*, pp. 117, 119.
63. D. Harrison, "Freemasonry, industry and charity: The local community and the working man," *Voluntary Action*, 5, 1, 2002, pp. 39–43, 45.
64. R. Humphreys, *Sin, organised charity and the Poor Law in Victorian England*, London: St Martin's Press, 1995, p. 94.
65. M. MacKinnon, "English poor law policy and the crusade against outrelief," *Journal of Economic History*, 47, 1987, p. 3.
66. A. P. Wadsworth, "The first Manchester Sunday schools," in M. W. Flinn and T. C. Smout, eds., *Essays in social history*, Oxford: Oxford University Press, 1974, pp. 101, 117, 119; P. H. J. H. Gosden, *The Friendly Societies in England, 1815–1875*, Manchester, UK: Manchester University Press, 1961, pp. 20–21; K. D. M. Snell, "The Sunday school movement in England and Wales: Child labour, denominational control and working-class culture," *Past and Present*, 164, 1999, pp. 130–1.
67. F. Prochaska, *The voluntary impulse: Philanthropy in Modern Britain*, London: Faber and Faber, 1988, pp. 55, 62, 74.
68. W. H. Beveridge, *Voluntary Action: A report on methods of social advance*, London: Allen & Unwin, 1948.
69. B. Harrison, *Peaceable kingdom: Stability and change in modern Britain*, Oxford: Oxford University Press, 1982.
70. N. Doran, "Risky business: Codifying embodied experience in the Manchester Unity of Oddfellows," *Journal of Historical Sociology*, 7, 2, 1994, p.134.
71. R. Campbell, *Rechabite history*, Manchester, UK: Independent Order of Rechabites, 1911, p. 21.
72. Anon., *The complete manual of Oddfellowship*, Manchester, UK: MUOOF, 1879, p. 94.
73. Owen, *English philanthropy*, p. 424. Owen notes the pattern among philanthropists of being either single or childless.
74. H. Newby, "The deferential dialectic," *Comparative Studies in Society and History*, 17, 1975, pp. 161–163.
75. A. P. Donajgrodzki, ed., *Social control in nineteenth-century Britain*, London: Croom Helm, 1977; Stedman Jones, *Outcast London*, pp. 267, 270.
76. Owen, *English philanthropy*, p. 227.
77. S. Horrell and D. Oxley, "Work and prudence: Household responses to income variation in nineteenth century Britain," *European Review of Economic History*, 4, 1, 2000, pp. 27–58.
78. D. J. Appleby, "Combination and control: Cultural politics in the management of friendly societies in nineteenth-century Essex and Suffolk," *Essex Archaeology and History*, 33, 2002, p. 325.
79. J. Obelkevich, *Religion and rural society: South Lindsey 1825–1875*, Oxford: Oxford University Press, 1976, p. 89.
80. John Thomas Becher, who ran the Southwell Friendly Society, Nottinghamshire, quoted in Cordery, "Friendly societies and the discourse," p. 42–4; Roberts, *Paternalism*, p. 132.
81. D. Weinbren, "The social capital of female friendly societies," in A. Prescott and M. Cross, eds., *Fraternalism and gender in Europe, 1300–2000*, Basingstoke: Palgrave, forthcoming.
82. Gorsky, *Patterns*, p. 128; see also p. 186; S. Cordery, "Friendly societies and the discourse of respectability in Britain 1825–1875," *Journal of British Studies*, 34, 1995, pp. 45, 58.

83. R. Colls, *The pitmen of the northern coalfield: Work, culture and protest 1790–1850*, Manchester, UK: Manchester University Press, 1987, pp. 70, 87, 246–8; E. P. Thompson, *The making of the English working class*, Harmondsworth, UK: Penguin, 1963, rev. ed. 1968, pp. 461, 459; J. K. Walton, *Lancashire: A social history 1558–1939*, Manchester, UK: Manchester University Press, 1988, pp. 148–150.

84. S. Cordery, "Friendly societies and the British labour movement before 1914," *Journal of the Association of Historians in North Carolina*, 3, 1995, p. 39; S. Cordery, *British friendly societies, 1750–1914*, Basingstoke: Palgrave, 2003, p. 135. See also Gosden, *Friendly*, pp. 55–56; M. Chase, *Early trade unionism, fraternity skill and the politics of labour*, Aldershot, UK: Ashgate, 2000, pp. 2–3, 107; G. Finlayson, *Citizen, state, and social welfare in Britain 1830–1990*, Oxford: Clarendon, 1994, p. 6; Z Bauman, *Between class and elite. The evolution of the British labour movement: A sociological study*. Translated by S. Patterson, Manchester, UK: Manchester University Press, 1972, p. 86.

85. J. Garrard, *Democratisation in Britain: Elites, civil society and reform since 1800*, Basingstoke: Palgrave, 2002, pp. 6, 184, 277, 282–83; T. Tholfsen, *Working class radicalism in mid-Victorian England*, New York: Columbia University Press, 1977, p. 246.

86. M. Savage, *The dynamics of working class politics: The labour movement in Preston 1880–1940*, Cambridge: Cambridge University Press, 1987, p. 126.

87. M. Fisher and D. Viner, "'Go thou and do likewise': The Ebington Friendly Society (1856–1920) and its banners," *Folk Life*, 37, 1998–99, pp. 64–79; J. Cooper, *The well-ordered town: A story of Saffron Walden, Essex 1792–1862*, Saffron Walden, UK: Cooper, 2000, p. 183; Neave, *Mutual aid*, pp. 1, 48–9, 68, 95, 97; N. Mansfield, *English farmworkers and local patriotism, 1900–1930* Aldershot, UK: Ashgate, 2001, pp. 47, 48, 198, 205.

88. Fisk, *Mutual self-help in Southern England, 1850–1912*, Southampton, UK: Foresters Heritage Trust, 2006, p. 135.

89. W. G. Rimmer, *Marshalls of Leeds, flax spinners, 1778–1886*, Cambridge: Cambridge University Press, 1960, pp. 104–5 194 216–17; S. Cordery, "Mutualism, Friendly Societies, and the genesis of railway trade unions," *Labour History Review*, 67, 2002, pp. 265–67; J. Benson, "Coalowners, coalminers and compulsion: Pit clubs in England, 1860–80, *Business History*, 44, 1, 2002; C. Bradbury, "The impact of friendly societies in north Staffordshire," *Staffordshire Studies*, 13, 2001, pp. 130, 134. On the dominance of the employers in a Wigan-based society, see *The Lancashire and Cheshire Miners' Permanent Relief Society Report of the 33rd AGM, 1906*, Wigan, UK: Wall and Sons, 1906, p. 9.

90. S. Lloyd, "Pleasing spectacles and elegant dinners: Conviviality, benevolence and charity anniversaries in eighteenth-century London," *Journal of British Studies*, 41, 2002, pp. 54–55; C. O. Reid, "Middle class values and working class culture in nineteenth century Sheffield," *Ph.D*, University of Sheffield, 1976, pp. 515, 539; I. Evans, "The Bishop's Castle and Lydbury North Female Friendly Society," *South West Shropshire Historical and Archaeological Society Journal*, 1, 1989, pp. 19–20; Weinbren, "The social capital"; Marland, *Medicine and society*, pp. 25, 190, 198–99.

91. Gorsky, *Patterns*, p. 167.

92. A. J. Kidd, "Civil society or the state?: Recent approaches to the history of voluntary welfare," *Journal of Historical Sociology*, 15, 3, 2002, p. 332; see also A. J. Kidd, "Philanthropy and the social history paradigm," *Social History*, 21, 2, 1996, p. 186.

93. Gosden, *Friendly*, pp. 88–93, 224–228.

94. E. Edwards, "The friendly societies and the ethic of respectability: Nineteenth century Cambridge," *PhD*, Cambridge College of Art and Technology, 1987, p. 499.
95. Fisk, *Mutual*, p. 131.
96. M. Bee, "A friendly society case study: The Compton Pilgrims Benefit Society," *Southern History*, 11, 1989, pp. 75–76.
97. Stibbins, "A highly beneficial influence," p. 46.
98. M. Home, *Autumn fields*, London: Metheun, 1944, p. 45. My thanks to Rex Russell for this reference.
99. N. Israel, "The Philanthropic Order of True Ivorites," *Glamorgan Family History Society Journal*, 11, 1986 pp. 22–23. For a similar example from Oxfordshire, see M. Bee, "Within the shelter of the old elm tree: Oddfellowship and community in North Oxfordshire, 1871–2002," *Family and Community History*, 6, 2, 2003.
100. Fisk, *Mutual*, pp. 19, 133, 161.
101. H. Levy, "The economic history of sickness and benefit since the Puritan Revolution," *Economic History Review*, 14, 2, 1944, p. 160.
102. G. Best, *Mid-Victorian Britain 1851–75*, London: Weidenfeld and Nicolson, 1971, pp. 291–92; J. E. Cronin, *The politics of state expansion: War, state and society in twentieth-century Britain*, London: Routledge, 1991, p. 25; D. Neave, *Mutual aid in the Victorian countryside 1830–1914*, Hull, UK: Hull University Press, 1991, p. 86; N. Kirk, *Change, continuity and class: Labour in British society, 1850–1920*, Manchester, UK: Manchester University Press, 1998, pp. 29–31 49–50, 60; A. J. Kidd, *State, society and the poor in nineteenth century England*, London: Macmillan, 1999, p. 112.
103. J. Haslam, "On the prescribing of accounting and accounting publicity by the state in early to mid-nineteenth century Britain: Accounting history as critique," *PhD*, Essex, 1991, 141–2.
104. For examples of the granting of such rate payments, see M. Barker-Read, "The treatment of the aged poor in five selected West Kent parishes from settlement to Speenhamland (1662–1797)," *PhD*, Open University, 1988, 60; S. B. Black, "Local government, law and order in a pre-reform Kentish parish: Farningham 1790–1834," *PhD*, Kent, 1991, 60. On the payment of arrears up to and after 1834, see R. P. Hastings, *Essays in North Riding history 1780–1850*, Northallerton, UK: North Yorkshire County Council, 1981, pp.117–118. On friendly societies as means of reducing the rates, see J. N. Baernreither, *English Associations of Working Men*, London: Sonnenschein, 1893, p. 371.
105. Gosden, *Friendly*, p. 17; H. M. Coombs and J. R. Edwards, "The evolution of The District Audit," *Financial Accountability and Management*, 1990; Simon Cordery, "John Tidd Pratt," *Friendly Societies Research Group Newsletter*, 10, May 2003.
106. J. R. Edwards and R. Chandler, "Contextualising the process of accounting regulation: A study of nineteenth-century British friendly societies," *Abacus*, 37, 2, 2001, p. 195.
107. S. Fowler and W. Spencer, *Army records for family historians*, London: PRO Publications, 1998; N. A. M. Rodger, *Naval records for genealogists*, London: HMSO, 1988. See also S. Fowler, *Tracing army ancestry*, Barnsley, UK: Pen and Sword, 2006.
108. Waddington, *Charity*, p. 32.
109. P. L. Garside, "The impact of philanthropy: Housing provision and the Sutton Model Dwellings Trust, 1900–1939," *Economic History Review*, 53, 4, 2000, p. 750.
110. E. Higgs, "Disease, febrile poisons and statistics: The census as a medical survey, 1841–1911," *Social History of Medicine*, 4, 3, 1991, pp .465–478;

C. Hamlin, *Public health and social justice in the age of Chadwick: Britain, 1800–1854*, Cambridge: Cambridge University Press, 1998, pp. 84–120.

111. E. Higgs, "Colloquium on *The information state in England: The central collection of information in citizens, 1500–2000*, London: Palgrave, 2004," *Journal of Historical Sociology* 18 1/2, 2005, p. 140.
112. M. S. Granovetter, "The strength of weak ties," *American Journal of Sociology*, 78, pp. 1360–80.
113. Strong ties are also associated with feuding and the marginalisation of fresh information by a clique.
114. Neave, *Mutual aid*, p. 95.
115. This paragraph is derived from A. Fisk, *Mutual*, pp. 67, 68, 70; R. J. Lee, "Encountering and managing the poor: Rural society and the Anglican clergy in Norfolk 1815–1914, *Ph.D*, University of Leicester, 2003, pp. 35, 125, 180, 184; A. Howkins, *Poor labouring men: Rural radicalism in Norfolk 1870–1923*, London: Routledge & Kegan Paul, 1985, pp. 12, 13, 28, 34, 35, 47, 48, 51, 52, 55, 56, 64, 66, 69, 72, 78, 79; 89–90, 104, 151, 169; Stibbins, "A highly beneficial influence," pp. 24, 48; *Oddfellows' Magazine*, April 1880, pp. 402–03.

5 Historical Welfare Economics in the Nineteenth Century

Mutual Aid and Private Insurance for Burial, Sickness, Old Age, Widowhood, and Unemployment in the Netherlands

Marco H. D. van Leeuwen

Utrecht University[1]

Mutual and private insurance against the vicissitudes of life, health, and work existed long before the beginning of the welfare state. This chapter briefly sketches the mixed economy of welfare that existed before the welfare state and outlines some of the classic problems that plagued mutual, commercial, and social insurance. It then discusses patterns, problems, and processes of burial insurance, old age and widows' pensions, unemployment insurance, and compensation for loss of income and the cost of medical treatment during sickness in the nineteenth century. Classic insurance problems, such as moral hazards and adverse selection, existed, but they could be overcome to a greater or lesser extent without the need for compulsory state arrangements. The chapter concludes by comparing these patterns, problems, and processes across the various types of insurance.

The historical literature on what has been termed mutual aid, mutual benefit, fraternal, friendly, or benevolent societies has mushroomed in recent years. These societies appear to have existed, and indeed still exist, in many countries across the globe over the past two centuries, and in some instances over a much longer period.[2] However, they have seldom been studied as insurance groups, with their classic problems and solutions, and they have not been studied in combination, and competition, with other insurers covering the same risks.[3] This chapter discusses both mutual and private insurance schemes. It will make a quantitative assessment of their coverage and, as far as possible, of their terms and conditions; it will also look at the qualitative evidence on factors explaining their success, survival, or decline. In doing so, it aims to answer the following questions:

> What proportion of the population was covered by an insurance for burial, sickness, old age, widowhood, and unemployment, and how did this coverage evolve over time?

Why did the insurance market grow?

What factors explain the variation in coverage risks?

How was the market divided between mutual and private insurers, and how did this division evolve over time?

The historical example described here relates to a mixed economy of welfare in the transition from the *ancien régime* to the welfare state, and a few words are in place to introduce it. Ever since the birth of the Dutch Republic at the end of the sixteenth century, a variety of risks had been covered by a variety of arrangements, including mutual insurance, private insurance, and charity. The dissolution of the Dutch Republic in 1795 did not put an end to charity, but it did, soon afterwards, put an end to guild-based mutual welfare.[4] Once the guilds had been abolished in 1820, guild welfare petered out. Commercial insurance existed before then, and continues to exist today. Indeed, in 2006 it took over health insurance from the state. State insurance was unknown until the enactment of the 1901 Industrial Accidents Act, the first social security law in the Netherlands. After that date, state insurance gradually expanded while leaving ample room for charity (until the enactment of the 1965 General Income Support Act) and mutual insurance, including that provided by trade unions.[5] In the case of health insurance, it was not until 1941, during the German occupation, that the Dutch state began to compel its citizens to be insured. There was nothing unusual about a mixed economy of welfare; indeed, such a mixed economy existed in many European countries. It is difficult to point to what was unique about the Dutch case, but it was certainly not the existence of a mixed regime, nor the nature of the problems plaguing welfare arrangements—such as adverse selection, moral hazards, and free-rider problems; nor were the options available to combat these problems unique either. For these reasons, the Dutch example might also be instructive for those scholars whose primary interest is not the Netherlands.

SOME INSURANCE PROBLEMS: MORAL HAZARDS, ADVERSE SELECTION, AND CORRELATED RISKS

Even if the overwhelming majority of the population desires to be insured against illness or other risks and can pay for it, and even if there are providers willing to insure, insurances against illness or other risks may not come into being. There can be several reasons for this unhappy situation. Some of the most pressing are those of moral hazards, adverse selection, and correlated risks, and these will be discussed now.

Profitable but risky human action is stalled if the risk is seen as too high. Individuals, firms, and other institutions, and society at large, might as a result suffer a loss of welfare. Insurance is a way to recover welfare by shifting the burden of risk to a party better able to bear it. This party might be a private firm, a mutual aid group, the state, or a group of states.[6] Insurance against risks, be it private insurance or organized mutual aid, is known to suffer from certain problems. Three classic problems are those of moral hazards, adverse selection, and correlated risks.

A moral hazard is behaviour that increases the occurrence of the risk for which one is insured. Insurance against loss of wages when ill or unemployed, for example, might increase the frequency of reported illnesses or lack of work. Some illnesses are partly subjective, and they are certainly not always easy to establish objectively. Whether there is suitable work available for an unemployed person might depend on what is deemed appropriate work or on how diligently work is sought. A person with insurance has less of an incentive to go to work than a person without insurance. Moral hazards range from simple fraud to the rightful exercise of a certain measure of personal discretion. Whatever their moral, contractual, or legal status, moral hazards raise expenditure and are thus a problem for an insurer, and to some extent for the insured because insurance premiums go up. If the insurer fails to combat these moral hazards sufficiently, no insurance can be offered. Both the individual and the society at large suffer a loss of welfare.

Solving moral hazards might take the form of good monitoring techniques or coinsurance (where the insurer is responsible for bearing only part of the risk, with the client bearing the remainder). A waiting period is an example of coinsurance. It is the length of time before which sickness or unemployment benefits can be claimed, and it shifts part of the loss of income due to ill health or lack of work on to the insured, in order to reduce the risk of their imagining ailments or setting excessive demands when considering whether to accept new employment. Good monitoring techniques are also a way to curb moral hazards. In small, homogeneous groups whose members are dependent on, and in frequent contact with, one another, monitoring is generally easier and cheaper than in large, heterogeneous groups whose members meet infrequently and who are not very dependent on each other.[7] Monitoring may be delegated to experts, such as a doctor or the agent of an unemployment office. However, there is invariably a limit to what can be monitored legally, feasibly, and without incurring prohibitive costs.

Moral hazards can be seen as a problem of hidden action—the insurer cannot prevent the insured from acting in a way that will raise expenditure. Adverse selection can be seen as the problem of hidden information: the insured has knowledge that increases expenditure, knowledge that the insurer does not have. When an insurer finds it impossible or too costly to distinguish "good" from "bad" risks, the latter may profit by insuring themselves, paying standard contributions with above-standard returns. As a consequence, good risks find it increasingly beneficial to leave, or not join, in order to avoid subsidizing bad risks. Without proper measures, this problem of adverse selection might thus preclude an insurance scheme being set up, even though there are providers interested in offering it to good risks and good risks able and willing to pay for it. Solutions for adverse selection include compulsory insurance for all risks, good or bad, better screening techniques before a risk is accepted, a differentiation in contribution level according to risk category, and stipulations that the insurer will not pay out if wilfully misled.

Insurers can predict expenditure and thus levy appropriate premiums if risks are uncorrelated. This is not always the case with illness or unemployment. Correlated risks occur, for example, when a contagious disease hits an area and the insurer has to meet claims from a large number of sick policyholders. Similarly, a trade union could be faced with high expenditure on unemployment benefits if, due to a depression in trade, many of its members are laid off at the same time. To make matters worse, this is also likely to be a time when members find it most difficult to pay premiums.

ESTIMATES

The estimates used in this chapter of the coverage for certain types of insurance are often based on backward projections from a fixed point in the late-nineteenth or early-twentieth century taken from a national survey. We know the number of insurance funds and the number of insured at such a point and thus also the average number of insured per insurer. From there, we can work backward, using the known total number of funds per decade in the nineteenth century and an estimate of the average number of insured per type of fund, taking into account any general information available on developments over time. To be on the safe side, and to enable us to better indicate the margins of error relating to the estimates, we have used both a low and a high average for the number of insured per fund. The actual figure will have been somewhere in between.

There is, however, one complication: the existence and growth of factory schemes. Sometimes, factory workers were insured through an insurance fund that covered only their factory or a group of factories in the same branch of industry (and usually in the same region). The number of workers insured though factory schemes can be estimated for the period 1888–1890, but no information on the number of factory schemes or on their membership exists before those years. We have addressed this problem by estimating the coverage excluding factory schemes and adding in an estimate of the numbers covered by factory schemes per decade. For the latter, we use the number of workers insured under factory schemes in 1890 and project backward on the assumption that factory schemes did not exist in 1810 and that they grew especially rapidly after 1860.[8]

Before making our backward projections, we will first discuss the nature and evolution of factory schemes. Having done that, we are able to discuss burial insurance in general and give a well-documented, interesting example in particular. Then we discuss old age and widows' pensions, unemployment provisions, and sickness insurance (both for loss of income and for the costs of medical treatment), to end with a general conclusion.

FACTORY SCHEMES

Although the earliest known factory scheme was that at a textile factory in 1812, most such schemes do indeed date from after 1860. Around that time, more than half of all textile employees in Twente—in the east of the country—were covered under a health-insurance scheme. Apart from textiles, there were other branches of industry with similar schemes, most notably the machine and metal industry, chemicals, mining, building, and the railways. Obviously, the employer was more powerful than the mutuals. The employer often bore part of the costs. Not only was he concerned to ensure that his money was not wasted; he also wanted to ensure that the fund could not be used against him, as a strike fund of sorts. In some instances, employees had no influence over their factory schemes. The employer acted as a benevolent dictator. In those cases, benefits were usually a little higher—funds operated in part by workers themselves tended to be somewhat more frugal—but the rules of the game were more arbitrary too. In his benevolence, the employer could be generous to a friendly employee; in a malevolent mood, he might be anything but. At the end of the nineteenth century, the labour inspectorate noted that factory owners were increasingly of the opinion that their employees should be covered by some kind of scheme. Some factory owners even advocated state health insurance.[9]

Some factory owners also used the existence of the funds as a way to attract, and retain, good workers. During the First World War there were even factory schemes covering unemployment.[10] These seem to have been set up in cases where it was too costly to dismiss a surplus worker and rehire him when demand picked up. This would have been the case where workers with a specific skill were relatively rare (there was the obvious risk that they might go to work for another factory), if their work necessitated a long period of on-the-job training (an investment that would be lost if they were dismissed), or if the skills they needed became apparent only after a time (the cost of supervising a new worker was relatively high).

During the period 1888–1890, the Dutch government carried out a survey of the degree to which workers in factories and workplaces with more than ten employees were insured against sickness and other risks.[11] As Table 5.1 shows, 42 per cent of all factory workers were not compensated at all for loss of wages in the event of sickness; 16 per cent might receive "something" from their employer; 11 per cent were insured through mutual or commercial funds, but might also receive a supplement from the factory; and 31 per cent received an allowance through a factory scheme. All in all, factory schemes covered about a third of all factory workers. A more or less similar situation existed with regard to medical costs. About a quarter of workers were insured through their factory scheme; a quarter might receive discretionary payments, perhaps to supplement an allowance under a policy taken out privately; half received nothing and were forced to apply

Table 5.1 Workers in Dutch Factories and Workplaces with More Than Ten Employees, Insured Against Risk of Sickness, 1888–1890

	Number Employees (000s)			Percentage of Employees	
	Any Coverage	Covered for Wages	Covered for Medical Costs	Covered for Wages	Covered for Medical Costs
Factory schemes	46	44	35	31	25
Other insurers	16	16	13	11	9
Ad hoc	22	22	17	16	12
None	56	58	75	42	54
Total	140	140	140	100	100

Source: van Leeuwen, De eenheidsstaat, 173.

for medical-poor relief. About a quarter of all factory workers had burial insurance through a factory scheme, and one in six was insured for the costs of childbirth (Table 5.2). By 1890, there were even around 30 funds offering old-age-pension schemes. They covered a mere 3,000 individuals, but they also formed the nucleus of a Dutch tradition that, by the start of the twenty-first century, had resulted in enormous capital sums being built up by company pension funds to fund old-age pensions.[12]

Table 5.2 Workers in Dutch Factories and Workplaces with More Than Ten Employees, Insured for Costs of Burial or Childbirth, 1888–1890

	Number Employees (000s)			Percentage of Employees	
	Any Coverage	Covered for Burial	Covered for Childbirth	Covered for Burial	Covered for Childbirth
Factory schemes	45	36	24	26	17
Other insurers	16	13	9	9	6
Ad hoc	22	18	12	13	9
None	56	73	95	52	68
Total	140	140	140	100	100

Source: van Leeuwen, De eenheidsstaat, 87.

BURIAL INSURANCE

Burial schemes were big business in the nineteenth century, with an ever-increasing multitude of mainly very small local funds covering more and more individuals. They may be regarded as life insurance in miniature. And miniature they were. At the end of the nineteenth century, almost every village had its own burial fund, and there would be several in a city. While the number of members could exceed 100,000 (in one instance), most had no more than 500 members, and some indeed had only a handful. Table 5.3 lists the number of burial schemes according to type; factory schemes are excluded. Around 1800, ordinary mutual societies, often associated with guilds, dominated the market almost totally, leaving room for only a few commercial insurers. From the middle of the nineteenth century, schemes were set up by trade unions and doctors. The number of schemes rose across the board, with the total number of burial schemes more than trebling over the century.

To estimate the proportion of the population covered by burial insurance (Table 5.4), we multiplied the known number of insurers by the estimated average number insured and added in workers covered by the factory schemes.[13] The tremendous growth in burial insurance in the nineteenth century is evident from the figures, with the proportion of the total population covered rising from a few per cent at the start to more than fifty per cent by the end. The rest had their burial paid from their savings or by friends and

Table 5.3 Burial Insurers in the Netherlands by Type, 1800–1890, Excluding Factory Schemes

Year	Mutual	Trade Union	Total Mutual	Doctors	Commercial	Total
1800	248	0	248	0	6	254
1810	279	0	279	0	13	292
1820	298	0	298	1	17	316
1830	373	0	373	1	35	409
1840	392	1	393	1	46	440
1850	426	8	434	3	72	509
1860	404	20	424	5	86	515
1870	392	79	471	5	106	582
1880	405	150	555	5	120	680
1890	448	240	688	6	128	822

Source: van Genabeek, Met vereende kracht, 112, 133, 145, 156, 191, and 200.

Table 5.4 Coverage of Burial Insurance in the Netherlands, 1800–1890

Year	Number of Insurers, Excluding Factory Schemes (000s)	Minimum Number of Insured, Excluding Factory Schemes (000s)	Maximum Number of Insured, Excluding Factory Schemes (000s)	Number of Insured with Factory Schemes (000s)	Minimum Number of Insured (000s)	Maximum Number of Insured (000s)	Population Covered, in % (Percentage)
1800	254	64	127	0	64	127	3–6
1810	292	73	146	0	73	146	3–7
1820	316	183	252	2	185	254	8–11
1830	409	371	447	4	375	451	14–17
1840	440	544	613	5	549	618	19–21
1850	509	797	860	7	804	867	26–28
1860	515	975	1,024	9	984	1,033	30–31
1870	582	1,293	1,330	18	1,312	1,348	36–37
1880	680	1,735	1,756	27	1,762	1,783	43–44
1890	822	2,367	2,367	36	2,403	2,403	53

Source: van Leeuwen, De eenheidsstaat, 81.

relatives; or they were buried free of charge, the cost paid by a poor-relief agency—something greatly to be avoided.

The percentages reported in Table 5.4 are for the total Dutch population. As both the geographical coverage and the rate of coverage between the sexes were uneven, in some instances coverage would have been much higher and in other cases much lower. It may reasonably be assumed, for example, that in the urban west of the country a higher-than-average proportion of the population would have been covered and in the east, north-east, and south a lower-than-average proportion. Although we lack data on membership by gender (and, also, by other characteristics such as age and ethnicity), it may safely be assumed that most of the insured were adult males, although we cannot tell how many women were insured or coinsured. The coverage rate among male adult workers must have been considerably higher than the coverage rate in Table 5.4, which refers to the total population (women and children included). Coverage among women must have been lower.

Burial insurance usually offered a modest sum to cover the cost of a modest funeral. Such insurance had originated long before the birth of the Dutch Republic—provided by guilds, whose members collected coins for the widow and carried the coffin to its final resting place. At the end of the eighteenth century, burial insurance was still largely guild-based, but by then it was more formally organized. After the dissolution of the guilds in 1820, both commercial and mutual insurance—no longer, in the latter case, limited to workers in the same trade in the same town—took over the business of insuring burials.

Avoiding a pauper burial was often said to be the prime reason why most Dutch workers committed themselves to the periodic savings that burial insurance funds required:

> The members of the popular classes attach great importance to being buried decently. Even if they are from the lowest ranks of society, including beggars and paupers, they wish to avoid "being buried as a pauper." Contributions to the mutual fund were paid if at all possible. In times of difficulty, membership of a sickness fund was more likely to be terminated than membership of a burial fund—and the latter only in times of dire necessity. Quite naturally, workers were less concerned about leaving something to their widow and children than about being buried properly. . . . On the contrary, the belief that "someone else would then profit from my money after my death" was one frequently voiced. It must be said, however, that burial funds did unwittingly accustom their members to the notion of insurance, of providing for the future, forcing even those with hardly anything to spare to save, on however modest a scale.[14]

Mutual funds had an advantage over commercial ones in that their premiums did not include a margin for profit. Furthermore, they were run for the insured themselves,[15] whereas commercial funds denied them any influence. On another point, though, commercial funds had a comparative advantage. The mutuals provided relatively low benefits. They prevented large segments of the population (women, for example) from joining and sometimes turned away potential new members once the number of members had reached a self-imposed limit. Mutuals probably did this to avoid time-consuming administration, and perhaps also because they felt that this would enable them to minimize the risk of bankruptcy due to their inability to calculate premiums correctly. Closing the scheme to new members once a certain maximum had been reached meant, however, that premiums had to be calculated accurately, with, in any case, higher premiums for those members who joined later on in life, since they would generally contribute to the fund over fewer years, while being entitled to the same benefits as younger clients. Premiums had to be calculated correctly since, if they turned out to be insufficient to cover costs, these costs could not easily be recovered from the premiums charged to new entrants. As mutual funds generally did not use life tables to calculate premiums, they sometimes levied premiums that were too low and were forced to increase premiums when their mistake became apparent. This increase had to be borne either by a fixed number of clients or by new entrants, hardly an attractive prospect for those young men and women. In some cases, the schemes went bankrupt.

Commercial funds did not have these limitations, and the allowances they provided were about double those of the mutual funds (Table 5.5). The commercial funds did not set a limit to the number of members, thus ensuring the possibility of a continuous inflow of new, young contributors. Furthermore, older members were charged higher premiums (to reflect their greater mortality risk) than younger members, and so the latter did not need to feel they were subsidizing the premiums of the former. Commercial

Table 5.5 Burial Allowance in the Netherlands, by Type of Insurer, 1812–1895

Year	Type of Insurer	Average Allowance (in Guilders)
1812	Mutual	28
1827	Mutual	39
1827	Commercial	68
1890	Mutual	49
1890	Commercial	185
1890	Trade Union	46

Source: van Genabeek, Met vereende kracht, 116, 139, and 206.

funds proved better able than their mutual competitors to expand regionally and then nationally. At first they tried to expand their membership by charging lower premiums and offering higher benefits in urban areas. However, this put pressure on profits without attracting sufficient new members. After the mid-nineteenth century, they therefore opted for a new approach and directed their energies to attracting participants in rural areas. It soon became apparent that there was a market here that could afford insurance while at the same time being so geographically dispersed as to prevent a mutual fund being established in each and every village.[16]

During the first few decades of the nineteenth century it was still customary for funds to be set up locally by a group of mutually interested individuals. Often, such initiatives took the form of formalizing preexisting informal and small-scale arrangements (which usually did not involve premiums being paid in advance) between members of the same trade, and most notably of a guild, or between inhabitants of the same neighbourhood. Such arrangements would include adorning the coffin, carrying it to the grave, and providing food and beverages for mourners. From the 1830s onward, commercialization set in. Undertakers began to take over the whole business of death and burial. So too did others, including innkeepers, barbers, and doctors, who had hitherto been active only in a certain segment but who, thus, already possessed some familiarity with the business of burying. They levied contributions in return for a burial allowance. To start such a fund, neither a great deal of money nor a great number of participants was needed; nor did the initiators need much more knowledge than they already possessed. This made it easy to set up a fund, and many new ones appeared during those years.[17]

The larger funds, operating in the major cities or regionally, worked with *bodes*, or insurance collectors. An insurance collector was the pivotal player in the burial-insurance business:

> Most members do not know to which fund they belong; they never see a policy, nor the scheme's regulations; nor are they particularly interested in seeing them. Instead, they simply consider themselves to be a member of the fund, with this or that collector. "They are with collector A or collector B." This they know, and it is enough to satisfy them. Neither the name nor the financial soundness of the fund is looked into; the only compass they sail upon is the insurance collector's assurance that the fund is reliable and its premium lower than that of other funds.[18]

This great trust could not be abused with impunity. Abuse meant ill repute and loss of custom: "The effect of a refusal to pay a benefit, or the irregular or partial payment of a benefit, was usually of great consequence for a fund, or a branch of it. Occasionally, a collector lost his whole branch as a result."[19]

Burial funds were big business. Around 1890, total annual premiums were 4.1 million guilders, and the funds received a further 0.4 million guilders in interest on their assets (of around 12.5 million guilders). They provided a total of 2 million guilders a year for some 50,000 funerals. In theory, they could predict future expenditure, and thus the level of the premium reserve from which future obligations would be paid, using a life table to calculate life expectancy. However, a national survey conducted in 1890 concluded that most funds did not calculate future expenditure, though it added that in many cases the reserves were sufficient. It was estimated that 300,000 of the 1.8 million insured were covered by actuarially unsound funds, representing obligations amounting to 22 million guilders, compared with total future obligations of 128 million guilders. A not insignificant part of the insurance market was thus rotten, though it is perhaps surprising that the situation was not worse given the seemingly arbitrary nature of the way in which premiums were often calculated.[20]

At the end of the nineteenth century, by which time the premium reserve was being calculated correctly, it often exceeded the value of future obligations. The Amsterdam branch of Groot-Noordhollandse had a surplus of 40 per cent in 1890; for the rural branch the corresponding figure was 200 per cent.[21] Prudent guesswork played a part in this fortuitous situation, as did sheer luck. Mortality rates were being calculated unsoundly—if at all. But adult life expectancy rose in the nineteenth century, so the insured lived longer and paid premiums for longer than past experience suggested. Another prime cause of the healthy financial situation of these funds was the widespread and profitable practice of cancellation.

It was generally remarked that "a fund could stay solvent on the proceeds of cancellation [alone]" . . . the necessity for a sound reserve is countered to some extent by the fact that it applied only if the insured continued with the same fund until they died. But often they did not. After several years, participants might switch to a different fund, and so their insurance should be considered temporary; as a result, the annual premiums are almost always sufficient, and it is not necessary to set part of these aside.[22]

What did one get in return for one's premium? A typical mutual burial-insurance scheme would

> provide a coffin for the deceased, toll the church bells, and organize a church service and transport to the cemetery. Often some members carried the deceased in a solemn procession to his or her final resting place, in the company of other members, whose presence at the service was generally assumed. The funds often possessed attributes such as a hearse and a bier. Some associations of typographers had a banner embroidered with the association's name, and this could be draped over the coffin during the funeral.[23]

In addition, many funds offered financial support. Around 1890, the average allowance provided was approximately 50 guilders.

Complaints were often voiced about the high level of premiums and the rules and regulations (which seemed to benefit the funds more than the insured). The Society for the Promotion of Medicine in particular was of that opinion. In retrospect, as has already been noted, premiums were generally more than sufficient to meet any claims, and in this sense could indeed be said to have been too high. On paper, the rules and regulations of the insurance funds did seem to allow them considerable scope to abuse their discretionary powers, but in reality the situation seems to have been less dramatic: "The rules are formulated in such a way as to allow the funds, as a guarantee against bad practices [on the part of the insured], to reject claims in all but a few cases. But it was also in the interests of the insurance funds and societies to offer an interpretation of the rules that was as generous as possible."[24] Customers flocked to funds with a good reputation and shunned those considered tight fisted.

Burial funds accepted clients without requiring them to first undergo a medical examination. Examinations were simply too expensive—around one and a half guilders, equivalent, in many cases, to the annual premium. Cheaper examinations were available, but they were less useful: "We vividly remember . . . how someone was witness to several examinations being carried out [by a doctor], without the doctor, who was also driving, leaving his carriage." A more efficient way to counter adverse selection was to instruct the insurance collector to be scrupulous: "In practice an honest collector who does not accept a member without having seen him can exercise stricter control than a doctor."[25] Many funds refused to pay out if they subsequently discovered that they had been misled and that a member had failed to report an existing illness when joining the fund. Of course, they first had to discover that they were being misled—by no means an easy matter. It was for this reason that some funds resorted to a classic remedy: either not paying out if a member died within a year of taking out burial insurance, or remitting the full amount only after a member had paid dues for several years.

Moral hazards were few. However, some funds explicitly stipulated that no payment would be made in cases of suicide, or if death resulted from a fight begun by the deceased, in cases of death while serving in the army, if the death took place in the workhouse, at sea, or, more generally but rarely, "in all cases decided on for serious reasons at the discretion of the directors." Funds terminated insurance if a member insulted either the collector or management. In general, however, "the regulations governing the monetary allowances do not give rise to disapproving criticism: on the contrary, the generosity of many funds deserves to be greeted with enthusiasm."[26]

LET OP UW EINDE[27]

At the end of the nineteenth century, the overwhelming majority of funds were still small—with fewer than 500 participants, and many with less than 100—but there were also a few large insurance companies operating nationwide. The evolution of Let op Uw Einde, or Memento Mori, is illustrative of the rise, flourishing, and then demise of burial insurance, though it was exceptional in its subsequent ability to rise from its ashes.

Let op Uw Einde was begun by D. Stolwerk and W. P. Ingenegeren in Utrecht in 1847. Stolwerk had been an insurance collector for a major mutual fund; he left, taking with him not only his expertise but also "his" members. Ingenegeren had been a dealer in secondhand goods and so was familiar with the funeral branch, as he often bought clothes and household effects from the families of the deceased. He also had a sharp mind and was quicker than most of his competitors to see where the future lay. The number of participants in Let op Uw Einde grew from 8,000 in 1848 to 264,000 in 1884, before declining to 217,000 in 1893. The company worked with insurance collectors, who collected premiums on a weekly basis. Such rapid growth was made possible by the system of collectors and their supervisors, the agents. The collector recruited new participants, collected premiums, paid out benefits, and was responsible for the paperwork. The agents were the middlemen, operating between the collectors and head office; they were responsible for ensuring that the collectors operated in exactly the same way, regardless of their location, and for detecting irregularities and fraud. Collectors came and went all the time; 40 per cent resigned within a year, and 70 per cent within two years. Their work was far from easy, and their success depended, in large measure, on their personal skills. The insurance collector kept a fairly modest set of records. He added the names of the newly insured on one list and marked those no longer insured on a separate one. Another list included the names of members who had moved locally, while those moving outside his district were listed separately. All this information was carefully copied into a *stamboek*, or register, for the agent to inspect. He also had a *loopboek*, or notebook, in which he ticked off the names of those he had visited in his district and whose premiums he had collected. Every week, he listed the premiums he had collected, and those still due, in a *rekeningboekje*, or accounts book, which he then sent to the agent, who signed it by way of endorsement before sending it on to head office.

It was for the agent to decide if and when to pay out any benefits. He would check the collector's work for mistakes—inevitable, given the frequent changes that had to be recorded—and for signs of fraud. Sometimes, for instance, the collector himself paid the premium for a sick adult or child, expecting, or even hoping, for an early death—in which case he might claim part or all of the insurance payout for himself, although the collector might also take pity on the deceased's family and pay them the full benefit. In both cases, the company lost out through what they regarded as fraud. Some collectors forged death certificates and claimed the insurance payout for themselves. Sometimes a collector "lent" the premium to a family unable to pay it, either out of compassion or because he expected to gain in the event of an early death in the family. The agent endeavoured not only to combat fraud; he also tried to prevent collectors leaving and either moving to another fund or beginning one of their own (taking with them their clients, whose loyalties, if any, were to the insurance collector rather than the company). Naturally, the directors of Let op Uw Einde decried such practices, though in fact they had started out the same way.

Let op Uw Einde was run by the two founders (directors) and four members of the supervisory board. The directors were in charge of day-to-day activities and received a salary which, until 1879, was based on the benefits paid out in any one year. A virulent epidemic was bad for clients and for the company, but it was a financial blessing for the directors. After 1897, directors' salaries were set at 3–4 per cent of annual premiums, the equivalent in 1882 of 8,000 guilders. Ingenegeren was in charge of the company's central administration and as such responsible for ensuring that the data in the collectors' registers and notebooks were recorded and processed. He had weekly reports drawn up on the number of insured, premiums collected, premiums in arrears, and benefits paid out. These weekly reports subsequently formed the basis of monthly and annual reports.

The fund was open to everyone. There were six classes of coverage, each with its own level of premium and benefit. Premiums were only partly determined by the applicant's age on joining. Around the mid-nineteenth century, premiums ranged from 1½ cents per week for a child aged 8 or older in the lowest class to 32 cents or more for elderly members in the highest class. Most weekly premiums were between 1½ cents and 10 cents. Premiums did not rise with age, even though the mortality risk did, especially among the elderly. On joining the fund, a young adult would therefore be paying a modest supplement, but he thereby avoided having to pay a higher premium later on.

Nonpayment was frequent and usually the result of insufficient income, especially in winter. Alcoholism was another cause. The more astute collectors tried to ensure premiums were paid before they could be spent on drink. There was also a group of professional defaulters, who switched from one collector to another, sometimes after changing their address. Since premiums tended not to vary with age, one could get away with frequently rejoining without paying a prohibitive penalty in the form of a higher premium. Cancellations for arrears were common: in 1882 ten per cent of policies were cancelled. Given the administrative costs involved and the initial commission (*aanbrengpremie*) that had to be paid, this might be an expensive practice for the company, particularly if the policy was fairly recent. In all other cases the company would profit, since the company could forfeit the premiums in full without having to pay for a burial.

The level of benefit depended on age at joining and class of insurance. In the mid-nineteenth century, benefits varied from 5 guilders for a 1-year-old child in the lowest class to 190 guilders for an adult in the highest class. Most of those insured could expect 5 guilders for a child and 30 guilders for an adult. Roughly half of total revenue was spent on benefits, and a quarter was used to meet personnel costs and other operating costs; the remainder was invested in stocks and bonds.

Like most burial funds, Let op Uw Einde had two characteristics that distinguished it from the so-called modern life-insurance companies that emerged at the end of the nineteenth century. First, it did not make acceptance conditional on a medical examination. This attracted a number of people who were seriously ill and who, realizing they were unlikely to live very long, hoped to help their families avoid having to pay for the funeral themselves. A medical examination could have prevented such adverse selection, but this would have been too expensive in relation to the premium. Instead, as we noted earlier, the fund relied on the intuition and common-sense of the collector, probably not an inappropriate alternative, given the rather limited predictive powers of medical tests at that time.[28] Furthermore, the insurance policy included a clause allowing the company to insist on a medical examination if it suspected fraud, for example, if it believed an applicant had failed to divulge details about a preexisting illness. This was not necessarily an effective solution though, since many doctors tended to sympathize with the relatives of the deceased.

Whereas modern insurers register children separately and can therefore calculate their premiums on a fairly sound actuarial basis, Let op Uw Einde (along with most other burial funds) did not. Children under the age of 8 were insured "free of charge." What this meant, of course, was that the costs of a child's funeral were met by the insured as a group, in the form of higher premiums. Given that the burial funds did not register children separately, neither the precise number of individuals insured nor the volume of potential claims could be accurately calculated. Nor, then, strictly speaking, could premiums. This problem was aggravated by adverse selection: families with young children were attracted to funds that did not charge a separate premium for children. However, as most funds did charge such a premium, the problem was relatively mild.

To circumvent these problems, in 1883 Ingenegeren founded De Utrechtse, a modern burial insurance company, which did register children separately. From then on, the board channelled most of its energies into the new company, to the detriment of Let op Uw Einde. In 1893, the latter was absorbed by De Utrechtse, a process that took ten years due to two complications. To begin with, it was unclear whether, legally speaking, the directors owned Let op Uw Einde or were merely employed by it as managers.[29] A solution to this problem was found by buying off any claims to ownership for 150,000 guilders. One final problem remained. It was also unclear whether Let op Uw Einde's assets exceeded its liabilities, in the form of future obligations. From 1881 onward, the young children insured premium-free were gradually included in the records of the fund, allowing a reliable statement of assets and liabilities to be drawn up a decade later. As a result, the number of insured was calculated at 210,000. Assets exceeded liabilities by 150,000 guilders: of this, 50,000 guilders was paid to the directors and 80,000 guilders to the company's employees, while the residue was repaid to policyholders in the form of slightly higher benefits.

OLD AGE AND WIDOWS' PENSIONS

Death may have been an insurable risk when it came to paying for the funeral, but paying for the widow was uncommon, as indeed was insurance for old age generally. Old-age-pension schemes cost considerably more than burial insurance, and very few people could afford them. Table 5.6 gives the number of funds offering old age pensions and provides estimates of coverage.[30] The number of funds doubled in the second half of the nineteenth century, but total coverage remained low: just 0.5 per cent of the population. By far the great majority of insurers were mutual funds; there were never more than a handful of commercial insurers.

Most funds were local and small. Their premiums were estimated on the basis of past experience. In the case of burial insurance, this worked rather well, since life expectancy rose and so too did the number of years during which premiums were paid. However, this same development must have created problems for mutual old age pension schemes since it also meant an increase in the number of pension years.

There were also a handful of "modern life insurers." Of those, the Hollandse Sociëteit van Levensverzekeringen (1807) is thought to have been the first to calculate premiums based on life tables.[31] The number of such

Table 5.6 Coverage of Old-Age-Pension Schemes in the Netherlands, 1800–1890

| Year | Number of Schemes, Excluding Factory Schemes | Number of Insured (000s) | | Percentage of Population Covered |
		Excluding Factory Schemes	Including Factory Schemes	
1800	49	13	13	0.6
1810	50	13	13	0.6
1820	39	10	10	0.4
1830	45	11	11	0.4
1840	47	12	12	0.4
1850	50	13	13	0.4
1860	50	13	13	0.4
1870	62	16	17	0.5
1880	72	18	20	0.5
1890	87	22	25	0.5

Source: Number of insured and coverage, van Leeuwen, De eenheidsstaat, 96; number of schemes, van Genabeek, "Onderlinges 1800–1890," 339; and van Genabeek, Met vereende kracht, 200.

life insurers remained very small until the end of the century; with relatively high premiums, they catered for the top segment of the market. In 1860, there were only three; in 1870 eleven; and in 1880 nineteen. Between 1880 and 1890 twenty-three new companies entered the market, most of them operating on a commercial basis.

Insurance to provide widows or widowers with a pension was even rarer. Guilds had provided such pensions in the seventeenth century, as did commercial companies in the eighteenth, albeit on a limited scale. Wealthy guilds could use some of their investment income to subsidize widowhood insurance, but the abolition of the guilds in 1820 put an end to this practice. Widows' benefits now had to be paid from the reserve set aside for this purpose and paid from the annual premiums. That required a rather high level of premium. Nonetheless, schemes to provide for widows (and orphans) were established after 1820. Initially almost all of them were mutual schemes, sometimes guild schemes resuscitated under a different name but with many of the same members. A decade later, there was a brief period that saw a significant number of new commercial funds being founded. But the proportion of the Dutch population covered by widowhood insurance never reached more than 1 per cent during the nineteenth century, with the exception of the peak around 1830 when, at most, 1½ per cent of all Dutch men and women were insured (Table 5.7).[32]

Such funds often made unrealistic promises. The Dutch historian Ben Gales has summarized the resulting problem as follows:

> The core problem was that if the premium were to be calculated correctly, it would be too high and the market as a consequence too small. It was tempting therefore to attract a larger market by charging lower premiums. . . . Insurers could try to ensure rapid growth by offering premiums that were too low and then trust to a miracle to meet their obligations. . . . The life-insurance branch thus demanded a rather large measure of self-discipline, and this was not always forthcoming during the nineteenth century. Companies operating on actuarially sound principles emerged only very slowly. Of the twenty-eight widows' funds established in the decade prior to 1830, only one, the Algemeen Meisjes-, Vrouwen- en Weduwenfonds, met with the approval of the government adviser.[33]

Many years could elapse, however, between the start of an unsound but expanding fund and its demise, since during this period rising expenditure could be financed from the expansion in revenue. Nonetheless, a series of bankruptcies in 1830 led to a Royal Decree that brought all widowhood, old-age, and general life-insurance funds under state supervision.[34] From then on, funds were required to submit their regulations to the Ministry of the Interior for approval. Never again during the nineteenth century did the total number of insurers reach its 1830 level.

Table 5.7 Coverage of Widowhood Insurance in the Netherlands, 1800–1890

Year	Number of Schemes, Excluding Factory Schemes			Number of Insured, Including Factory Schemes, as Percentage of Total Population
	Mutual	*Commercial*	*Total*	
1800	21	0	21	0–1
1810	22	2	24	0–1
1820	26	5	31	1–2
1830	30	23	53	0–1
1840	31	9	40	0–1
1850	32	7	39	0–1
1860	19	7	26	0–1
1870	24	6	30	0–1
1880	34	5	39	0–1
1890	48	4	52	0–1

Source: Coverage, van Leeuwen, De eenheidsstaat, 96 and 381; number of schemes, van Genabeek, "Onderlinges 1800–1890," 339; and van Genabeek, Met vereende kracht, 200.

UNEMPLOYMENT

Unemployment insurance schemes were rare before the twentieth century. Commercial insurers did not offer them, nor did factory owners, though a few mutual funds did (Table 5.8). At their "zenith," these funds insured 0.2 per cent of the Dutch labour force against unemployment.[35] In addition, two out of seven national trade unions offered unemployment insurance of sorts in 1890. Again, few workers were insured, and we can thus conclude that unemployment insurance was only a marginal phenomenon during the nineteenth century. Moreover, those schemes that did offer such insurance were not really very generous. In 1895, a trade unionist could claim unemployment benefit for at most nine weeks,[36] during which time he would receive up to five guilders per week, about half his wage. After that, he would have to resort to poor relief, which, though less, could last much longer. Furthermore, the trade union paid no benefit during the first week of any unemployment.

Unemployment schemes were notoriously difficult to operate due to the problems of adverse selection, moral hazards, and correlated risks.[37] Those who worked in a sector of the economy plagued by periodic unemployment, such as the building industry, would be among the first to take out

Table 5.8 Coverage of Unemployment Insurance in the Netherlands, 1800–1890

Year	Number of Funds Providing Unemployment Insurance	Percentage of the Labour Force Covered
1800	0	0.0
1810	0	0.0
1820	0	0.0
1830	0	0.0
1840	0	0.0
1850	0	0.0
1860	4	0.2
1870	10	—
1880	15	—
1890	39	0.1

Source: van Genabeek, "Onderlinges 1800–1890," 339; van Leeuwen, De eenheidsstaat, 231.

unemployment insurance, since it would certainly repay itself. Apart from such adverse-selection effects, the problem of moral hazards was also a major hindrance to unemployment insurance. While it was most unlikely that a pension claimant could fake old age or a severe handicap, unemployment was something of a grey area, one whose boundaries were liable to be thoroughly tested by the more unscrupulous. Indeed, in Western Europe, today's national unemployment schemes often allow claimants some discretion in refusing work for which they are overqualified. It can be argued, however, that national trade unions have a comparative advantage over commercial insurers in offering unemployment insurance because they are better able to cope with adverse selection—partly by making it compulsory for their members—and moral hazards—given their extensive familiarity with both the labour market and their members. In fact, the first few decades of the twentieth century were the heyday of trade union unemployment insurance; it came to an end with the enactment of the 1949 Unemployment Insurance Act. Well before then, however, the Dutch government had had to step in. During the Great Depression, so many workers suddenly became unemployed that the unions were faced with both huge costs and a decline in contributions. This is an example of the problem of correlated risks, which had also plagued unemployment insurance in the nineteenth century and for which even the unions had no solution.

The political climate in the nineteenth century was hostile to the notion of a national unemployment-insurance scheme. During the Dutch Republic there had at least been the notion that local authorities, employers, and patrician families were responsible for the well-being of workers in their locality, although workers' organizations were often regarded with suspicion. However, the nineteenth century witnessed the flourishing of laissez-faire liberalism and a weakening of that sense of local responsibility, while the hostility to workers' organizations continued. Under French rule, the *Code Pénal* was implemented in the Netherlands in 1811, and it explicitly denied workers the right to unite in order to strike or demand higher wages. Although this part of the code seemed to be contradicted by the rights granted to workers under the Dutch Constitution of 1848, it was not abolished until 1872, after an amendment by a Social Liberal member of parliament. Indeed, it was only toward the end of the century that social liberalism, which was less averse to workers' organizations, truly gained ground. Social liberals believed that the state had a duty to intervene in serious social problems that would otherwise be left unsolved. For most of the century, however, laissez-faire liberalism predominated, and this did nothing to advance the emergence of unemployment insurance by trade unions, as laissez-faire liberals considered trade unions as much an obstacle to the well-being of society as the guilds of the *ancien régime*

SICKNESS: COMPENSATION FOR LOSS OF INCOME

The *ziekenfonds*, or health insurance fund, was a feature of the Netherlands right up until 2006. The ziekenfonds insured its members against the costs of medical treatment (such insurance became compulsory in 1941). As a term, however, ziekenfonds has a much longer provenance, and did not acquire its present meaning until well into the twentieth century. Around 1800, ziekenfonds primarily meant insurance against loss of income during periods of sickness.[38] A national survey of 1892 listed every ziekenfonds in the country. Half of these covered loss of income—they were, to be more precise, *ondersteuningsfondsen*, or benevolent funds; a third covered the costs of medical treatment—the *medicijnfondsen*; and the remainder covered both. Half of the insurance funds called themselves mutual funds, which in principle meant that they were owned by their members and that these members could dismiss the director (though this rarely happened); in some cases the term was exploited by companies with an entirely different legal structure because it evoked a sense of trustworthiness. In addition to the mutuals, there were *doktersfondsen* (operated by a single general practitioner), *directiefondsen* (commercial-based schemes run by boards of directors), and *artsenfondsen* (run by a group of general practitioners). There were also factory-based schemes covering employees at a single factory or a group of factories in a specific branch of industry.

Table 5.9 gives the number of insurers (excluding factory schemes) covering loss of income due to sickness; Table 5.10 presents an estimate of the proportion of the population covered by all insurers (including factory schemes).[39] Around 1810, between 4 and 7 per cent of the labour force was insured against loss of income in the event of sickness; by the end of the century the corresponding figure was 27 per cent. This growth, which was particularly apparent after 1860, can be attributed to two factors: first, women and farmers too began to take out insurance; secondly, rates of coverage rose among industrial male labourers—the traditional target group. All types of insurer, but especially the commercial, profited from this growth. Commercial insurers had a negligible share of the market around 1800; a century later they had almost a third.

In 1812, average weekly sick benefits were around 2 guilders, in 1890 3 guilders, approximately half the average wage (Table 5.11).[40] These benefits were significantly higher than those paid by poor-relief agencies, but they were paid for a shorter period. Poor relief continued for the duration of the sickness, while health-insurance benefits were generally restricted to a maximum of three months—though there was much variation here. The pattern was clear: the longer the maximum duration, the lower the level of benefit.[41]

In 1890, the standard premium was 5 cents, which entitled one to a weekly benefit of 3 guilders for thirteen weeks. Members joining after the

Table 5.9 Number of Insurers in the Netherlands Covering Loss of Income Due to Sickness, by Type of Insurer, 1800–1890, Excluding Factory Schemes

Year	Mutual	Trade Union	Total Mutual	Doctors	Commercial	Total
1800	194	0	194		1	195
1810	211	0	211		1	212
1820	203	0	203		2	205
1830	253	0	253		8	261
1840	268	1	269		13	282
1850	270	9	279	3	19	301
1860	237	25	262	3	23	288
1870	229	89	318	6	25	349
1880	252	191	443	7	23	473
1890	343	374	717	8	29	754

Source: van Genabeek, Met vereende kracht, 112, 133, 145, 156, 191, and 200.

Table 5.10 Coverage of Insurance for Loss of Income Due to Sickness in the Netherlands, 1800–1911

Year	Number of Insurers Excluding Factory Schemes	Number of Factory Schemes	Total Number of Funds	Minimum Number of Insured (000s)	Maximum Number of Insured (000s)	Percentage of the Labour Force Insured	Percentage of the Population Insured
1800	195	0	195	29	59	.	1–3
1810	212	0	212	32	64	4–7	1–3
1820	205	33	238	40	72	.	2–3
1830	261	67	328	61	101	.	2–4
1840	282	100	382	79	119	.	3–4
1850	301	134	435	98	137	8–11	3–4
1860	288	167	455	111	145	8–11	3–4
1870	349	268	617	161	198	.	4–5
1880	473	368	841	236	274	.	6–7
1890	754	468	1222	366	402	21–23	8–9
1900	992	569	1561	502	519	.	10
1911	1229	669	1898	639	639	27–27	11

Source: van Leeuwen, De eenheidsstaat, 175.

Table 5.11 Average Weekly Sick-Benefit Levels in the Netherlands, 1812–1895

	Type of Insurer	Average Weekly Benefit (Guilders)	As Percentage of Wages	As a Multiple of Poor Relief
1812	All	2	44	—
1827	All	2.1	47	9
1890	All	3.1	45	—
1895	Trade Union	4.5	52	—

Source: van Genabeek, Met vereende kracht, 116, 139, and 157; van Genabeek, "Onderlinges 1800–1890," 342; van Leeuwen, De eenheidsstaat, 175.

age of around 35 to 45 generally paid a higher premium, with premiums being increased 50 per cent for every five years beyond that age; they were sometimes obliged to pay a substantial joining fee too.[42] This differentiated premium structure reflected the fact that the elderly were more likely than young workers to become (or be) ill; it was felt only fair that they should therefore pay more. Once a member had joined, the premium was fixed. Young members thus bore part of the cost of insuring the risk of sickness among older members, and this is still the case in the Netherlands today.

Often the level of premiums was calculated on the basis of a young insurance base; this led to difficulties as members aged. It was a problem familiar to all nineteenth-century benevolent funds. Though any annual surplus was transferred to a reserve, a practice also followed by the burial funds, after a time this reserve became deceptively large and, as a national commission noted at the end of the century, "[the size of this reserve] was thought, particularly by the mutual funds, to warrant either a reduction in premiums or an increase in benefit levels, or to justify making other provisions for members, such as organizing festivities, monetary distributions, introducing death or retirement benefits," without the fund really knowing whether, actuarially speaking, it could afford to.[43] Having a 67,000-guilder reserve, one (unspecified) fund was particularly "generous"; an actuarial calculation, employing morbidity tables, suggested that the reserve actually needed a further 56,000 guilders to meet its commitments. A national commission stated: "Many schemes live literally from hand to mouth, each year paying out more or less as much as they receive; often, they can carry on like this for a long time since deficits are ruled out. After a while though, benefits for the growing number of elderly decline until they are inadequate in relation to premiums; the young no longer join at all, and so a scheme like this goes under."[44]

The finances of the smaller funds, and most of them were small, were of particular concern. First, because "a year in which the number of sick is just slightly above average completely exhausts the reserve and can force the fund to increase premiums or reduce benefits out of all proportion to what members are accustomed."[45] This problem reflected a combination of a small insurance base and correlated risks. Many funds were vulnerable in times of widespread sickness; during the cholera epidemics of 1832–1833, 1848–1849, 1855, and 1866, and the smallpox epidemic of 1871, for instance, bankruptcies were frequent.[46] Second, because of the "life cycle" of the funds: "First there are several favourable years with surpluses, then several years of deficits and failings; finally the fund has to be dissolved—in some cases being reincorporated immediately by the younger members, the elderly being regarded as a burden."[47] There was another problem: "It is by no means uncommon for the operator of a benevolent fund to continue collecting the premiums, using these to create a good impression or simply saving them, and then, in the first case, to terminate the fund the moment significant numbers apply for benefits . . ., or, in the latter case, to vanish as soon as he has collected enough."[48] The commission urged "a degree of government regulation, to avoid abuse and ensure confidence among the general public."[49]

Benefit levels were not always fixed. If the reserves were insufficient, premiums would be raised or benefits reduced.[50] Under the Dutch Republic, the guilds too found this an effective way of managing risks that were difficult to predict. For many funds, the alternative was bankruptcy, or such high premiums—or such low benefits—that few workers could or would consider joining. In addition, the funds generally used the same means to limit the moral risk of malingering: "As a rule, the benefits paid by a fund could never exceed the weekly wage, and sometimes three-quarters, a measure to counter malingering."[51] Benevolent funds that accepted women often required a surcharge of 50 per cent, "a measure apparently necessary due to the higher rates of morbidity among women (whether actual or due to malingering)."[52] This practice could be explained, the commission claimed, by the fact that in winter these women were unable to find sufficient work and hoped the insurance would compensate for this.[53] Another measure to limit moral risk—and preclude bankruptcy—concerned the duration of the benefit. Insurers often limited the benefit duration to between thirteen and eighteen weeks. This limit sometimes depended on the nature of the illness: four weeks for an external sore, twelve for a broken arm or leg, and fifty-two weeks for a serious illness. Nonmutual funds often restricted the total number of weeks recipients could claim benefits to about 40–60 during the lifetime of the policy. The *Karenztijd*, or waiting period (the initial period of sickness during which members were not eligible for benefit), was between three and fourteen days.[54] Often, a doctor's certificate was required. Many funds also required applicants to have been a member for a minimum number of months or years before they were eligible for benefits. Some funds refused to pay benefits if the sickness "is due to: contributory negligence, attempted suicide, fighting, rioting, war, excesses, or if the sickness is an undisclosed regular tertian fever, rheumatic disorder or madness."[55]

SICKNESS: COSTS OF MEDICAL TREATMENT

Whenever a doctor had to be paid, or medicines or bandages bought, there were generally three options: having one's health insurance pay—if one were fortunate to have a policy; turning to the medical branch of a charity; or paying out of one's own pocket—even if that meant dissaving, borrowing, or pawning. There was a bewildering variety of health insurers, of various types, setting various conditions, and it is by no means easy to distil an over-all impression from the historical sources. We will start, though, as before, by looking at the number of insurers by type, excluding factory schemes. We then provide estimates of the total number and proportion of the Dutch population covered by insurers (including factory schemes) and summarize the various conditions set by the funds and how these funds operated. We conclude with an interpretation of the data. This time, we begin our quantitative analysis in 1901, the year of a comprehensive national survey. Projecting back from our data for that year, we construct estimates of rates of coverage in the nineteenth century, using the known number of health insurers and the estimated average number of insured per insurer.

In 1800 there were some sixty providers of health insurance, almost all of which were mutual (Table 5.12). In 1890 there were 461 providers (excluding factory schemes), half of which were ordinary mutuals, while a

Table 5.12 Number of Health Insurers in the Netherlands by Type, 1800–1890, Excluding Factory Schemes

Year	Mutuals	Trade Union	Total Mutual	General Practitioners' Funds	Doctors' Funds	Commercial Funds	Total
1800	55	0	55	0	0	5	60
1810	69	0	69	0	0	10	79
1820	97	0	97	0	0	13	110
1830	160	0	160	1	2	21	184
1840	187	0	187	2	3	32	224
1850	207	0	207	9	10	44	270
1860	180	2	182	13	11	51	257
1870	168	8	176	18	14	57	265
1880	177	15	192	24	64	59	339
1890	235	37	272	27	96	66	461

Source: van Genabeek, Met vereende kracht, 112, 133, 145, 156, 191, and 200.

further thirty-seven were run by trade unions. The total number of mutual funds rose between four- and fivefold during the century, but they still lost ground to commercial insurers (the number of which showed a thirteenfold increase) and to funds operated by the medical profession. The latter funds were of two sorts: the *doktersfondsen*, run by the physician who also treated the patient; and the *artsenfondsen*, operated by groups of medical practitioners. Both types flourished in the second half of the century.

Table 5.13 provides estimates of the percentage of the Dutch population covered by health insurance. We have a fairly accurate figure (18%) for 1901. But there is a margin of error before that date since we have no precise figures for the average number of insured. The best we can do here, as in our previous estimates, is to offer minimum and maximum percentages.[56] The overall pattern of growth is clear, however: a more or less continuous increase in coverage from very low levels—around 1 per cent—at the beginning of the nineteenth century.

Insurance to cover the consequences of sickness tended to target the middle classes. By and large, the poor were catered for by medical poor relief, while the rich bore the costs themselves. Sickness funds were primarily

Table 5.13 Coverage of Health Insurance in the Netherlands, 1800–1901

	Number of Funds, Excluding Factory Schemes	Number of Factory Schemes	Total Number of Funds	Minimum Number of Insured (000s)	Maximum Number of Insured (000s)	Percentage of the Population Insured
1800	60	0	60	9	18	0–1
1810	79	0	79	12	24	1
1820	110	3	113	34	49	1–2
1830	184	7	191	86	108	3–4
1840	224	10	234	141	165	5–6
1850	270	13	283	214	237	7–8
1860	257	17	274	248	266	7–8
1870	265	29	294	311	326	9
1880	339	42	381	460	473	11–12
1890	461	54	515	700	709	15–16
1901	.	67	616	930	930	18

Source: van Leeuwen, De eenheidsstaat, 179.

meant for those poorer sections of society that desired no charity and could afford a modest weekly contribution; these included day labourers, artisans, factory workers, servants, low-paid workers in offices, civil servants, and those of lesser social ranks who had retired.

Over the course of the century, two new types of health-insurance schemes emerged alongside the factory schemes: doctors' funds and trade union funds.[57] In the countryside, doctors set up their own schemes, with members paying a fixed premium. The doctor acted as manager of the fund, gave medical treatment, and supplied medicines, which he also often prepared himself. For doctors, this arrangement was attractive because it enabled them to draw patients who would otherwise normally never consult a doctor. Hitherto, when such patients did consult them, the doctor was faced with the option of either not helping them or of forgoing payment, which, so it was said, was not uncommon. Furthermore, rural doctors could hardly expect to make a living from their few private patients.

In addition to these initiatives by individual doctors, groups of medical practitioners also began to set up health-insurance funds. One of the first was the Algemeen Ziekenfonds Amsterdam (AZA), founded in 1846. The AZA targeted the middle classes. Membership was restricted to workers earning less than a set limit. Those earning above this threshold had to sign up with a commercial insurer. An innovative feature of the practitioners' funds was that members could choose from among the AZA-affiliated doctors and that the doctors had the right to refuse patients. The choice of doctor had no effect on the level of contribution, which was the same for everyone. This way, the AZA tried to combine the advantages of a private practice with those of a health insurance scheme. The fund offered insurance against the costs of medical treatment as well as sickness benefit and life insurance, with separate premiums and benefits for each. The AZA grew rapidly, and by 1850 4 per cent of the Amsterdam population was insured by the AZA; by 1900 the figure was 18 per cent. That growth was not at the expense of the mutual and commercial health-insurance funds. The total proportion of Amsterdam's population insured rose from 25 per cent in 1842 to 42 per cent in 1898. The AZA's success inspired initiatives elsewhere, and similar health-insurance funds emerged in the towns and cities of Middelburg (1849), Zeist (1856), Gouda (1857), Rotterdam and Haarlem (1858), Den Helder (1862), Beverwijk (1865), Delft (1873), Almaar and Gorkum (1874), Hoorn (1880), Breda (1885), Arnhem (1866), and Nijmegen (1888).[58] None of these was as successful as the AZA though.

The emergence of funds for craftsmen and workers at the end of the nineteenth century reflected the rise of labour organizations and the degree of organization among workers: it was not until after the middle of the century that labourers were permitted to set up trade unions and join anything other than nonpolitical mutual funds.

In the course of the nineteenth century, health-insurance coverage rose significantly. The scale of activities also increased, especially among the commercial funds and the doctors' funds. To join a fund, an applicant had to supply a health certificate; this was usually issued either by the patients themselves (oddly enough) or their doctor. Not surprisingly, this form of selection was not very effective: "It led to abuse on a number of occasions, with people joining only once they were sick and leaving soon after they had recovered." This phenomenon we now term adverse selection. In the nineteenth century it was tolerated for a reason: "... for doctors, especially in rural areas, where they were also charged with poor relief, this practice was often the lesser of two evils, since they would otherwise have to offer help free of charge or simply not get paid."[59] In fact, there was a process of double adverse selection: the sick applied to join in return for a premium calculated on the assumption of their being healthy and left the fund when they were better again.[60] The funds did, though, exclude the elderly—those aged 50 to 70—and those who applied to join during an epidemic (or they insured them only on restrictive terms). Risk selection was managed in other ways too. For instance, new members might have to wait between eight days and thirteen weeks before being entitled to benefits. Moral risks were also restricted: "Very many funds provide no help in the case of venereal or syphilitic diseases, unless the patient is younger than fifteen or unless it can be shown that the disease had not been contracted as the result of contributory negligence. This question of contributory negligence is applied in a broader sense, too, and includes being wounded as the result of one's negligence, in a duel, due to wilfulness, a dissolute life, or the abuse of alcohol."[61] The older funds especially had many such restrictions.[62]

The weekly premiums were almost always identical across age groups, with the exception of very young children.[63] As with the burial funds, it was relatively easy, therefore, for the elderly to switch to another fund if they found themselves unable to pay their premiums or if they moved elsewhere, since the new premium would be scarcely any higher than that charged by their existing insurer. On average, each family paid a premium of 15 to 35 cents. In practice, there was some leeway, and the rural doctors' funds in particular might charge less; the alternative in some cases was having no members at all.[64]

The benefits provided by the insurer included reimbursing the costs of consulting a doctor. The costs of minor treatment, medicines, and bandages, for example, were also reimbursed. Maternity care was rarely covered; nor was hospital admission. Many of the risks that health-insurance funds now cover were thus excluded in the nineteenth century. In general, the funds provided only very narrow assistance, restricted to what one might term "ordinary sickness."[65] The duration of that assistance was almost always unrestricted. However, the funds did exclude people who had been sick for too long or too often—perhaps for over two consecutive months or over thirteen weeks in a six-month period.[66] This practice was more common among funds that paid their doctors or pharmacists on a consultation or prescription basis rather than a fixed annual sum per insured, since in the former case a lengthy sickness could prove to be expensive.

How can one explain the existence, let alone the growth, of medical insurance during the nineteenth century, despite the existence of classic insurance problems and the dissolution of guild-based medical insurance in 1820? The mutual funds were the oldest of the funds, dating from the early-modern period, and predating even the medieval guilds. The prime function of the early-modern funds had been to cover loss of income, and that is probably why, at the start of the nineteenth century, the word *ziekenfonds* referred to that type of insurance rather than the medical costs insurance that came to predominate in the twentieth century. This shift in meaning was accompanied by shifts in numbers. Around 1800, four times as many insurers covered loss of income than medical costs; around 1860, the corresponding figures were more or less equal; 30 years later, at the time of the national survey of 1892, the pattern was similar to that in 1800 (Tables 5.9 and 5.12). These shifts can be explained as follows. The main providers of health insurance in 1800 were guilds, whose expertise and concern lay primarily with work rather than medical care. Over the century, medical practitioners too began to offer health insurance as a way to supplement their income, and they were more oriented toward paying the costs of medical care. At the end of the century, however, trade unions became active in the insurance market, and their focus was similar to that of the guilds. These unions had the advantage that their administrative work was carried out largely by unpaid union members—and was thus relatively cheap compared with commercial companies, costing about the same as the mutual funds. But they were also familiar with the labour market and their members. At relatively low cost, they could obtain information on the earnings capacity of a particular claimant, since other union members could be relied on to provide information; after all, these members had to meet the cost of any claims, so they had a stake in keeping costs low.[67] Trade unions therefore had a comparative advantage both when it came to insuring loss of income due to sickness and when it came to providing unemployment insurance. Indeed, they were the only party able to offer such insurance.

The centuries-old tradition in the Netherlands of insuring against loss of income and the cost of medical treatment in the event of sickness survived the abolition of the guilds, from which that tradition emerged. Other occupational mutuals, but also the general, nonoccupational, mutuals set up especially after about 1750, assumed the role previously undertaken by the guilds. Commercial insurers, factory schemes, and doctors' funds developed that tradition further. For both types of health insurance, coverage rose significantly throughout the country. The relative importance of commercial insurers and general practitioners' funds also grew. Average fund size in terms of membership rose for all types of fund, though least in the case of the mutuals. By origin, mutuals were local and often fairly small organizations.

They were able to operate successfully due to their low administrative costs. They had a good knowledge of their local market and were able to monitor their members carefully; they were relatively well placed thus to counter moral risks. They believed that their small size gave them a competitive edge, and with the exception of the problem presented by an ageing membership this was probably true. Commercial insurers—but also the general practitioners' funds—appointed full-time managers, and when innovative forms of communication (i.e., the telephone, tram, and train lines), as well as insurance collectors and agents, reduced the problem of communicating information over long distances, the information gap between the commercial insurers and the mutuals narrowed, while the organizational advantages of upscaling activities continued to benefit the commercial insurers. Gradually, the advantages of the local mutuals in terms of knowledge and costs began to disappear, and economies of scale became increasingly important, especially perhaps at the end of the nineteenth century.

The nineteenth century saw an epidemiological transition in the Netherlands. Epidemic-related mortality gradually declined and yielded to a new pattern of mortality and morbidity, dominated by noninfectious diseases. At the same time, there was a gradual shift in age-related mortality from infants and children to the elderly. This epidemiological transition can be attributed only partly to progress in medical sciences. That there was such progress is not disputed, but for a time it had only a limited effect. Of greater importance for the epidemiological transition were the rise in living conditions from the middle of the century, greater access to clean drinking water, and improved disposal of sewage and household waste. The hygienists were the driving force behind these developments.

Whatever its causes, the epidemiological transition gradually increased the ability of insurers to predict morbidity and mortality and made it easier for them to design schemes to cover these risks. As noted earlier, correlated risks, such as those of epidemics, are a problem for insurers, and the decline of epidemics enabled insurers to cover illnesses better. As a result, many workers were now able to insure themselves with the mutuals, and later with commercial insurers, for the cost of medicines and loss of income. In the nineteenth century, as before, health insurers endeavoured to limit the classic insurance problems of adverse selection and moral risks. Adverse selection was not normally countered by requiring a full medical examination or by making participation compulsory. The first was too expensive, and, given the lack of diagnostic equipment, not entirely useful. The second was vetoed by laissez-faire liberals. With the abolition of the guilds in 1820—as a much criticized mainstay of the corporatist republic—compulsory guild membership and the guild funds were also swept away. It was not until the end of the nineteenth century that support began cautiously to be voiced for a compulsory, this time national, health-insurance scheme, one that really only began to take shape during the following century.[68] Adverse selection was in fact often countered by requiring a superficial medical examination (applicants appearing to be critically ill were not accepted), by setting age limits (because morbidity risks among the elderly were relatively high), and by paying benefits only to those who had been members for a minimum period. More importantly, the maximum benefit-duration period was restricted to thirteen weeks, after which the insurer was no longer liable to pay for the chronically sick—including those who had failed to disclose an illness on joining. Moral risks were countered through doctors and work colleagues, who, it was felt, could be relied on to identify malingerers and by refusing to pay benefits in cases where the applicant was culpable. The costs of treating an accident arising from drunkenness were not therefore normally reimbursed; nor were the costs of treating venereal disease. Furthermore, there was a Karenztijd of around one week, during which no benefits were payable.

These strategies were insufficient to prevent some funds going bankrupt. These bankruptcies resulted from premiums being set too low and inadequate reserves being built up. There was also the problem of correlated risks: an epidemic could easily hit so many fund members that the fund went bankrupt. In the nineteenth century, insurers probably tried to mitigate this problem in the same way as their predecessors during the Dutch Republic: by increasing premiums and cutting benefits.

The maritime provinces of Noord and Zuid Holland in the west of the country had the most funds. Drenthe, Limburg, and Zeeland had the fewest. This geographical pattern was evident as early as 1795 but can actually be dated to 1700 and even to 1600. It was a continuation of a phenomenon seen not only during the Dutch Republic but also in medieval times, and it survived right up until the very end of the nineteenth century. One should not assume that it reflected the development of medical poor relief, with those provinces offering better medical poor relief having fewer health-insurance funds. Indeed, the reverse was probably the case: in Holland's cities poor relief was also well developed. A number of more convincing factors have been adduced to explain this pattern and its survival over time. They include the relative prosperity of Holland and its comparatively high degree of urbanization (which set it apart from other Dutch provinces). These fostered a modern occupational structure and the expansion of guilds—an important development since, in the Netherlands, health insurance originated with the guilds. These same factors explain why a geographical pattern rooted in medieval times continued for several centuries. Furthermore, over time the existence of funds itself became a factor perpetuating this geographical pattern, since it was easier for a well-established and reputable fund to continue than it was for a new (and thus unfamiliar) fund to become established and successful. It is remarkable that this medieval legacy continued to influence the dissemination of health insurance in the Netherlands for centuries.

MEDICAL POOR RELIEF

Poor relief in the Netherlands was organized at the local level by both the church and the municipality, and—unlike the situation in England and Wales—there was no central supervisory authority.[69] Dutch poor-relief agencies helped those who were ill or infirm with food, fuel, and funds. They saw to it that doctors treated the sick and paid for certain medicines, including nutrients such as milk, eggs, and bouillon. From 1830 onward there was even a volume containing standard recipes for poor patients: the *Pharmaco-poea Pauperum*. Some organizations employed a doctor or an apothecary. Others paid the costs of a visit or had a contract under which they paid a small fee per pauper per year in advance. Some gave money directly to a sick pauper so that he or she could pay these costs, wholly or in part. In rare cases, poor-relief agencies supplied the doctor with a list of those in receipt of relief who were ill, so that the doctor could decide to charge them less at his own expense. Poor-relief agencies sometimes encouraged recipients to join a mutual insurance scheme while they were healthy and offered to pay part of the premium.

As medical poor relief was organized in such a kaleidoscopic way, it is not easy to generalize about how many individuals were assisted. It was certainly a significant proportion of the population. In the southern city of Maastricht, for example, during the nineteenth century between a fifth and a third of the population were helped in this way. Health-insurance and factory schemes helped just a few per cent.[70] Although the new Poor Law of 1854 reaffirmed the municipality's role as one of last resort (if the church failed to help), church-based relief was already on the retreat. As time went by, municipal relief helped increasing numbers (including the sick and the infirm). Even around the middle of the century, in half to two-thirds of cases it was the municipalities, not the church, that appeared to be helping.[71] Over the years, this proportion grew, and, first in the major cities and later in the smaller ones too, ecclesiastical agencies withdrew altogether. At the end of the century, medical poor relief was the preserve almost wholly of municipal poor-relief agencies. They in turn transferred the sick to the new municipal health service, the Gemeentelijke Geneeskundige Diensten.

In the development of schemes to counter the risks of life, death, and work, the nineteenth century built on the legacy of the Dutch Republic. While one legacy of the republic, the health-insurance funds, expanded and innovated, another legacy, medical poor relief, stagnated, as did poor relief in general. During the nineteenth century, an increasing proportion of the Dutch population began to take out insurance against sickness, a response to a rise in living standards, as a result of which increasing numbers could afford such insurance. The insured tended to belong to the middle classes. They earned too little to pay doctors' fees or to cover loss of earnings during sickness from their savings, but they also earned too much to be eligible for poor relief.

CONCLUSION AND DEBATE

Having discussed the world of insurance in the nineteenth century according to type of insurance (life, health, and work), we can now draw some general observations and return to the questions posed at the start.

What proportion of the population was covered, and how did this coverage evolve over time? As Table 5.14 makes clear, coverage varied widely at the beginning of the nineteenth century, and these variations increased over the next 100 years: some types of insurance grew rapidly; other did not. The growth in burial insurances (initially covering just a few per cent, later covering over half the population) is remarkable. So even before the Industrial Accidents Act of 1901, a majority of the Dutch population had become accustomed to paying a small, periodic premium for social welfare. Of the two types of health insurance, insurance against loss of income was the most popular around 1800; less so around 1890. Both types expanded, but insurance to cover medical costs expanded more rapidly. Insurers paid the doctors' bills of one in six Dutchmen around 1890 and compensated one in twelve workers for loss of earnings. Medical heath insurance continued to grow. National legislation in 1941 making health insurance compulsory did not in fact raise rates of coverage much: a similar proportion of the population were already insured under voluntary schemes. It is important to note

Table 5.14 Percentage of the Population Insured Against Various Risks in the Netherlands, 1800–1890

	Burial	Medical Costs	Loss of Income When Ill	Widowhood	Old Age	Unemployment
1800	3–6	0–1	1–3	0–1	0–1	0
1810	3–7	1	1–3	0–1	0–1	0
1820	8–11	1–2	2–3	0–1	0–1	0
1830	14–17	3–4	2–4	0–2	0–1	0
1840	19–21	5–6	3–4	0–1	0–1	0
1850	26–28	7–8	3–4	0–1	0–1	0
1860	30–31	7–8	3–4	0–1	0–1	0
1870	36–37	9	4–5	0–1	0–1	0
1880	43–44	11–12	6–7	0–1	0–1	0
1890	53	15–16	8–9	0–1	0–1	0

Source: See previous tables.

that our coverage rates for burial and health insurance are national averages. In some regions—notably the west of the country and in cities, and *a fortiori* in cities in the west—coverage was higher than the national average. Elsewhere it was lower. The same was true of the other types of insurance listed in the table (old age, widowhood, and unemployment), though in all three cases the national average was so low as to be barely detectable.

Why did the insurance market grow? One factor was the growth in the standard of living after the middle of the nineteenth century, which allowed many more men and women to take out insurance against the most common risks of life. At the same time, poor relief—in a sense an alternative form of protection against those risks—became less attractive. Poor relief had just about managed to avoid collapse during the difficult times around 1800, but the allowances granted after that period never equalled those prior to 1800. Another factor was the long tradition of mutual insurance—an institutional heritage of the Dutch Republic. Experience and trust can accumulate over time: joining a new insurance scheme might seem less attractive than joining an existing one. Remarkably, the dissolution of the guilds' mutual funds in 1820 did not create a discontinuity: mutual organizations continued under new names, and probably with many of the same members, administrators, and procedures as before; in a sense they perpetuated an age-old mutual tradition. Mutual insurers had much experience in administering burial and health insurance and even widowhood and old-age insurance. There were techniques in operation to combat adverse selection and moral hazards. A little luck also contributed to the success of insuring a large part of the population against common risks. The rise in life expectancy meant that even though (or perhaps because) burial insurers did not calculate premiums in an actuarially sound way, using life tables, their revenues were higher than expected—in many cases more than necessary to pay the costs of burying their clients.

What factors explain the variation in coverage risks? Surely, one prime factor explaining why burial insurance was so popular and pension schemes were not was the price. Burial insurance was relatively cheap. Everyone faced having to be buried, while many people could afford the premium. Not everyone would survive to old age, and premiums for an old-age pension were simply unaffordable for many. The classic insurance problems of moral hazards and adverse selection played a part in raising premiums for certain types of insurance to high levels. These problems were either of little significance or nonexistent, in the case of burial insurance, and of much greater significance for unemployment and health insurance. There was also the problem of correlated risks associated with both unemployment and illness, though in the case of illness the degree of correlation declined over time due to the epidemiological transition. There was the institutional heritage of the Dutch Republic too. Guilds were the prime providers of health insurance at the beginning of the century. They were work-based and their primary concern was in compensating loss of income among their sick members, and this was where their expertise lay. Even before the dissolution of the guilds, from the mid-eighteenth century onward, other insurers entered the market for health insurance. Many more did so in the course of the nineteenth century, including funds operated by doctors. Their primary concern was to cover the costs of medical treatment, and this was where their particular expertise lay. It was only at the end of the nineteenth century that trade-union insurers entered the market, and they were perhaps better equipped to deal with the problem of loss of earnings than the problem of paying doctors' bills.

How was the market divided between mutual and private insurers, and how did this division evolve over time? This is a difficult question to answer because our data cover only the number of funds by type, and we have no precise figures on the average membership of mutual and private insurers. Nonetheless, it seems safe to say that commercial insurers acquired an increasing share of the market. The number of private insurers grew more rapidly than the number of mutual insurers, at least until the final decades of the century, and some private insurers became very large at the end of the century. As a percentage of all funds, the private insurers continued to grow until at least the 1870s. They subsequently lost ground—in terms of numbers of funds, though not *per se* in terms of membership—to trade-union funds as well as to doctors' funds, some of which can be considered private, though most were nonprofit. Although it is difficult to be precise, it seems likely that private insurance was expanding throughout most of the century. This was due perhaps to the fact that as the century progressed it became easier for commercial insurers to profit from economies of scale: they were able to offer insurance to large numbers, fairly cheaply, without suffering a concomitant loss of control. Covering a large part of the country had previously meant relatively high administrative costs, a loss of power both to combat moral hazards and adverse selection among clients, and limit fraud among employees. Improvements in transport, communication, administration, and medical tests may have opened up larger markets.

Mutual aid reached its zenith in the Netherlands in the nineteenth century—almost five centuries after it originated in the medieval guilds. By then, half of the total population had become accustomed to the savings regime of the burial societies, in which mutual insurance played such a prominent role. This self-imposed discipline of saving for a better future not only provided some protection against the vicissitudes of life; in mitigating dependence on others for assistance, it also boosted the self-esteem of a multitude of workers. Although private insurance did cover part of the market, and possibly an ever-increasing part, there were many signs suggesting that mutual aid was the road to human progress. And these signs were visible all over the world.

It is perhaps hardly surprising then that the Russian anarchist Prince Kropotkin saw mutual aid as a factor in human evolution. With special reference to the situation in the Netherlands, he wrote:

The mutual-aid tendency in man has so remote an origin, and is so deeply interwoven with all the past evolution of the human race, that it has been maintained by mankind up to the present time, notwithstanding all vicissitudes of history. . . . All these associations, societies, brotherhoods, alliances, institutes and so on, which must now be counted by the ten thousand in Europe alone, and each of which represents an immense amount of voluntary, unambitious, and unpaid or underpaid work—what are they but so many manifestations, under an infinite variety of aspects, of the same ever-living tendency of man towards mutual aid and support? . . . In the practice of mutual aid, which we can retrace to the earliest beginnings of evolution, we thus find the positive and undoubted origin of our ethical conceptions; and we can affirm that in the ethical progress of man, mutual support—not mutual struggle—has had the leading part. In its wide extension, even at the present time, we also see the best guarantee of a still loftier evolution of our race.[72]

So it seemed to many at the time, and it continued, perhaps, to seem like that during the first few decades of the twentieth century. Had Kropotkin (1842–1921) lived longer, he would have been disappointed. Not because the First World War shattered his belief in mutual support—and not struggle—as a constant in human history. Strangely, it did not. But because mutual insurance against life's risks was, in many countries, ousted by private insurance and compulsory state insurance. The rise of state insurance, however, is a different story.[73]

NOTES

1. This article has benefited from research at the International Institute of Social History in Amsterdam on the history of mutual aid, and in particular from data on the number of insurers between the sixteenth and twentieth centuries collated as part of that research. Some of the earliest results were published in J. van Gerwen and J. Lucassen, "Mutual societies in the Netherlands from the sixteenth century to the present," in M. van der Linden, ed., *Social security mutualism: The comparative history of mutual benefit societies* (Berne: Peter Lang, 1996), pp. 431–79. Comprehensive data on the number of insurers by type is presented in J. van Genabeek, *Met vereende kracht risico's verzacht. De plaats van onderlinge hulp binnen de negentiende eeuwse particuliere regelingen van sociale zekerheid* (Amsterdam: Internationaal Instituut voor Sociale Geschiedenis, 1999). For my study of the history of risks in the Netherlands during the nineteenth century I used van Genabeek's data to estimate the proportion of the population insured: M. H. D. van Leeuwen, *De eenheidsstaat. Onderlinges, armenzorg en commerciële verzekeraars 1800–1890* (vol. 2 of *Zoeken naar zekerheid. Risico's, preventie, verzekeringen en andere zekerheidsregelingen in Nederland 1500–2000* [Amsterdam: NEHA/Verbond van verzekeraars, 2000]). In reworking material from my book for this article, I have tried to add observations of a more general nature while omitting some of the particular or technical details included in the notes to the book.

2. See, for example, the essays in van der Linden, *Social security mutualism*, covering Europe, the Americas, and Asia over the past two centuries; A. de Swaan, *In care of the state: Health care, education and welfare in Europe and the USA in the modern era* (New York: OUP, 1988); A. de Swaan and M. van der Linden, eds., *Mutualist microfinance: Informal savings funds from the global periphery to the core?* (Amsterdam: Aksant, 2006); S. B. Bacharach, P. A. Bamberger, and W. J. Sonnenstuhl, *Mutual aid and urban renewal: Cycles of logics of action* (Ithaca and London: Cornell University Press, 2001); D. T. Beito, *From mutual aid to the welfare state: Fraternal societies and social services, 1890–1967* (Chapel Hill and London: The University of North Carolina Press, 2000); G. Emery and J. C. Herbert Emery, *A young man's benefit: The Independent Order of Odd Fellows and sickness insurance in the United States and Canada, 1860–1929* (Montreal: McGill-Queen's University Press, 1999); D. G. Green and L. G. Cromwell, *Mutual aid or welfare state: Australia's Friendly Societies* (Boston: Allen and Unwin, 1984); M. D. Sibalis, "The mutual aid societies of Paris, 1789–1848," *French History*, 3 (1989), 1–30.

3. With some notable exceptions. See H. Emery, "Fraternal sickness insurance," *EH-net encyclopedia*, March 2006; M. Hechter, *Principles of group solidarity* (Berkeley: University of California Press, 1987), ch. 6; M. van der Linden, "Introduction," in van der Linden, Social security mutualism; idem, "Varieties of mutualism," in de Swaan and van der Linden, *Mutualist microfinance*, ch. 7; L. Siddeley, "The rise and fall of fraternal insurance organizations," *Humane Studies Review*, 7 (1992); as well as M. H. D. van Leeuwen, "Trade unions and the provision of welfare in the Netherlands 1910–1960," *Economic History Review*, 50 (1997), 764–791.

4. On guild insurance and welfare, see S. Bos, *"Uyt liefde tot malcander." Onderlinge hulpfondsen binnen de Noord-Nederlandse gilden in international perspectief* (Amsterdam: Internationaal Instituut voor Sociale Geschiedenis, 1998); idem, "Beroepsgebonden onderlinges 1500–1800: Gilden- en knechtsfondsen," in J. van Gerwen and M. H. D. van Leeuwen, eds., *Studies over zekerheidsarrangementen. Risico's, risicobestrijding en verzekeringen in Nederland vanaf de Middeleeuwen* (Amsterdam: Internationaal Instituut voor Sociale Geschiedenis, 1998), pp. 91–140; S. Bos and I. Stamhuis, "Begrafenis- en weduwenfondsen en prebende sociëteiten," ibid., pp. 175–182; M. H. D. van Leeuwen, *De rijke Republiek. Gilden, Assuradeurs en armenzorg 1500–1800* (vol. 1 of *Zoeken naar zekerheid. Risico's, preventie, verzekeringen en andere zekerheidsregelingen in Nederland 1500–2000* [Amsterdam: NEHA/Verbond van verzekeraars, 2000]).

5. On trade union insurance, see van Leeuwen, "Trade unions," pp. 764–91.

6. The economic literature on insurance, and the problems associated with it, is abundant. Some of the classic articles by K. J. Arrow have been reprinted in K. J. Arrow, *Essays in the theory of risk-bearing* (Amsterdam and London: North-Holland Publishing Company, 1970). On moral hazards, adverse selection, correlated risks, and the notion of coinsurance to combat these problems, see especially Chapters 5 ("Insurance, risk and resource allocation"), 6 ("Economic welfare and the allocation of resources for invention"), and 8 ("Uncertainty and the welfare economics of medical care"). On moral hazards, see also C. A. Heimer, *Reactive risk and rational action: Managing moral hazard in insurance contracts* (Berkeley: University of California Press, 1985); on adverse selection, see G. A. Akerlof, "The market for 'lemons': Qualitative uncertainty and the market mechanisms," *Quarterly Journal of Economics*, 84 (1970), 488–500. Historical studies on moral hazards and adverse selection include Siddeley, "The rise and fall"; van Leeuwen, "Trade unions"; and H. R. Southall, "Neither state nor market: Early welfare benefits in Britain," in B.

Palier, ed., *Comparing social welfare systems in Europe: Vol. 1. The Oxford conference* (Paris: MIRE, 1995), pp. 59–92. Historical studies on risk and social insurance include P. Johnson, "Risk, redistribution and social welfare from the poor law to Beveridge," in M. Daunton, ed., *Charity, self-interest and welfare in the English past* (London: UCL Press, 1996), pp. 225–248; and M. H. D. van Leeuwen, "Histories of risk and welfare in Europe during the 18th and 19th centuries," in O. P. Grell, A. Cunningham, and R. Jütte, eds., *Health care and poor relief in 18th and 19th century Northern Europe* (Aldershot, UK: Ashgate, 2002), pp. 32–66. Sociological works on insurance and solidarity include Hechter, *Principles of group solidarity*, ch. 6, and the studies by van der Linden and de Swaan mentioned in note 2.

7. Dependency and visibility are stressed by M. Hechter and S. Kanazawa, "Group solidarity and social order in Japan," *Journal of Theoretical Politics*, 5 (1993), 455–93, especially pp. 460–61.

8. For further information on how the estimates of the number of insured in Table 1 have been calculated, see van Leeuwen, *De eenheidsstaat*, 404 (note 53) and 409–10 (note 114). For the estimates in Table 2, it has been assumed that factory schemes had no members in 1810, in 1860 a quarter of the number they had in 1888–1890, while the number of insured in other years has been calculated using linear interpolation.

9. Van Genabeek, *Met vereende kracht*, pp. 221–36; H. Smissaert, *Voorzieningen bij ziekte van werklieden in 96 ondernemingen* (The Hague: Mouton, 1902), p. x.

10. J. H. de Wildt, "Wachtgeldregelingen in het particuliere bedrijfsleven in de eerste helft van de twintigste eeuw," *Sociaal Maandblad*, 41 (1986), 452–68.

11. The results were not straightforward due to both over- and underregistration. Tables 5.1 and 5.2 contain the corrected results, see Van Leeuwen, *De eenheidsstaat*, pp. 410–11 note 116.

12. On company pension funds, see J. van Genabeek, "Collectieve pensioenregelingen 1800–2000," in van Gerwen and van Leeuwen, *Studies over zekerheidsarrangementen*, pp. 883–905.

13. For further information on how the estimates have been calculated, see van Leeuwen, *De eenheidsstaat*, pp. 81 and 404–05 (note 57), where an explanation is given of how the total number of has been derived. The average number of insured per fund in 1810 is assumed to have been between 250 and 500. The average number of insured between 1810 and 1890 has been calculated using linear interpolation.

14. W. L. P. A. Molengraaff, *De begrafenisfondsen in Nederland: Rapport uitgebracht door de commissie van onderzoek van de Maatschappij tot Nut van 't Algemeen* (n.p., 1891), p. 133. This detailed report contains some of the information referred to later in our text. See also van Leeuwen, *De eenheidsstaat*, p. 89, and van Genabeek, *Met vereende kracht*. B. P. A. Gales, "L'assurance de la vie populaire aux Pays Bas," *Risques*, 31 (1997), 57–71, estimates that total expenditure by burial funds on allowances for burials was much higher than that by poor-relief agencies.

15. In principle at least, there is too little information to judge how this worked in practice in the Netherlands.

16. Van Genabeek, *Met vereende kracht*, pp. 205–07.

17. J. L. J. M. van Gerwen, "De levensverzekeringsbranche in de negentiende eeuw," in van Gerwen and van Leeuwen, *Studies over zekerheidsarrangementen*, pp. 371–402, especially pp. 378–81.

18. Molengraaff, *De begrafenisfondsen in Nederland*, p. 90. Such lack of information implies that not all insured will have chosen funds that indeed were reliable or had a lower premium.

128 *van Leeuwen*

19. Molengraaff, *De begrafenisfondsen in Nederland*, p. 90.
20. Ibid., pp. 31, 35, and 157; van Gerwen, "De levensverzekeringsbranche," p. 385.
21. B. P. A. Gales, *Tot de dood ons scheidt* (Groningen: Instituut voor Economisch Onderzoek, 1992), p. 11.
22. Molengraaff, *De begrafenisfondsen in Nederland*, pp. 51–2, see also p. 165.
23. J. van Genabeek, "Onderlinges 1800–1890," in van Gerwen and van Leeuwen, pp. 317–48, especially p. 341.
24. Gales, *Tot de dood ons scheidt*, pp. 2–3 and 15.
25. Molengraaff, *De begrafenisfondsen in Nederland*, pp. 104 and 105.
26. Ibid., pp. 86 and 87.
27. J. B. J. Bollerman and J. N. J. Broenink, *Het begrafenisfonds "Let op Uw Einde" 1847–1893* (Leiden: Nijhoff, 1983).
28. K. Horstman, *Public bodies, private lives: The historical construction of life insurance, health risks, and citizenship in the Netherlands 1880–1920* (Rotterdam: Erasmus Publishing, 2001), ch. 2.
29. The problem of establishing who the owner was occurred more generally in the life-insurance business in the nineteenth century. See van Gerwen, "De levensverzekeringsbranche," p. 384; Gales, *Tot de dood ons scheidt*, pp. 22–25.
30. The number of insured, excluding factory schemes, has been estimated by multiplying the number of funds in the table by an assumed average number of insured per fund of 250, which, if anything, might be rather high. The number insured by factory schemes has been estimated using the 1888–1890 survey of factory schemes, in the same manner as we did earlier for burial insurance.
31. Van Leeuwen, *De eenheidsstaat*, pp. 97–99.
32. The number of insured, excluding factory schemes, has been estimated by multiplying the number of funds in the table by an assumed average number of insured per fund of 800, which, if anything, might be rather high. The number insured by factory schemes has been estimated using the 1888–1890 survey of factory schemes, in the same manner as we did earlier for burial insurance.
33. B. P. A. Gales, "Ontstaan en ontwikkeling van het levensverzekeringsbedrijf tot 1914," in B. P. A. Gales and J. L. J. M. van Gerwen, *Sporen van leven en schade: Een geschiedenis en bronnenoverzicht van het Nederlandse verzekeringswezen* (Amsterdam: NEHA, 1998), pp. 9–38; the quotation is taken from p. 15. The government adviser in question was Rehuel Lobatto (1797–1866). For more information on Lobatto, see van Leeuwen, *De eenheidsstaat*, pp. 104–05.
34. Van Genabeek, *Met vereende kracht*, 204.
35. The number of insured has been estimated by multiplying the number of funds in the table by an assumed average number of insured per fund of 500. For more details, see van Leeuwen, *De eenheidsstaat*, p. 413 (notes 58 and 59).
36. Van Genabeek, *Met vereende kracht*, pp. 139–40.
37. Van Leeuwen, "Trade Unions"; van Genabeek, *Met vereende kracht*, pp. 135 and 157. See van Leeuwen, *De eenheidsstaat*, pp. 188–219, especially p. 199, for a discussion of seasonal underemployment in certain sectors of the economy.
38. W. Stoeder et al., *De ziekenfondsen in Nederland: Rapport uitgebracht door eene commissie van onderzoek van de Maatschappij tot Nut van 't Algemeen* (Amsterdam: Maatschappij tot Nut van 't Algemeen, 1895), p.103. The next general survey, in 1908, used *ziekenfonds* only in the modern sense of the word. See C. F. Schreve et al., *Rapport van de Nederlandsche Maatschappij [tot bevordering der Geneeskunst] omtrent den toestand der ziekenfondsen*

in Nederland. Deel 2. Algemene beschouwingen (Amsterdam: Nederlandsche Maatschappij tot bevordering der Geneeskunst, 1908), p. 84 passim.

39. Briefly, the following procedure was adopted to produce the estimates given in Table 5.10. Data on the number of funds per decade were available from van Genabeek, *Met vereende kracht*. Multiplying those figures by the average number insured yields total numbers insured per decade. But how does one calculate this average? The total number of insured in 1911 as reported in surveys was corrected for underregistration. This yields a figure of 639,000 insured in 1911. The average number of insured per fund could then be calculated for 1911. For previous years it had to be estimated. We assumed an average of 150–300 insured per fund in 1800 and 1810 and interpolated linearly for the period after 1810 and before 1911. One complication is that the number of factory schemes is known for 1890 and 1911 but not for earlier years. For 1900, we used the average of the figures for 1890 and 1911. We also assumed that the figure for 1860 was a quarter of that for 1911 and that there were no factory schemes in 1810. The number of factory schemes in the intervening years was estimated using linear interpolation. See van Leeuwen, *De Eenheidsstaat*, p. 410 (note 115), for more details.

40. For a critical discussion of the sources see ibid., p. 410 (note 116).

41. Stoeder, *De ziekenfondsen in Nederland*, p. 28.

42. Ibid., p. 29.

43. Ibid., pp. 54 and 85.

44. Ibid., p. 55.

45. Ibid., p. 55.

46. Van Genabeek, *Met vereende kracht*, pp. 101 and 177.

47. Ibid., p. 55.

48. Ibid., p. 85.

49. Ibid., p. 90.

50. "As a general rule, the fund pays 3 guilders a week; but if its capital falls to less than 1200 guilders this is reduced to 2 guilders, and to as little as 1 guilder if the fund's capital is less than 300 guilders; another fund suspends payments completely if its capital is less than 1000 guilders; in this case an appeal is made to members on behalf of the sick." Ibid., pp. 30–31.

51. Ibid., p. 31.

52. Ibid., p. 29.

53. Ibid., p. 31.

54. Van Genabeek, *Met vereende kracht*, pp. 139, 157, and 177. For the early twentieth century, see the 1911 survey: Directie van den Arbeid, *Onderzoek naar de in Nederland bestaande fondsen tot ondersteuning van arbeiders bij ziekte* (The Hague: Trio, 1912). For 1910, there are also detailed data on socialist trade unions. See van Leeuwen, "Trade unions," p. 772. These unions required one to have been a member for at least 32 weeks before one became eligible for sickness benefit. The level of benefit was set at 4 guilders a week, the equivalent perhaps of 38 per cent of the average labourer's wage. After a year or more, members became eligible for sickness benefit for up to 69 days.

55. Stoeder, *De ziekenfondsen in Nederland*, p. 33.

56. Data on the number of funds (excluding factory schemes) per decade were available from van Genabeek, *Met vereende kracht*. The number of factory schemes in 1901 is known. The number for previous years was estimated by assuming that the figure for 1860 was a quarter of that in 1901 and that there were no factory schemes in 1810. The number of factory schemes in the intervening years was estimated using linear interpolation. Once the total number of funds, including factory schemes, is known, the total number of insured can be calculated by multiplying the number of funds by the average number of

insured per fund. This average is known for 1901. We assumed an average of 150–300 insured per fund in 1800 and 1810 and interpolated linearly for the period after 1810 and before 1901.

57. See, for example, ibid., pp. 175–91; K. P. Companje, *Over artsen en verzekeraars: Een historische studie naar de factoren die de relatie ziekenfondsenartsen vanaf 1827 op landelijk en regionaal niveau hebben beïnvloed* (Utrecht, 1997); Henk van der Velden, *Financiële toegankelijkheid tot de gezondheidszorg in Nederland, 1850–1941* (Amsterdam: Stichting Beheer IISG, 1993); B. Widdershoven, *Het dilemma van solidariteit: De Nederlandse onderlinge ziekenfondsen, 1890–1941* (Amsterdam: Aksant, 2005).

58. Van Genabeek, *Met vereende kracht*, pp. 185–90; similar schemes existed before then in Dordrecht (1845), Nijmegen (1844), Schiedam (1819), Vlaardingen (1845), and Zierikzee (1840).

59. Stoeder, *De ziekenfondsen in Nederland*, p. 14.

60. Ibid., pp. 15, 17, and 25; see also Schreve, *Rapport*, p. 27.

61. Stoeder, *De ziekenfondsen in Nederland*, p. 25.

62. Schreve, *Rapport*, p. 37.

63. Stoeder, *De ziekenfondsen in Nederland*, pp. 15–17.

64. Ibid., p. 17.

65. Ibid., pp. 22–24; Schreve, *Rapport*, p. 36.

66. Stoeder, *De ziekenfondsen in Nederland*, p. 26.

67. Van Leeuwen, "Trade unions."

68. Exceptions to this were the compulsory factory schemes and company pension schemes, including those for government employees.

69. See, M. H. D. van Leeuwen, "Armenzorg 1800–1912: Erfenis van de Republiek," pp. 276–316, in J. van Gerwen and M. H. D. van Leeuwen, eds., *Studies over zekerheidsarrangementen: Risico's, risicobestrijding en verzekering in Nederland vanaf de Middeleeuwen* (Amsterdam: NEHA).

70. B. P. A. Gales, *Het Burgerlijk Armbestuur: Twee eeuwen zorg voor armen, zieken en ouderen te Maastricht 1796–1996* (Maastricht: Stichting Historische Reeks Maastricht, 1997), p. 272.

71. Van der Velden, *Financiële toegankelijkheid*, pp. 33, 35, and 55.

72. P. Kropotkin, *Mutual aid: A factor of evolution*, edited with an introduction by P. Avrich (New York: New York University Press, 1972), quotations on pp. 194, 237, and 251.

73. For a general discussion, see van der Linden, "Introduction," pp. 11–40, especially pp. 34–38, and de Swaan, *In care of the state*. On the demise of trade-union insurance in the Netherlands, see van Leeuwen, "Trade unions," pp. 764–91, especially pp. 784–85. For other countries, see Beito, *From mutual aid to the welfare state*; W. Beveridge, *Voluntary action: A report on methods of social advance* (London: George Allen & Unwin, 1948); Green and Cromwell, *Mutual aid or welfare state*; B. B. Gilbert, "The decay of nineteenth-century provident institutions and the coming of old age pensions in Great Britain," *Economic History Review*, 17 (1965), 551–63; B. B. Gilbert, *The evolution of national health insurance in Great Britain: The origins of the welfare state* (London: Michael Joseph, 1966); D. Green, *Working class patients and the medical establishment* (New York: St Martin's Press, 1985).

6   Welfare-State Formation in Scandinavia

The Political Significance of Third-Sector Organisations for the Emergence of Sickness-Insurance Programs in Norway and Sweden

Peter Johansson

Institute for Futures Studies

How and why did different countries organise programs of cash support for people who were unable to work at the turn of the last century? In this chapter, I focus on Norway and Sweden where the so-called Workers' Question began to attract attention in the early 1880s.[1] By that time, the Workers' Question was established on the political agenda, and parliaments in both countries decided to appoint public inquiry commissions in order to investigate possible social-policy initiatives. By the beginning of the 1890s, the commissions had presented proposals for sickness-insurance legislation. However, the two proposals differed widely. In line with the German sickness-insurance law, the Norwegian commission suggested mandatory insurance for the working class, while the Swedish commission suggested a voluntary sickness-insurance program financed through state subsidies to existing sickness and burial funds.[2] The proposal presented by the Swedish commission was discussed in the Parliament in 1891, and, in the same year, a law on voluntary sickness insurance was enacted in Sweden. In contrast to Norway, the question was solved in a unanimous spirit. In Norway, the proposals made for mandatory class-based sickness insurance caused severe political conflict in 1897, and no insurance legislation was to be enacted until 1909.

The parallel developments in Norway and Sweden raise questions on why the two Nordic countries chose different solutions to what was in essence a common problem. Why did the Norwegian commission propose mandatory sickness insurance while the Swedish commission proposed a voluntary state-subsidised sickness-insurance program? What caused the acrimonious political debate in Norway, where a law could not be agreed upon until 1909—16 years after the first proposal—while the Swedish proposal could be enacted in substantial multiparty agreement already in 1891? What were the preconditions for a quick and "smooth" enactment of a first law on sickness insurance? Through these subsidiary questions, I want to investigate the emergence of the Swedish and Norwegian sickness-insurance programs with respect to the importance of "third sector organisations."

PERSPECTIVES AND HYPOTHESES

These questions, concerning the emergence of sickness-insurance programs in Sweden and in Norway, can also be asked with reference to a more comprehensive complex of problems on why states engaged in social policy and why and how social policy programs have emerged in different institutional shape and at different times.[3]

Questions on the timing and character of first social-insurance legislation have been discussed from a multitude of perspectives. In contrast to scholars who have emphasised the "logic of industry" or "processes of modernity" as underlying first social laws, research within a power-resource perspective has put forward political power relationships in society as crucial for the understanding of welfare-state development. The critical remarks addressed by these scholars especially concern the convergence hypothesis and the study of welfare-state expansion in terms of social expenditure. Studies from a power-resource perspective usually emphasise and analyse the diverging patterns of welfare states in the Western world.[4] Further, from this perspective the working-class organisations are held to be crucial in bringing about the welfare state, and first social policy initiatives are perceived as a response to a potential "threat" from the organised working class.[5]

Also, the role of the farmers and the middle class has been emphasised in analyses of the emerging welfare state. It has been claimed, in particular for Scandinavia, that farmers have played a crucial role for the design of social-insurance programs, being the major advocates for encompassing models. With respect to this perspective, farmers are treated as a specific-risk category rather than as a social class, whose support to establish encompassing programs is interpreted against the backdrop of their risks as well as their ability to counter these risks by their own means.[6] However, other scholars have questioned whether this also means that farmers actually have been a driving force actively bringing about social policy along such lines.[7] And, as has been pointed out by several scholars, the emergence of welfare states also can be perceived as a kind of state-building process. With reference to this ambition to "bring the state back in" into policy analyses, the organisational and institutional aspects of the emergence of social-policy programs have been emphasised. The design and timing of emergent welfare-state programs here also become questions concerning states' divergent capabilities to produce or reorganise administrative capacity.[8]

In this chapter, the interaction of political-power relationships in parliament and states' capability to engage administrative capacity are held to matter for the development of the first sickness-insurance programs. It is first suggested that the emergent Workers' Question in both Norway and Sweden—however important for the development of social-policy initiatives in both countries—did not crucially depend on the rise of a domestic organised working class. In the shadow of contemporary developments in Europe, especially in Germany, the major motive for social-policy initiatives among political elites in Norway and Sweden was to anticipate and prevent a potential threat from the organised working class, which was envisioned to emerge with the approaching industrialisation. The threat, so to speak, did not come from the still poorly organised working class in Scandinavia but from central Europe and from "the future" that seemed to be dawning there.

However, the fact that the contemporary political elite found it important to do something in order to avoid the societal unrest they expected to emerge in the wake of the ongoing industrialisation did not in itself imply a specific design of sickness-insurance programs. In order to account for the different paths taken by the two countries, and to develop an argument concerning the political significance of third-sector organisations for welfare-state formulation in Scandinavia, the Swedish and Norwegian states' differing ability to enact a voluntary sickness-insurance program is emphasised. From this angle, both the different choices made and the early, and smooth, enactment of a sickness-insurance law in Sweden is accounted for by reference to these states' diverging preconditions of addressing the Workers' Question by the potential means of creating a voluntary state-subsidised welfare. It is here suggested that third-sector organisations had political significance in at least two ways: with respect to their prevalence and to their organisational character.[9]

While the Norwegian "third-sector" capacity for administering welfare was not as developed, Sweden had the potential means. This provided Swedish politicians with the option to introduce a voluntary sickness-insurance program. Against the backdrop of the political conflict concerning social-policy initiatives at that time, this opportunity is here held to account for why a sickness-insurance program could be accepted without political strife in Sweden. But equally important was the character of the funds, and it is here argued that their smallness and local orientation suited major political interests to prevent the building of a highly risk-redistributive sickness-insurance program.

Theoretical questions on the nature of the relationship between civil society and the state will not be of major interest in this chapter. Rather, the purpose is to present and discuss empirical evidence, suggesting that the differing development of sickness and burial funds mattered for both the timing and the character of the emergence of sickness-insurance programs in the two countries. However, the two cases of Norway and Sweden also seem to illustrate what the American political scientist Lester M. Salamon has termed "third party government" and "voluntary failure." The two concepts are central to his attempt to formulate a theory on the relationship between governments and nonprofit organisations, suggesting that a focus on the cooperation between the two is of great importance for the understanding of the development of third-sector organisations.[10]

In line with his argument, the Norwegian case might be interpreted in terms of "voluntary failure," where the state had to take on greater responsibilities for the enactment of a nationwide sickness-insurance scheme due to the less-developed sickness and burial funds. However, this study also provides evidence that the weakness of the voluntary sector in Norway made it more difficult to implement a state scheme because of the absence of an existing voluntary infrastructure on which to base it. The need for the state to take on greater responsibilities in Norway was a source of the political conflict that delayed the enactment of a sickness-insurance scheme. In contrast, the Swedish case rather illustrates "third party government," where the reform of 1891 can be said to exemplify how governments can make use of already existing third-sector organisations in order to implement social-policy programs. As will be clear in the following, the funds are here treated in terms of their administrative capacity with varying prevalence and specific character rather than as being political actors trying to influence, advocate, or prevent legislative initiatives by the state.[11]

THE WORKERS' QUESTION AND THE APPOINTMENT OF COMMISSIONS IN NORWAY AND SWEDEN

Both in Sweden and Norway, means of social provision before the 1880s mainly consisted of state-organised poor relief. In both countries, programs for poor relief developed during the early nineteenth century. It was mainly targeted at people, such as elderly and orphans, who had no ability to work and lacked someone to provide for them. Regulations for outdoor poor relief were stipulated by the state, but financing and administration were in essence made a local concern. In order to avoid abuse of the poor relief, anyone receiving such relief lost his right of self-determination, such as the right to vote or the right to go to court. However, from the late nineteenth century, poor relief faced increasing criticism because of the humiliating regulations that characterised this form of social provision.

In the mixed economy of welfare that characterised this period, voluntary organisations were also of some importance. Third-sector organisations consisted mainly of voluntary funds for mutual benefit, often organised in workplaces, as well as philanthropic assistance from the church or on private initiative. Several voluntary organisations emerged during the late nineteenth century concerned with social issues and involved in various forms of charity. From the 1880s, modern means of social provision such as sickness-, accident-, and pension-insurance programs were discussed. Initial state initiatives preceding the emergence of a modern welfare state responded to the ongoing industrialisation and consisted mainly of general industrial-safety regulations as well as regulation of child labour and of women industrial labour.[12]

In Sweden, as well as in Norway, labour parties were established during the late 1880s.[13] However, the fact that labour party foundings preceded the enactment of the sickness-insurance programs in both countries does not imply that the organised working class has been an influential political actor in this matter. When the 1909 law finally was enacted in Norway, the labour party representatives actually voted against the government proposal since they wanted the costs for the insurance to a higher degree to be covered by taxes and to a lesser degree by the insured themselves. From their point of view, the proposal laid an unjustified financial burden on people already in financial stress.[14] In 1891, the Swedish Labour Party, due to electoral rules then in force, had no representation in the parliament at all.[15] Besides, at this time the newborn party, still in its infancy, was more concerned with questions of suffrage and labour-market regulations, such as the demand for eight-hour workdays, than social-insurance issues.[16] In practice, the political management of the emerging Workers' Question during the 1890s was a matter for the conservative and liberal political elite represented in the Parliament.

This does not necessarily imply that the rise and the organization of the working class have been of no importance at all for the emergence of a modern welfare state. On the contrary, it seems fruitful to view the emergence of the working class as one of the motives for social-policy initiatives taken by the conservative and liberal political elite. However, this argument does not presuppose a broad and extensive national organisation of labour parties or unions, but it does entail the existence of a political elite deeply concerned with the Workers' Question.[17] It is the argument here that this concern was founded more on foreign experiences and future expectations than domestic developments.

Certainly, the societal tensions caused by the so-called *Thranittbevegelsen*[18] in Norway during the mid-nineteenth century were held in mind during the 1880s and brought forward by reform advocates as a terrible warning of what might be expected if the government failed to handle the Workers' Question in a proper way.[19] It is also true that, in Sweden, a major strike in the town of Sundsvall at the centre of the area of sawmill industries in the northern part of Sweden already in 1879 might have heralded increasing levels of social antagonism in the wake of the ongoing industrialisation. However, the rise of the Workers' Question, and the discussion on how to respond to real as well as perceived potential threats following from the ongoing industrialisation and the emergence of a working class, was to a great degree outlined by the contemporary political elite under influences from central Europe. Especially Bismarck's social-policy initiatives during the early 1880s appear as central for how the Workers' Question was established on the political agenda in Scandinavia. That the first writing to be published in Sweden on this matter was a translation of the German *Katheder-Sozialist* Gustav Schönbergs work on the social aspects of industrialisation is one example of how the German experiences were introduced into a Scandinavian context. A few years later, the Swedish professor in national economy, Mr Gustav Steffen, who played an important role in the Swedish discussions on social issues at the turn of the last century, spent some time in Germany, where he got in touch with the so-called *Katheder-Sozialisten* and their ideas. Mr Steffen published a pamphlet in 1889, "The Industrial Working Question—the Most Important Issue of Our Times," in which he focused on the countries in central Europe, primarily Germany.[20] The German example also played an important role in the lectures given by the Norwegian county governor Bredo Morgenstierna in the spring of 1886.[21] The interest for foreign legislation was also expressed in the public inquiry commission reports in which they were studied and discussed extensively. In Sweden, the commission published a comprehensive study in which both the German and Austrian social-insurance legislations were studied in detail.[22] The Norwegian commission began its work in October 1885 by studying the German sickness-insurance program.[23]

The tendency at the time to turn south for inspiration in attempts to resolve the Workers' Question did not mean that the Scandinavian reform advocates or commissioners blueprinted the German way to organise sickness-insurance programs in their own countries. On the contrary, it was with a critical attitude they studied the foreign precedents, and the emergence of sickness insurances in Scandinavia cannot be regarded as cases of policy diffusion.[24] Still, by taking this focus on the Bismarckian legislative efforts into consideration, it appears as no surprise that concern with the unifying working class characterised the discussion on social-policy initiatives in both countries. What the political elite in Scandinavia learned by studying the German precedent was, among other things, that social-policy initiatives could be utilized with social-pacifist purposes. In Germany, both the prohibition of the Social Democratic Party in 1879 and the establishment of insurance programs might be seen as part and parcel of a Bismarckian social-pacifist approach to the Workers' Question that, by the establishment of social insurance along corporatist lines, made a unification of the German working class more difficult.[25]

However, in the early 1880s the Bismarckian social-pacifist approach to the Workers' Question had to be adapted in order to appear relevant for Norwegian and Swedish circumstances, where industrialisation had not yet had its complete breakthrough and where the Labour Parties were not to be established until the late 1880s. Even though the problems observed in industrialised countries such as Germany were not occurring at home for the time being, both Swedish and Norwegian parliamentary representatives used the foreign precedents as a point of reference and as an argument as to why the state should play a more active role in social-policy issues. This was, for example, the case in the successful 1884 motion to the Swedish Parliament for the appointment of a workers' insurance commission, by the liberal MP Adolf Hedin. Here he argued that even though the social "inconveniences" that fuelled the Workers' Question in Europe were not occurring to the same extent in Sweden for the time being, it was wrong to draw the conclusion that nothing needed to be done. On the contrary, he argued that the developments abroad made a call for social policy initiatives since they heralded future developments about to take place also in Sweden. He argued that "we still have time, with the experience of others in mind, to try to avoid these problems."[26] In this sense, the threat that made a call for social-policy initiatives came from the experiences made in Europe and from likely domestic future developments.

In this discourse, social-policy initiatives appeared as a means to forestall future social eruptions by increasing the living conditions for the working class. In the parliamentary discussion that followed, Mr Hedins's motion, Mr Baron Leijonhufvud talked about the working-class movement and how to react to it. According to his speech, he supported the proposal to establish a commission since he believed that social-policy initiatives could "disarm the bitter elements" in the working-class movement, a movement he found powerful.[27] In a motion to the Swedish parliament in 1882, Mr Erik Westin, a representative for the Farmers Party, claimed that it would be wise to regulate the relationship between employers and the employed in order to avoid social antagonism. Mr Westin argued that it was important to "meet all justified demands" made by the working class in order to avoid serious future breaches that might have a "negative influence on the well-being of the societal body." He claimed that state initiatives were necessary in order to establish a "sound development" through which "socialistic currents" could be avoided. With a clear reference to the ongoing situation in Germany he reminded the reader that such currents had "raised justified apprehension and called for severe regulations" in other countries.[28]

The parliamentary debates in 1882 and 1884 also reflect how the Swedish political elite, in the late nineteenth century, took on a somewhat new strategy to deal with social-protest movements in comparison with the middle of the nineteenth century. During the rebellious year of 1848 and in its aftermath, both the Norwegian and Swedish political elite, as in most of Europe, choose to suppress dissent by military means and by imprisoning the leaders of the protest movements. Also, the Swedish strike in 1879 was regarded as a point of order, rather than a political issue. In the late nineteenth century, however, the Scandinavian Social Democratic Parties were never declared illegal, as in Germany. When the new potential threat seemed to rise in the wake of industrialisation, the strategy rather was to prevent agitation and to forestall such disruptions.

This is also expressed in the proposition for the enactment of a public inquiry commission in Norway. In his 1885 proposal to the Norwegian Parliament to establish the public inquiry commission, the Minister of Interior established that the Workers' Question was "nurtured" by the differences in the living conditions between capitalists and the proletariat that followed from the ongoing industrialization. For the time being, such differences were more common in the industrialized countries in Europe than in Norway, he argued, and for this reason, Norway had thus far been spared eruptions of social disagreement. However, the minister added, from that it could not be concluded that it would be wise to reject the challenge that this question would pose also on Norway in due course. The minister argued that the ideas that heightened this question abroad would, sooner or later, also spread to Norway and be internalised and utilised by "devout agitators." If the Norwegian state stood inactive, there was an obvious risk for the emergence of an "unreasonable and one-sided agitation that will make the [public] opinion uncivilized."[29]

This line of reasoning was similar to that of the Swedish Parliament, and, needless to say, the Norwegians were well aware of the proposals discussed in their neighbour country. Besides, the proposal by the Minister of Interior was originally brought about by the Norwegian Prime Minister, Mr Johan Sverdrup, who in December 1884, in a letter to the Department of Interior, advocated the enactment of a social-policy commission. He, in his turn, had discussed the matter in a mail correspondence with the Swedish-Norwegian king, Oscar II, during the autumn of 1884. In November, the king wrote to Sverdrup and told him that he was absolutely right about "my warm interest in the Workers' Question." In late November, Oscar II wrote that he was looking forward to see "the announced confidential letter on the Workers' Question," which he, in a new letter in December, declares that he had read.[30] The king's engagement in the Workers' Question has been interpreted as an attempt to win the initiative in social-policy matters from his liberal political opponents.[31] Later on, in 1888, the king also published a dictation on the Workers' Question. Behind the dictation stood Swedish Prime Minister Mr Gillis Bildt, who, during the early 1880s, was a Swedish minister in Berlin, where he on location followed the legislative measures taken by Bismarck. During his time in Berlin, Mr Bildt sent reports to the Swedish commission about the situation in Germany. In a letter to Oscar II in May 1888, he claimed that it was important to deal with the Workers' Question. Otherwise, he warned the king, it would be difficult to handle the political situation that would evolve, because sooner or later "these questions will break through by agitation."[32]

In both countries, the Workers' Question was discussed with reference to the ongoing situation in Europe, especially in Germany. Reform advocates claimed that the foreign experiences heralded future developments in Scandinavia and thus also called for social policy initiatives in Norway and Sweden. This way of reasoning appeared convincing, and both parliaments agreed on the necessity to investigate new possible social-policy initiatives by the state. A Swedish commission was appointed in 1884 and a Norwegian commission was appointed in 1885.

WHY TWO DIFFERENT PROPOSALS?

Although the emergence of the so-called Workers' Question did put the issue of social-insurance policy on the political agenda, it did not in itself point at a specific design of social-insurance programs. The fact that the Workers' Question was brought forward and defined in a similar vein in both Norway and Sweden did not mean that similar solutions were found. Instead, the two governments eventually decided to choose two different ways to handle the establishment of sickness-insurance programs. The different approaches to the enactment of a sickness-insurance program became first evident in the two public inquiry commission reports, both delivered to the national governments in 1889 and 1890, respectively. The 1890 Norwegian proposal suggested the establishment of a state-run compulsory sickness-insurance program targeted towards working-class constituencies, while the Swedish commission proposal instead suggested state subsidies to preexisting voluntary sickness and burial funds.

It is the argument of this chapter that the diverging previous development of the third-sector organisations in the two countries was of importance for the formulation of the two different proposals. Third-sector organisations were of interest to the commissions in both countries. In Norway, the minister of the interior especially pointed at the existing funds in his proposition for the enactment of a public inquiry commission.[33] This might also be seen against the background of the interest among policy-reform advocates in Parliament as well as the members of the commissions for the German legislation. When studying the German sickness-insurance program, they learned that existing sickness and burial funds played an important role for the organisation of a sickness-insurance program in Germany in 1883.[34] This was also true for other countries, such as Austria and, later, Denmark.[35] Considering this, it appears logical that the prevalence of third-sector organisations became of major interest for the two commissions. In both countries the commissions undertook full-scale investigations of all existing sickness and burial funds, obviously in order to evaluate their capacity to "carry" a sickness-insurance program on nationwide scale.

How the options for mandatory voluntary sickness-insurance schemes were made up in close reference to the development of insurance funds is in particular illustrated by the reasoning of the Norwegian commission during the early autumn of 1886. The commission had been established in 1885, and in October the same year the principles of the sickness-insurance program were discussed on at least two occasions.[36] There is no clear empirical evidence that the commission, by this time, had reached an agreement on what kind of sickness-insurance program it wanted to propose. Besides, the question of whether the forthcoming sickness-insurance program should constitute compulsory or voluntary membership was raised again in October 1886, when all the commissioners suddenly were convened. It was the subgroup responsible for the proposal for a sickness-insurance program that assembled the commission for new meetings. The reason for this sudden call was that a prior investigation of the Norwegian sickness and burial funds, made by the Norwegian statistician Zakarias Hermanssen, finally was completed. According to the report, the preexisting Norwegian sickness and burial funds were not particularly widespread, and they had no more than 37,000 members in total.[37] The subgroup now argued that Mr Hermanssen's preliminary report called for a new discussion on the principles of the sickness-insurance program that was to be proposed by the commission, and the appointees began to discuss a state-organised mandatory sickness insurance wherein the state itself would organise the local administration.[38] This turn towards a mandatory principle entailed by state engagement in managing the administration was in essence built on a sceptical perception of the working class' willingness or ability to engage voluntarily in sickness and burial funds. According to the commission report, a further expansion of the voluntary funds seemed unlikely and it was held to be true that the establishment of a sickness-insurance scheme encompassing the working class called for a mandatory solution.[39]

Although the conclusion differed, this way of reasoning had evident similarities with the reasoning of the Swedish commission. The Swedish commission also expressed some doubts concerning the strength and the ability to persist among the Swedish sickness and burial funds, and it claimed that only a mandatory insurance scheme would make it possible to cover the entire working class. According to the commission, the funds were small and they had primitive systems of financing as well as of benefit regulations. This was held to be especially problematic for elderly members of the funds. However, the commission concluded its report in a positive spirit with regard to their interpretation of the future of the funds. The number of funds, the commission claimed, did increase by the year, and as far it was concerned the funds had to be regarded as "promising results of voluntary initiatives." In their conclusion, the appointees expressed little doubt that the existing mutual funds were to expand further, especially when given the help of state subsidies. For the time being, they argued, it was too early to make a call for a mandatory insurance program.[40]

In retrospect, it thus appears that the interpretation of the voluntary sickness funds' development and of their ability to expand made by the commissions in each country played a crucial role for the decisions eventually made by the governments. Nevertheless, in accounting for the establishment of cases of "voluntary failure" and "third-party government" in the two countries, it must be held as possible that the conclusions drawn by the two commissions might be the result of political considerations as much as from conclusions made only with sheer respect to the results of statistical investigations.[41] Therefore, the empirical evidence presented by the commissions, as well as the ideological and political aspects of their work, will be subject to further discussion in the following.

THE DEVELOPMENT OF SICKNESS AND BURIAL
FUNDS IN SWEDEN AND NORWAY

Given the emphasis laid upon the prevalence of funds by commissioners themselves, it appears natural to explain the different proposals by emphasising the diverging prevalence of funds in the two countries.[42] However, a comparison of the number of fund members as a proportion of the total population in each of the two countries around the 1880s does not yield a clear difference. In both countries the respective number of fund members in proportion to the total population in 1880 and 1890 varied between 2 and 3 percent.[43]

Certainly, the small differences of number of members in proportion to total population at the end of the nineteenth century do not, in a satisfying manner, support the idea that the difference in policy choice had some correspondence to actual differences in prevalence of voluntary funds in the two countries at that time. However, given the fact that both commissions addressed the Workers' Question and thus singled out members of the working class as the actual prioritised recipients of the sickness insurance, the national prevalence of funds might not be the most interesting measurement. Potentially more important to the commissioners should have been the tendency among the working class to join the funds and the concentration of funds into the cities where the working class primarily lived and worked.[44] As envisioned in Tables 6.1 and 6.2, industrialisation as well as urbanisation had come a bit further in Norway than in Sweden at this time.[45]

Both commissions showed that the development of funds was mainly an urban phenomenon and that many funds were organised in close relationship to the developing industries. According to the report presented by the Swedish commission, 1049 sickness and burial funds existed in Sweden in 1884, and they had altogether 138,726 members.[46] In 1884, about 70 per cent of all the members belonged to the funds located in the cities. From a

Table 6.1 Level of Industrialisation in Norway and Sweden About 1890 (in Thousands)

	Sweden 1890	Norway 1891
Number employed in manufacturing industry	263	177
Total employed population	1865	774
Manufacturing population as percentage of total employed population	14.10	22.87

Source: B. R. Mitchell, *European historical statistics 1750–1970*, Basingstoke: Macmillan, 1975, pp.159, 162.

Table 6.2 Level of Urbanisation in Norway and Sweden, 1880 and 1890
(in Thousands)

	Sweden 1880	Sweden 1890	Norway 1880	Norway 1890
Urban population	690.4	899.7	414.3	474.1
Total population	4565.7	4784.9	1923.3	2000.9
Urban population as percentage of total population	15.12	18.80	21.54	23.69

Sources: _Statistisk aarbok for kongeriket Norge 1914_, Kristiania 1915, table 2; _Historical statistics for Sweden I. Population 1720–1950_, Stockholm 1955, table A 4.

geographical point of view, this meant that about 12 per cent of the population in the cities were fund members but only 1 per cent in the countryside.[47] The relationship between the development of funds and the ongoing industrialisation is especially underlined by the fact that more than one-third of all the members in Sweden in 1884 belonged to the so-called factory funds—these were funds located at specific factories and often organised and initially financed by the factory owner. According to the Swedish commission report, the almost 300 factory funds alone organised more than 40,000 members in 1884.[48] The relationship between industrialisation and expansion of funds is also emphasised when industrialised cities are singled out and studied in detail. For example, in the Swedish town of Norrköping, with major textile industries, almost 19 per cent of the inhabitants were fund members already in 1884. In Sundsvall, a town with sawmill and paper industries, and in Eskilstuna, a town with manufacturing industries, the corresponding proportions were almost 20 and 25 per cent, respectively, in the same year. The funds in Stockholm had almost 35,000 members, or 17 per cent of the inhabitants.[49]

Also in Norway, a similar relationship among industrialisation, urbanisation, and the development of funds is traceable. In his report, Zakarias Hermanssen stated that the number of funds was about 220–240 in 1885, and they had approximately 37,000 members.[50] Unfortunately, the Norwegian report is much less detailed than the Swedish and does not provide the same kind of specified information about individual funds. It seems that about fifty of the Norwegian funds were factory funds, and it is also clear, as in Sweden, that the sickness and burial funds were concentrated in the urban areas. According to the report, more than 40 per cent of all members belonged to funds located to the two major cities of Kristiania and Bergen.[51] However, this did not mean that a great proportion of the working class was members. According to later estimates made by Norwegian scholars, about one-third of around 45,000 Norwegian factory workers were members of a fund in the middle of the 1880s. However, if manual labourers are taken into account as well, only about one-seventh of the working class was members.[52]

As is demonstrated in Table 6.3, a study of the total membership numbers in proportion to the population living in the cities and to the number employed in manufacturing industry reveals a more distinct difference between the two countries. It must be kept in mind that both the urban population as a proportion of the total population and the manufacturing population as a proportion of the total employed population were higher in Norway than in Sweden. This suggests that both urbanisation and industrialisation had come further in Norway. If there ever was a causal relationship between industrialisation, urbanisation, and development of funds, we would expect the Norwegian funds to be more developed in relative terms. But they were not.

The preceding discussion suggests that industrialisation and urbanisation in Norway did not entail the same development of sickness and burial funds as in Sweden. This is also in line with previous findings on the development of trade unions during the late nineteenth century and the development of voluntary unemployment funds in the two countries.[53] One possible determinant for the different development of voluntary funds in the two countries might have been the different nature of the industrialisation processes in Norway and Sweden. Swedish industrialisation around this time was based on the textile industry, the sawmills, and the ironworks; and it has been argued that the emergence of the permanent and relatively larger production sites in Sweden provided a more fruitful soil not only for unions but also for the creation of sickness and burial funds than the more small-scale Norwegian industries.[54]

OTHER REASONS FOR THE TWO DIFFERENT PATHS?

Although the definition of "voluntary failure" that was made by the Norwegian commission seems to have had some correspondence with the actual development of mutual funds in Norway, such a definition must be suspected to be politically biased. However, it is difficult to account for the diverging options made by the commissions with respect to possible differences in

Table 6.3 Relative Development of Funds in Norway and Sweden

	Sweden	Norway
Number of fund members* as % of manufacturing population around 1890	52.75	20.90
Number of fund members* as % of urban population 1890	15.43	7.81

Sources: See Table 6.1: *in 1884 for Sweden and in 1885 for Norway.

general notions of third-sector organisations among the political elite in the two countries. On the contrary, both in Sweden and in Norway a positive view of the voluntary sector was expressed by the political elite by the late nineteenth century.

Previous research has established that among the members of the Norwegian Parliament a voluntary solution was perceived as more desirable to promote than a mandatory solution.[55] Besides, the Norwegian commission also paid attention to the conditions for the voluntary funds when designing their proposal for a mandatory sickness-insurance program administered by state-run official funds. In order to protect the voluntary funds from being driven out of business by the state-run funds, the commissioners suggested that the latter would provide only sickness insurance and the voluntary funds would provide for additional benefits such as medical treatment.[56] The commissioners' concern with the relationship between state-run and voluntary funds does not disclose a principled stance against self-help and voluntary organisation. Thus, it does not seem fruitful to point to ideological differences between the countries as an explanation for the different options.

This might also be illustrated by how a minority in the Norwegian commission at first did disagree with the proposition for a mandatory sickness and insurance scheme. They claimed that it would have been more advisable to support the working class' organisation of voluntary funds, as in Sweden or in Denmark. On principled grounds, they opposed the idea to single out a specific group and oblige them to pay for their membership in a mandatory program. However, due to the limited prevalence of funds in Norway, they were forced to abandon their position, and the proposal for a mandatory sickness-insurance program was finally presented by a united commission.[57]

Two of the three members of the Norwegian commission that initially opposed a proposal for mandatory sickness-insurance program were members of the liberal workers movement in Norway, which had a tradition of self-help and of organising voluntary sickness funds. The appointees' initial protests, as well as their final approval of the proposal, also put into question the eventual importance of group interest for the differing decisions made in Sweden and Norway.

In previous attempts to account for the decisions made by the governments in Sweden and Norway, as well as in Denmark, it has also been suggested that funds themselves were important actors that, to differing degrees, were successful in their attempts to influence decisions on the design of sickness-insurance programs.[58] However, the composition of the commissions seems not to account for the differing proposals. In the Swedish commission, only one member did represent the liberal labour movement, and still it proposed a voluntary scheme.[59] Besides, a hypothesis emphasising the political influence of group interest for decisions made by the commissions or the governments does not sufficiently appreciate the late establishment of funds' interest organisations in the two countries. It was not until after the legislation had been enacted that the funds began to organise themselves in national-interest organisations. In Sweden, a national-interest organisation for funds was not established until 1905—fourteen years after the enactment of the 1891 law on sickness and burial funds. In Norway, such an organisation did not appear until 1912.[60] Finally, it might be put into question whether the voluntary funds actually did resist the enactment of mandatory sickness-insurance programs. In Norway, the liberal labour movement, at an early stage, approved with the proposals for mandatory sickness insurance. In the late 1910s also, Swedish funds did support suggestions for a mandatory sickness-insurance program.[61]

As will be clear in the following, parliamentary political-power relationships did matter for the handling of the two proposals. Whether the political-power relationships in the two parliaments also affected the proposals made by the commissions for sickness-insurance programs seems, however, less certain. In both countries, farmers played a crucial role in the parliamentary decision-making process, and, as will be clear in the following, their support was needed for the establishment of social-policy initiatives. Members of both the Swedish and Norwegians commissions were presumably well aware of the farmers' standpoints in the parliaments. However, the farmers' position did not rule out the possibility for the commissions to propose either an encompassing mandatory sickness-insurance program with low-risk redistribution or a continued voluntary insurance. In Norway, the commission did not suggest either form of scheme but put forward a proposal that raised farmers' discontent.

Thus, even though the definition of "voluntary failure" must be regarded as a process whereby the interpretation and adaptation of empirical findings are politically biased, it does not seem likely that the different propositions made by the commissions in Sweden and Norway can be easily accounted for with respect to differences in terms of ideology or group-interest organisation. It appears more likely that the diverging prevalence of funds in the two countries actually did matter for the proposals made by the commissions.

THE TWO PROPOSALS FOR SICKNESS-INSURANCE POLICY

To establish that funds were relatively more developed in Sweden than in Norway is not sufficient when elaborating the political significance of third-sector organisations for the political treatment of the Workers' Question. It is also necessary to interpret how these differences constituted different conditions for policymaking in the two countries with respect to how the political actors themselves defined their political options. This is done here in a study of how the proposals for sickness-insurance programs, and their reception in parliament, were treated. Two aspects of the proposals that proved to be politically controversial will be emphasised: that of state engagement in administrative/financial questions and that of risk redistribution. The latter will also highlight the importance of the organisational character of the funds for the relatively conflict-free enactment of a sickness-insurance program in Sweden. Thus, the Norwegian case illustrates how the lack of preexisting funds, which, on a voluntary basis, could administer a voluntary sickness insurance that also covered the working class in the cities meant that the state itself had to take on a larger degree of responsibility for financing as well as implementing a sickness-insurance program. It was this responsibility that was debated and caused political disagreement. The Swedish case illustrates both how the policy opportunity that stemmed from more prevalent funds was utilised by the Parliament and how the character of the funds further made such a solution easy to enact.

The Norwegian policy might be regarded as a kind of enforced self-help by which the political elite in Norway "from above" made the working class engage themselves in state-organised funds. In line with the commission report, the proposal suggested a program mainly targeted at the working class that would be administered through local funds that on a national level were economically connected through a national fund, the so-called *Landssykekassan*. According to the proposal, the program would cover all Norwegian citizens with permanent employment who had annual earnings of less than 1200 NKr. The income limit guaranteed that most of the working class in the cities would be covered, and at the same time it prevented state subsidies from being given to the "better off." However, groups such as farmers, as well as leaseholders, were not covered by the proposal, although their annual earnings might have been below the income limit. The program was suggested to be financed mainly through contributions by the members of the program—in essence this was the meaning of "self-help."[62] The administration costs for the local funds were to be financed by the municipalities, but the state would cover all costs for the national fund. Any deficits in the program would be covered by the municipalities together with the state. Municipalities would cover their part in relationship to the number of members in the local fund. Contributions from the members would be paid via deductions on wages by employers and collected by the local funds, which also administered payments and control of the insured.[63] This arrangement explains why only workers with more permanent occupations could be covered by the program.

Although the commission, established in 1885, already in its report from 1890 complained about the fact that a voluntary sickness-insurance program could not be developed in Norway, it also pointed at the many advantages with the suggested program. First of all, the establishment of a nationwide administration of interconnected local funds made it possible for members to bring along their membership when moving within the country, for example, in search of employment. Another advantage of the interconnected local funds, it was claimed, was the possibility for redistribution of risks and resources among the different local funds. From a nationwide system of interconnected funds would follow the possibility to level out economic differences between different parts of the country. In contrast to free-standing local funds that had to carry their losses on their own and had to endure periods of economic constraint without extra help, the proposal for the so-called *Landssykekassan* would provide a greater scope of economic safety for the members.[64] Against the backdrop of the Norwegian proposals for a sickness-insurance program, the Swedish proposal stands out as quite different both with respect to risk redistribution and to state responsibility for implementing a sickness-insurance program. The sickness and burial funds in Sweden were voluntary, and local funds did not redistribute risks and resources on a regional or a national scale. On the contrary, the sickness and burial funds were mostly independent and voluntary risk pools, where members themselves were to decide upon whom to share their risks with. Members would pay their fees to their fund and state subsidies were inversely related to the number of members. Apart from the financial subsidies, the state took on no responsibility for financing the administration of the sickness-insurance program, nor would it cover any deficits eventually occurring in the funds. The specific nature of the proposals meant that no attempt was made to regulate these aspects of the scheme to any greater extent.[65]

Thus, in Sweden, the funds remained small and local and questions on membership, financing, and benefits were still to be decided upon by the funds themselves. With respect to the Norwegian law, the Swedish law did not presuppose any far-reaching state involvement. In comparison, the proposal in Norway suggested a "big step," including the creation of new funds, the regulation of their activities, and a risk-redistributing element, while the Swedish law is characterised by its modest intervention in the activities of the free-standing local funds. The two cases clearly represent two different approaches to sickness-insurance policy.

RESISTANT FARMERS IN NORWAY AND SWEDEN

When studying the political reception of the two diverging proposals, it must be noted that one major political obstacle for the accomplishment of social-policy initiatives in both countries by this time was put up by the politically influential farmers.[66] With a marked countryside perspective on political issues, they successfully opposed reform proposals that they held to favour the working class in the cities at the cost of farmers and others in the countryside. In Norway, this became evident in 1897. The proposal, then put forward by a member of the Liberal cabinet, faced strong political resistance. However, the intense political debate did not follow party lines but divided the two major parties in half. Farmers from the Liberal Party joined members of the Conservative Party in a successful attempt to block the proposal.[67]

In brief, Norwegian farmers in parliament opposed the legislation proposal with a view to two intervening issues in the political debate: *coverage* and *costs*. According to farmers' opinion, a mandatory sickness-insurance program financed partly by the state and municipalities and mainly covering the working class meant that capital would be transferred from taxpaying farmers in the countryside to the insured working class in the cities. One of the leading farmers in the Norwegian Parliament, Mr Wollert Konow, claimed that the working class in the cities was not the only group to need such insurance, and he strongly rejected the idea that farmers, constituting the majority of taxpayers, would pay for an insurance program mainly targeted at the working class.[68] Furthermore, farmers claimed that a class-based insurance would increase the depopulation of the countryside. This was especially important during the 1890s, when farmers, due to increasing industrialisation and urbanisation, experienced a shortage of cheap labour force in the countryside.[69] In consonance with this line of argument, farmers also rejected the idea of increasing social costs for the state that would stem from eventual financial deficits in the program. This became obvious in the long parliamentary debate on "the actual costs" of the sickness-insurance program and on whether these costs really would reduce costs for outdoor poor relief in the municipalities. Two lines of argument here emerged; critics of the proposal feared that the calculations on the actual costs of the sickness-insurance program were misleading, and it was suggested that the annual deficit would be as much as 800,000 NKr, to be compared with the estimated 388,000 NKr in annual costs for the Norwegian state. In contrast, reform advocates such as the leading member of the Liberal Party *Venstre*, Mr Gunnar Knudsen, claimed that against the backdrop of the benefits for the members of the program, possible deficits were not that important. Farmers also opposed the major administrative efforts that would follow from implementing the proposal for mandatory sickness insurance.[70]

In Sweden, as mentioned above, these points of disagreement never seem to have come up. The 1891 proposal for a voluntary sickness-insurance program with state subsidies to already existing sickness and burial funds went through without much ado. In both chambers the proposal received overwhelming support.[71] However, this does not suggest that Swedish farmers had another point of view on the questions debated in Norway than the Norwegian farmers. For example, when the convening of the 1884 commission was discussed in the Swedish parliament, farmers in the lower chamber strongly opposed an investigation that only considered the industrial working class in the cities. From a perspective identical to that of the Norwegian farmers, Swedish farmers emphasised that people living in the countryside shared the same need for support as the working class in the cities.[72] In brief, farmers wanted the countryside to be considered as part of the Workers' Question. In parliamentary debate in 1884, the MP A. P. Danielsson, a leading member of the Farmers Party, claimed that he agreed on the "main purpose" of the idea of launching a commission but that he strongly opposed that the commission would consider only the working class in the cities. The most important thing of all, said Danielsson, was that the Parliament did not overlook the situation for workers and small farmers in the countryside and gave the workers in cities, especially factory workers, a "monopoly" on social questions. In his speech, he particularly emphasised the needs of the yeomen, and Danielsson announced that he was ready to vote against convening the commission if his (and other farmers') criticisms on this matter were not taken seriously enough.[73]

However, issues of coverage and of costs that triggered farmers' dissent in Norway in 1897 were never to be politicised in Sweden in 1891. These questions were in essence to be solved by the funds themselves. A voluntary sickness-insurance program did not exclude farmers from the subsidised funds in the same vein as the Norwegian mandatory insurance. Farmers in Sweden were free to join the subsidised voluntary funds. In addition, state subsidies were not expensive for the state. According to the 1891 proposition, 59,000 SKr was deposited for the first year, which can be compared to Norway, where the total cost for the state was estimated at 388,000 NKr, and just as much for the municipalities.[74] Besides, in Sweden, administration was to be handled by the local funds, and there was at first no perceived need for the Swedish state to build a national administration in order to implement sickness-insurance legislation.

The development in Norway and Sweden also underlines that farmers, if the possibility was at hand, prioritised voluntary solutions that did not include elements of risk redistribution on a national level, rather than formulating their interests in terms of being a specific risk category struggling for an encompassing program. It was only when they encountered proposals for mandatory sickness-insurance programs targeting the working-class constituencies that they campaigned for universal solutions.[75] When they, as in Sweden, due to relatively well-developed third-sector organisations, had the possibility to opt for a voluntary sickness-insurance program, they did so. In contrast to what has been suggested by scholars who put emphasis on the role played by farmers in the emergence of the universal Scandinavian welfare state, it cannot be concluded that farmers, being a specific risk category, did campaign for universal solutions as such. Rather, they acted as being rational actors formulating their interests with reference to their economic preferences rather than as a risk group.[76]

THE IMPORTANCE OF FUNDS' ADMINISTRATIVE CHARACTER

This interpretation of farmers' policy choices emphasises the importance of redistributive questions, and at the same time it highlights the importance of the organisational character of the funds in Sweden. Here, organisational character refers to the smallness and local orientation of most funds. The funds in both countries might be characterised in different ways—by their concentration in the cities, by their male dominance or membership regulations—but in this particular context their relative smallness, with reference to the number of members in each and every fund and their local orientation, stands out as being of greatest importance.[77]

To the public inquiry commissions, the organisational character of funds, especially their smallness, appeared as problematic. However, from a political point of view, where risk redistribution is not desirable, their smallness and local orientation might rather appear as an advantage. Through their specific character as local risk-pools the funds did not promote distribution from people living in the countryside to the more risk-prone urban working class. This was in the farmers' interest and crucial for their political support in Parliament, something which assisted a smooth enactment of the 1891 reform.

That the organisational character of the Swedish funds did matter for farmers content with the 1891 legislation on sickness and burial funds is supported further by their political action in the wake of the 1891 reform. Once the law was enacted, the Swedish Parliament was soon to realise that the voluntary funds did not choose to register with the state as extensively as expected. Previous research, however limited, on the funds' tendency to register with the state has suggested that funds in general were reluctant to do so, but that this trend was more emphasised among the trade-organised funds. In these funds, which had a close relationship with the emerging unions or even were organised by the unions, the financial assets could be used in the struggle against employers as strike funds. This was not allowed by the 1891 law on sickness and burial funds.[78]

A discussion in the parliament soon arose when demands were put forward to raise the financial subsidies to the funds. It was argued that higher subsidies and an overall reformation of the rules for the subsidies would encourage the funds to register with the state. These demands were not agreed upon easily, and now political disagreement arose in the Swedish Parliament. Reform advocates suggested that raised subsidies would encourage the funds to register with the state. Opponents, on the other hand, referred to the 1891 law, where it was stipulated that the financial subsidies would be considered not as economic encouragement to the funds but as a contribution to the costs that stemmed from the fulfilling of the responsibilities laid upon the funds by the law.[79] This discussion eventually led to two reforms, in 1897 and 1898, when the Parliament agreed upon proposals especially favouring small funds. The driving force behind such policy was the *Statsutskottet*,[80] in which farmers dominated. The question at stake was how to relate the state-financed subsidies to the funds. The Standing Committee of Supply opted for a solution along the lines of inverse proportionality with respect to the number of members in the funds. This meant—with respect to other proposals made by the government as well as other MPs—that the Standing Committee of Supply lowered the subsidies for funds with more than 300 members and raised them for funds with less than 100 members. Besides, a subsidy limit, already decided upon in 1891, was kept despite demands for its abolition. This meant that state subsidies were paid at the rate of 1.5 SKr for every member in funds with at the most 100 members, 1 SKr per member in funds with up to 300 members, and with 0.50 SKr for each member in funds with more than 300 members. The subsidy limit was 1500 SKr.[81] This policy of regulating the subsidies gave no, or very weak, incentives for funds to grow with respect to their membership. Besides, it was strongly in favour of funds located on the countryside, which in general had fewer members per fund than the funds located in the cities.[82] Thus, farmers' willingness to promote a nonrisk-redistributing insurance program eventually led to a policy in favour of small and local funds.

CONCLUSION

In this chapter, the two different ways of approaching the Workers' Question, by means of enacting sickness-insurance programs, are studied. It is here suggested that the political preconditions were similar in both countries: The Workers' Question was defined in a similar vein in both Norway and Sweden and in both countries farmers played a crucial role in the political decision-making process. According to this study, the emergence of a domestic organised working class seems to have played a limited role for the rise of the Workers' Question in Sweden and Norway. Rather, developments in central Europe were used as a pretext for national social-policy initiatives.

In both countries, farmers had an important position in parliament and social-policy initiatives could not prevail if they raised farmers' discontent. Thus, political power relationships in parliament and the definition of the Workers' Question in the two countries cannot alone be held to account for either the design or the timing of the sickness-insurance programs established. Instead, it is here argued that the combination of the prevalence and the character of third-sector organisations, together with political power relationships in parliament, are of importance for the understanding of the two paths of welfare-state formation taken in the two countries.

The two commissions drew different conclusions with respect to the possibilities to utilize the preexisting funds for a voluntary sickness-insurance program. I have argued that these diverging interpretations seem to correspond with actual development in the both countries. The Norwegian public inquiry commission proposed a mandatory sickness-insurance plan for the working class. In contrast, in Sweden, where the funds were relatively more developed, the Swedish commission proposed a voluntary sickness-insurance program. Against the backdrop of contemporary political relationships in parliament, the ability to propose a voluntary sickness-insurance program seems to have gone together with the possibility of enacting a reform that did not cause political disagreement. Thus, by making use of the voluntary funds as administrative local resources, a political solution was found in Sweden by which crucial questions could be removed from the political agenda. In Norway, however, questions on coverage, costs, and even administration had to be dealt with by the state, and these questions caused political disagreement in the parliament. In particular, farmers opposed proposals for mandatory and class-based insurance in favour of a more encompassing model, arguing that the need for a sickness-insurance program also existed in the countryside. In Sweden, these questions were to a large extent resolved by the mutual funds themselves and thus were never disagreed on in parliament.

The two cases discussed here illustrate a central part of the Salamon theory on the relationship between governments and third-sector organisations. The Norwegian case provides an example of how "voluntary failure" paved the way for, or made necessary, a greater degree of state involvement. This might be compared to Sweden, where the more developed sickness and burial funds offered the government an additional, less controversial, policy option: that of subsidising already existing funds. In Salamon's terms, the Swedish case illustrates how "third party government" can be established in areas where "non-profit organizations were on the scene before government arrived."[83]

However, this does not mean that the existence of relatively prevalent funds did facilitate the enactment of whichever form of sickness-insurance program. Given their organisational character, they were in particular suited for a voluntary scheme with no risk redistribution. This happened to be in line with farmers' ambitions to avoid the enactment of sickness-insurance programs that did redistribute risk and resources from the countryside to the working class in the cities. During the 1920s, the dependency on the sickness and burial funds eventually, and in tandem with new political ambitions due to changes in political power relationships in the Swedish Parliament, became an administrative and political obstacle to further sickness-policy reform in Sweden.[84]

The ability to opt for a voluntary sickness-insurance program in 1891 meant that Swedish farmers never found reason to oppose the enactment of a sickness-insurance program in the same vein as farmers did in Norway. In contrast to the situation in Norway, this paved the way for a smooth enactment of a sickness-insurance program. Neither did they, like the Norwegian farmers, propose a mandatory and encompassing sickness-insurance program. Hence, it is here argued that farmers' support for encompassing sickness insurance appears as part and parcel of resistance against mandatory class-based insurance, rather than as a consequence of strategic action to implement principled universalism. Due to the character of the Swedish sickness and burial funds, it was easy for Swedish farmers to vote in favour of the 1891 proposal. This was further emphasised by their policy in the wake of the 1891 reform when they in particular favoured the small funds. In so doing, their actions disclosed their awareness of the importance of the character of third-sector organisations. The farmers not only took advantage of the funds being small and local risk pools; they also stood up for funds to continue to be that way by engaging political means such as the regulation of state subsidies to registered funds.

Finally, given the political power relationships in parliament, the results indicate that the importance of states' capabilities to produce skills and administrative capacity for social-policy development also includes their capability to make use of administrative capacity in civil society. It would thus be suggested that it is fruitful to complement the ambition to "bring the state back in" to policy analysis with an examination of the state's capacity to engage third-sector organisations in the implementation of policy. In doing this, it also seems important to study not only the prevalence, but also the character, of the administrative resources presented by the third-sector organisations.

NOTES

1. An early draft of this chapter was reviewed by Professor Jane Lewis, London School of Economics, at the European Social Science History Conference in The Hague, Netherlands, 2002. I would like to thank her for insightful and encouraging comments. I also would like to take the opportunity to thank Eero Carroll, Institute for Social Research, Stockholm University; Lena Eriksson, Department of History, Stockholm University; and especially the editors, Paul Bridgen and Bernard Harris, University of Southampton, for valuable comments on previous drafts of this chapter.
2. Swedish (and Norwegian) sickness and burial funds can, to some extent, be compared with friendly societies in Great Britain. Each member frequently paid a fee to the fund, and upon occurrence of inability to work due to illness or accident, a small compensation was paid to the member. However, the funds were small, local, and often had few members. For an investigation of mutual-benefit societies, see M. van der Linden, ed., *Social security mutualism: The comparative history of mutual benefit societies*, Bern: Peter Lang, 1996.
3. W. Korpi, "Contentious institutions: An augmented rational-choice analysis of the origins and path dependency of welfare state institutions in Western countries," *Rationality and Society*, 13(2); A. Hicks, *Social democracy and welfare capitalism: A century of income security politics*, New York: Cornell University Press, 1999, chapter 2.
4. G. Esping-Andersen, *The three worlds of welfare capitalism*, Cambridge: Polity Press, 1990; W. Korpi and J Palme, "The paradox of redistribution and strategies of equality: Welfare state institutions, inequality and poverty in the western countries," *American Sociological Review*, 63(5).
5. E. Carroll, *Emergence and structuring of social insurance institutions: Comparative studies on social policy and unemployment insurance*, Stockholm: Swedish Institute for Social Research, 1999, chapter 2; G. Esping-Andersen and W. Korpi, "From poor relief to institutional welfare states: The development of Scandinavian social policy," in R. Erikson, E. Hansen, S. Ringen, and H. Uusitalo, eds., *The Scandinavian model: Welfare states and welfare research*, New York: Sharpe, 1987.

6. P. Baldwin, *The politics of solidarity: Class bases of the European welfare state 1875–1975*, Cambridge: Cambridge University Press, 1990; "Scandinavian origins of the interpretation of the welfare state," *Comparative Study of Society and History*, 31(1).
7. O. Kangas, *The politics of social rights: Studies on the dimensions in sickness insurance policy in OECD countries*, Stockholm: Swedish Institute for Social Research, 1990, chapter 5.
8. E. Amenta and T. Skocpol, "Taking exception: Explaining the distinctiveness of American public policies in the last century," in F. G. Castles, ed., *The comparative history of public policy*, Cambridge: Cambridge University Press, 1989; P. B. Evans, D. Rueschemeyer, and T. Skocpol, eds., *Bringing the state back in*, Cambridge: Cambridge University Press, 1985.
9. The argument is developed in P. Johansson, *Fast i det förflutna: Institutioner och intressen i svensk sjukförsäkringspolitik 1891–1931*, Lund, Sweden: Arkiv, 2003.
10. L. M. Salamon, "Of market, voluntary failure, and third-party government: Toward a theory of government–nonprofit relations in the modern welfare state," *Journal of Voluntary Action Research*, 16(1 & 2), 36–43.
11. Cf. S. Kuhnle, "The growth of social insurance programs in scandinavia: Outside influences and internal forces," in P. Flora and A. J. Heidenheimer, *The development of welfare states in Europe and America* (New Brunswick, NJ, and London: Transaction Publishers, 1982). Also see J. H. Treble, "The attitudes of friendly societies towards the movement in Great Britain for state pensions 1878–1908," *International Review of Social History*, 15(2).
12. S. E. Olsson, *Social policy and welfare state in Sweden*, Lund, Sweden: Arkiv, 1990, pp 47–54; U. Lundberg & K. Åmark, "Social rights and social security: The Swedish welfare state 1900–2000," *Scandinavian Journal of History*, 26(3), 157–60.
13. The Swedish Social Democratic Labour Party (SAP) was organised in 1889 and the Norwegian Labour Party (NAP) was organised in 1887.
14. A. L. Seip, *Socialhjelpstaten blir til: Norsk socialpolitikk 1740–1920* (Oslo: Gyldendal, 1984), pp. 103–05. Also see P. Thane, "The working class and state "welfare" in Britain 1880–1914," *Historical Journal*, 27(4); B. Harris, *The origins of the British welfare state: Social welfare in England and Wales 1800–1945*, Basingstoke: Palgrave, 2004, pp. 153–55.
15. It was not until 1898 in Norway and 1907 in Sweden that the right to vote was enlarged. However, the right to vote was still limited along class as well as gender lines, and a full democratic breakthrough did not appear until 1913 in Norway and 1919 in Sweden. First social democratic MP, Mr Hjalmar Branting, chairman of the SAP, was elected in 1897 on a liberal mandate. In the year 1900, the Norwegian Labour Party got 16 per cent of all votes; however, due to election rules, they did not get any representation in the parliament. It was not until 1903 that they got four seats in the parliament.
16. G. Therborn, "Arbetarrörelsen och välfärdsstaten," *Arkiv för Studier i Arbetarrörelsens historia*, 41–42, 3–8.
17. E. Carroll, *Emergence and structuring of social insurance institutions*, pp. 78–85.
18. A strong popular movement—similar to the Chartist Movement in Great Britain—making a call for modernisation and democratisation of the Norwegian society. See E. Bull, *Arbeiderbevegelsens historie i Norge, bd 1, Arbeiderklassen blir til*, Oslo: Tiden, 1985, pp. 204–06.
19. Norwegian Parliament, Proposal no. 82, 1885, pp. 5–7.
20. G. Steffen, *Den industriella arbetarfrågan: Nutidens förnämsta sociala spörsmål*, Stockholm: Verdandi, 1889.

21. National Archive of Norway (NRA): The Archive of Arbeiderkommissionen, printed matter, B. Morgenstierne, *Om arbeiderforsikringer: Foredrag af amtmand Morgenstierne den 12te og 18de Martz 1886*, pp. 1–20; A. L. Seip, *Socialhjelpstaten blir til*, pp. 88–9.
22. Arbetarförsäkringskommittén, *Arbetarförsäkringen i Tyskland och Österrike*, Stockholm: public inquiry report 1889.
23. NRA, The Archive of Arbeiderkommissionen, Box 2, Minutes 6 October 1885.
24. S. Kuhnle, "The growth of social insurance programs in Scandinavia," pp. 126–31.
25. W. Korpi, "Contentious Institutions," pp. 250–51. For a critical remark on Bismarck's "social-pacifist" motives, see P. Hennock, "Social Policy under the empire—myths and evidence," *German History*, 16(1), 68–69.
26. Swedish Parliament: Second Chamber, Motion 1884:111, p. 1; for a similar way of reasoning in Norway, see Norwegian Parliament: Proposal no. 82, 1885, p. 5.
27. Swedish Parliament: Second Chamber: Minutes 1884:14, p. 19–20.
28. Swedish Parliament: Second Chamber, Motion 1882:76, p. 14.
29. Norwegian Parliament: Proposition no. 82, 1885, p. 5.
30. NRA, The archive of Johan Sverdrup, vol. 150.
31. S. E. Olsson Hort, "Före Bengt Westerberg: Adolf Hedin och det nyliberala ursprunget till den socialliberala välfärdspolitiken i Sverige," *Arkiv för Studier i Arbetarrörelsens Historia*, (58–59), 8–14.
32. K. Englund, *Arbetarförsäkringsfrågani svenskpolitik*, Uppsala: Acta Universitatis Upsaliensis, 1976, s. 38.
33. Norwegian Parliament: Proposition 1885:82, pp. 11–12.
34. G. Stollberg, "Hilfskassen in nineteenth-century Germany," in M. van der Linden, ed., *Social security mutualism*Bern: Switzerland: Peter Lang; D. Zöllner, "Germany," in P. A. Köhler, H. F. Zacher, and M. Partington, eds., *The evolution of social insurance 1881–1981: Studies of Germany, France, Great Britain, Austria and Russia*, London: St. Martin's Press, 1982, p. 25.
35. This argument is further explored in E. Carroll and P. Johansson, "Mutualism, institutional design, and early sickness insurance: A comparative analysis of six European nations," unpublished paper presented at the FISS Research Seminar, "Issues in Social Security," Sigtuna, Sweden, 17–20 June 2000; For Denmark, see D. Levine, "Conservatism and tradition in Danish social welfare legislation 1890–1933," *Comparative studies in Society and History*, (20)1, 68; *Poverty and society: The growth of the American welfare state in international comparison*, New Brunswick, NJ: Rutgers University Press, 1988, chapter 7.
36. NRA, The Archive of Arbeiderkommissionen, Minutes 6 and 8, October 1885.
37. Z. Hermanssen, *Oversigt over de norska Syge- og Begravelsekassers Virksomhed i 1885*, Oslo: public inquiry report 1886, p. 17.
38. Ibid., pp. 14–19, October 1886.
39. Arbeiderkommissionens Indstilling II, pp. 12–13.
40. Arbetarförskringskommittéts betänkande I:4, pp. 33–34.
41. S. Kuhnle, "International modelling, states and statistics" Scandinavian social security solutions in the 1890's," in D. Rueschemeyer and T. Skocpol, eds., *States, social knowledge and the origins of modern social politics*, Princeton, NJ: Princeton University Press, 1995.
42. Ø. Björnsson and E. Haavet, *Langsomt ble landet et velferdssamfunn*, pp. 55–59; S. I. Angell, *Den svenske modellen og det norske systemet: Tilhøvet mellom organisering og identitetsdanning i Sverige og Noreg ved overgangen til det 20. hundreåret*, Oslo: Det Norske Samlaget, 2002, p. 196.

43. P. Johansson, *Fast i det förflutna: Institutioner och intressen i svensk sjukför-säkringspolitik 1891–1931* (Lund, Sweden: Arkiv, 2003), p. 77. In 1909 the total number of fund members in Sweden was about ten times higher than in Norway.

44. In the proposition for enacting a public inquiry commission to the Norwegian Parliament in 1885, the problem of pauperism was mentioned with specific reference to the growth of the cities. Norwegian Parliament, Proposition No. 82, p. 1.

45. The result in Table 6.2 must be interpreted with some caution. In both countries the term "city" was a political and administrative concept meaning that a town had been given the formal rights of a city. This meant that some populated areas in both countries where not defined as cities. In table 6.1, also gas, water, electricity, and sanitary workers are included for both countries. See B. R. Mitchell, *European historical statistics 1750–1970*, p. 164.

46. This is not to say that 138,726 individuals were fund members in Sweden. Some persons might have been a member in more than one fund. This was probably the case also in Norway.

47. Arbetarförsäkringskommitténs betänkande III:6, pp. 26–28. Also see footnote 45 for information about the definition of the term "city."

48. Arbetareförsäkringskommitténs betänkande III:6, p. 21.

49. Arbetareförsäkringskommitténs betänkande III:6, pp. 26–28.

50. Z. Hermansson, *Oversigt*, p. 17.

51. Z. Hermansson, *Oversigt*, pp. 4, 17.

52. Ø. Bjørnsson and E. Haavet, *Langsomt ble landet et velferdssamfunn: Trygdens historie 1894–1994*, Oslo: Gyldendal, 1994, pp. 55–57.

53. S. I. Angell, *Den svenske modellen og det norske systemet*, p. 186

54. S. I. Angell, *Den svenske modellen og det norske systemet*, p. 196.

55. Norwegian Parliament, Minutes, 30 April 1897, pp. 516–18. See also A. L. Seip, *Sosialhjelpstaten blir til*, p. 99; Ø. Bjørnsson and I. E. Haavet, *Langsomt ble landet et velferdssamfunn*, pp. 56–59.

56. Arbeiderkommissionens Indstilling II, pp. 13–15.

57. Arbeiderkommissionens Indstilling II, p. 13. Also see Ø. Bjørnsson and E. Haavet, *Langsomt ble landet et velferdssamfunn*, p. 57.

58. S. Kuhnle, "The growth of social insurance programs in Scandinavia," pp. 141–45; Ø. Bjørnsson and E. Haavet, *Langsomt ble landet et velferdssamfunn*, p. 57.

59. K. Englund, *Arbetarförsäkringsfrågani i svensk sjukförsäkringspolitik 1884–1901*, (Uppsala: Acta Universitatis Upsaliensis, 1976, pp. 45–47.

60. P. Johansson, *Fast i det förflutna*, pp. 63–64.

61. Norwegian Parliament, Proposal no. 23, 1893, pp. 21–22; Norwegian Parliament, Minutes, 30 April 1897, pp. 517–18; P. Johansson, *Fast i det förflutna*, p. 63.

62. Arbeiderkommissionens Indstilling II, p. 53; Norwegian Parliament, Proposition 1893:23, p. 30–32.

63. Arbeiderkommissionens Indstilling II, pp. 21, 35.

64. Arbeiderkommissionens Indstilling II, pp. 21–22: Norwegian Parliament, Proposition 1896:30, p. 4

65. Swedish Parliament, Propostion 1891:25.

66. In both countries, the voting rules were in favour of the farmers. In Sweden, they held a strong position in the Second Chamber, and, since the Swedish constitution established that both chambers had to agree upon political decisions, farmers could easily stop proposals they disliked.

67. W. Mjånes, *Sjukeforsikringssaka i det politiske ordeskiftet*, Hovedfaguppgave, University of Bergen, 1975, pp. 134–40.

68. Norwegian Parliament: Minutes: 30 April 1897, p. 500
69. Norwegian Parliament: Minutes: 30 April 1897, p.546; slso see Trond Nordby, *Det moderne gionnombruddet i bondesamfunnet: Norge 1870–1920*, Oslo: Universitetsforlaget, 1991, pp. 131–33.
70. Norwegian Parliament: Minutes: 30 April 1897, pp. 502–03.
71. Swedish Parliament: Second Chamber: Minutes, 8 May 1891, pp. 17–20; First Chamber: 8 May, pp. 21–32.
72. Swedish Parliament: Statsutskottets utlåtande no. 12 a, 1884, p. 51.
73. Swedish Parliament: Second Chamber: Minutes, 27 February 1884, pp. 20–21.
74. Swedish Parliament: Proposition 1891:25, p. 1; Norwegian Parliament: Indst. O. XIII. 1896, p. 12. The rate of exchange was 1:1.
75. In Sweden, this was also the case in the pensions question, see Å. Elmér *Folkpensioneringen i Sverige: Med särskild hänsyn till ålderdomspensioneringen*, Lund, Sweden: Arkiv: 1960, pp. 18–23.
76. For a similar conclusion for Finland, see O. Kangas, *The politics of social rights*, pp. 154–155.
77. P. Johansson, *Fast i det förflutna*, pp. 39–47.
78. P. Johansson, "Självstyre och statligt inflytande: Relationen mellan sjukkasserörelse och stat under 1890-talet," *Arbetarhistoria*, 23(1), 17.
79. E.g., collecting statistics.
80. Standing committee of supply.
81. Swedish Parliament: Statsutskottets utlåtande, no. 7: 1897, p. 91. However, in 1899 the subsidy limit was increased.
82. P. Johansson, *Fast i det förflutna*, p.121.
83. L. M. Salamon, "Of market failure," p. 38.
84. P. Johansson, "Haunted by the past: Continuity and change in Swedish sickness insurance policy from the 1880s to the 1930s," in E. Carroll and L. Eriksson, eds., *Welfare politics cross-examined: Eclecticist analytical perspectives on Sweden and the developed countries*, Amsterdam: Aksant Academic Publishers, 2006.

7 Housing Charities and the Provision of Social Housing in Germany and the United States of America, Great Britain, and Canada in the Nineteenth Century

Thomas Adam

University of Texas at Arlington

PHILANTHROPY IN A TRANSATLANTIC WORLD

Daniel T. Rodgers reminds us that "historical scholarship bends to the task of specifying each nation's distinctive culture, its peculiar history, . . ."[1] Following this tradition, sociologists and historians concerned with the emergence of private and public social-welfare systems all too often claim that there are distinct paths taken by Germany, Great Britain, the United States, and Canada. While Germany is widely identified with a state-centered approach, the United States is considered to be the epitome of private responsibility. Such assumptions are based on studies that focus on the post–World War II era but exclude the nineteenth and early twentieth centuries.[2] This chapter will suggest that on both sides of the Atlantic, philanthropy was an essential force in dealing with the social challenges of industrialized presocial-welfare-state societies. Furthermore, it will be shown that London developed the first models of social-housing provision and, therefore, became the destination for German and American social reformers throughout the second half of the nineteenth century.[3]

While English historians, in particular, are accustomed to the notion that British social reform was based upon German precedents,[4] the role Great Britain played in the formulation of German housing reform has long been overlooked. However, long before British social reformers began to look towards Imperial Germany for ideas about social-welfare reform, German and American social reformers travelled to the British metropolis to study its social housing enterprises. When they returned home, they took with them ideas, detailed descriptions, plans, and transcripts of interviews, thereby "exporting" these models to German and American cities. In the process of this transnational and transatlantic transfer of social housing models, transformations and mutations occurred due to the preconceptions of the individuals involved, the legal system back home, and already existing indigenous institutions.[5] Furthermore, Henry I. Bowditch's investigation of London's philanthropic housing enterprises was highly selective in that he considered only the housing enterprises of Sir Sydney Waterlow and Octavia Hill as appropriate for replication back home in Boston but not the housing trust of his fellow American George Peabody. German reformers, such as Paul Felix Aschrott, followed suit and highly exaggerated the success and importance of Waterlow's housing enterprise in order to convince their fellow citizens back home to follow in Waterlow's footsteps.[6]

Although American, German, and Canadian cities certainly differed with regard to their political organization, cities such as Boston, New York, Toronto, Leipzig, and London shared a common social-political culture, in which social housing was considered a private responsibility. In all three countries, state officials were involved in housing reform by advocating private action; state legislatures intervened in the housing market by creating legal provisions that allowed the creation of limited-dividend companies in the United States and Canada and cooperatives in Germany.[7] However, local and federal governments did not become agents of housing construction before World War I. It was groups of philanthropists that formed limited-dividend companies and cooperatives in order to provide affordable housing for working-class families. Such enterprises could include anywhere between ten and two hundred male and female philanthropists who shared an understanding of philanthropy: that it was to benefit both the giver and the recipient. They insisted, however, that the return should be limited. George Smalley, in his biography of Sir Sydney Waterlow, pointed out that the "usual return for house property" was not "5 but 7 or 10 per cent."[8] And Volker Then argued, in his study of the development of German and English train companies and railroad systems during the industrialization, that two-digit dividends were normal until the 1860s.[9] The decision of a capitalist to invest his money into a company that decided to pay him a maximum of three to seven percent dividends indicates that he voluntarily gave up the claim to a potentially higher return.

Since such limited-dividend companies would not fit modern models of philanthropy, for instance, the definition of the nonprofit sector proposed by Helmut K. Anheier and Lester Salamon,[10] it is essential for this chapter to clarify my understanding of philanthropy. Anheier and Salamon's structural-operational definition of the nonprofit sector, as Susannah Morris points out, "conflates organizational form with purpose so that organizations which can distribute surpluses to their members, such as friendly societies or model dwellings companies, are assumed by definition to be unable to operate in the public interest."[11] Even though these nineteenth-century model-housing companies were considered philanthropic enterprises by contemporaries, social scientists, at the end of the twentieth century, consider them for-profit companies. These model housing companies, however, "were "philanthropic" in so far as their primary aim was not profit maximization per se but the development of a system of provision which could solve the housing problem."[12] Since the philanthropists/shareholders involved in limited dividend companies were convinced that, within a capitalist economy, the only promising way of helping the poor was to create economically self-sustaining enterprises that provided healthy and affordable housing, I have chosen to conceptualize the integration of market mechanisms into social housing enterprises (limited-dividend companies and cooperatives) as a form of collective philanthropy. In these cases, wealthy citizens provided funding for the purpose of house construction on the premise that they would receive a small return on their invested capital. They further had to relinquish their control over the invested resources to a board that, in consultation with all philanthropist-investors, decided about the economic activities of the company. Collective philanthropy involved often a hundred and more bourgeois citizens who had limited financial resources but wanted to be included into the philanthropic establishment of their respective municipalities. Philanthropy was certainly useful for establishing social contacts and relationships, but it furthermore was an essential tool for the making of the bourgeoisie.[13] Participation in philanthropic institutions, showing concern for the common good, and involvement in social betterment were important elements of climbing the social ladder and of being included into the local bourgeoisie. For women, furthermore, involvement into philanthropic activities opened doors into the public sphere and allowed them to escape the narrow world of the middle- and upper-class household. Philanthropy thus provided a basis for women's integration into nineteenth-century male-dominated bourgeois society. It offered niches in which women could become board members, run enterprises, and represent these enterprises to the outside world, all under the guise of philanthropic and charitable work that was considered a women's sphere for most of the nineteenth century.[14]

HOUSING THE URBAN POOR

The provision of affordable and hygienic (physically and morally) working-class housing was perceived by contemporary social reformers and philanthropists as the most important aspect of the social question. Living in unhealthy conditions was seen as not only leading to disease but also to the very destruction of the foundations of society. Therefore, the amelioration of housing standards was necessarily connected with the improvement of society as a whole. To put it simply, in the perception of nineteenth-century upper-class citizens, a well-housed worker was a happy worker and, as such, was unlikely to join radical, working-class movements.[15] This perception was not unjustified, at least in Germany, given the dreary living conditions of the working class. Answering Minna Wettstein-Adelt's challenge, "Tell me where you live and I'll tell you who you are," Alfred Kelly has suggested that, "most of the workers could not even be called human."[16] However, for a long time bourgeois and upper-class citizens were not even aware of the conditions of working-class housing. A nineteenth-century German conservative newspaper remarked that "we were better acquainted with the condition of life of the half savage African tribes than with those of our own people."[17] Thus, in order to solve the social housing question, American, British, and German reformers had to enter the world of the urban working class. Before travelling abroad, all individuals involved in the social housing reform in Boston, New York, and Leipzig travelled into parts of their own city they had never visited before—the slums and the working-class districts. Collecting information about the actual living conditions of working-class families and then publishing it was the first step towards a solution to the social question. Impressionistic accounts of the living conditions of the lower classes, often written by aspiring social reformers, social critiques, and volunteers or "friendly visitors," who would visit working-class families in their homes and make decisions about granting financial assistance, represented the first step in identifying the problem.[18]

Shortly after, statistical studies, first on the level of the municipalities and later on the federal level, complemented these impressionistic accounts and clarified the scope and extent of the housing problem. In 1886, Ernst Hasse, professor of statistics at the University of Leipzig and director of the Statistical Office of the city of Leipzig, published his major study *Die Wohnungsverhältnisse der ärmeren Volksklassen in Leipzig* (*The Housing Conditions of the Lower Classes in Leipzig*).[19] This path-breaking study was one of the first comprehensive analyses of the housing market in a major city of the German Empire. Hasse provided extensive material regarding the limited availability of small single-family apartments, the increase in rent over a period of fifteen years, a comparative analysis of incomes earned by workers and the rent for working class apartments, and so on. This study gave Leipzig's philanthropic establishment a statistical basis for action.

Furthermore, Hasse's study was included in the impressive two-volume edition *Die Wohnungsnoth der ärmeren Klassen in deutschen Großstädten* (*The Shortage of Tenements for the Lower Classes in German Cities*), which was published as volume XXXI of the *Schriften des Vereins für Socialpolitik* (*Publications of the Society for Social Policy*) in 1886.[20] This volume provided, for the first time, on the national level an empirical basis for any future steps of philanthropists and social reformers to solve the housing problem for the lower classes. Chapters on the living conditions of working-class families in Bochum, Chemnitz, Osnabrück, Crefeld, Dortmund, Essen, Berlin, Elberfeld, Breslau, and Leipzig offered insight into topics such as rent increases, hygienic standards, architectural structures, and density of the population. "The importance of this investigation for housing reform throughout Germany can," as Jan Palmowski rightly pointed out, "hardly be overestimated, for it ended over a decade of silence" on the topic of housing reform.[21] However, this volume did not cause state action but instead encouraged private engagement in the housing field. Housing foundations, limited-dividend companies, and housing cooperatives sprouted all over Germany as a result of this initiative. Yet the articles compiled in this volume were written by social scientists and socially concerned civil servants, not by architects. In 1902, the *Handbuch der Architektur* (*Handbook of Architecture*) dedicated one volume to the construction of *Arbeiterwohnungen* (apartment buildings and houses for working-class families).[22] This handbook became the standard work for architects and historians of architecture ever since. In more than 30 volumes, architects and city planners discussed every element of urban life, from the organization of waste disposal to the construction of sidewalks. Using various examples of already existing philanthropic housing foundations and companies as well as housing cooperatives and factory settlements, the authors of this particular volume discussed all aspects of housing the poor: size of the apartments, placing of the apartment buildings and houses in relation to the place of work and the cities, hygienic organization of the apartments, including different technologies for waste disposal and lavatories, etc.

In the beginning, American bourgeois citizens were as unaware of the dreadful living conditions in the immigrants and working-class neighborhoods as their German counterparts. New York and Boston's social reformers and philanthropists' first expedition was to tour the slums and collect data regarding the housing of the lower classes. In the 1870s, the newly founded Board of Health of the City of Boston took a lead in investigating the living conditions of the city's poor. In April 1873, the board began a large-scale inspection of tenement housing in Boston that provided public awareness of the housing problem.[23] Already in early 1870, Henry Ingersoll Bowditch, after he was elected chairman of the Massachusetts State Board of Health, toured the slums of Boston. The tenements he saw left him appalled and he resolved to achieve betterment. On December 1, 1870, Bowditch embarked on a second trip into Boston's slums. Bowditch reported this second encounter with lower-class housing in his published "Letter from the Chairman of the State Board of Health" hoping that wealthy Bostonians would feel compelled to engage in housing reform.[24] To underline the importance of such reform, Bowditch included a graphic description of one particular Boston home:

> This cellar room is scarcely high enough for us to stand erect. One can easily almost touch each of the four sides while standing in the centre of it. The floor is dark, dirty and broken; apparently wet also, possibly from the tide oozing up. Two women are there, commonly, yet rather tawdrily dressed, and doing nothing but apparently waiting, spider-like, for some unlucky, erring insect to be caught in their dusty but strong meshes. Tubs, tables, bed-clothes and china ware, are huddled incongruously together. Our guide strikes a match by the stove, and then opens

a door into a so-called bed-room. It is a *box*, just large enough to hold a double bed. No window is in it, no means of ventilation, save through the common room up the cellar steps. The bed is of straw, covered only by a dirty blanket. Everywhere is the picture of loathsome filth. The stench, too, of the premises is horrible, owing to long accumulated dirt, and from the belching up of effluvia from solutions of dark mud, reeking with sewage water from the city drains and water-closets. It is difficult for us to breathe in the tainted atmosphere.[25]

Bowditch's next move was to call for a housing reform under the guidance of philanthropically minded Bostonians. Since he did not know exactly how to proceed in reforming the housing of the working class, he made an extensive trip to London, where he spent six months.[26] In the last quarter of the nineteenth century, the British metropolis attracted a large number of social reformers from various countries, including the United States and Germany, who wanted to study the economic organization and architectural design of the city's working-class housing projects as well as their impact on social and moral standards.[27] London's social housing enterprises were held in high regard among German and American housing reformers. Between 1841 and 1914, wealthy Londoners had created about 43 social housing enterprises, which by 1914 provided about 36,000 tenements for the poor. The Peabody Trust and Waterlow's Improved Industrial Dwellings Company were in a top position among these enterprises with regard to the number of constructed apartment units.[28]

Peabody and Waterlow's housing enterprises represent examples of individual and collective philanthropy, respectively, and differing societal visions. George Peabody, a U.S. businessman, donated £500,000 for the creation of a social housing trust, which was to direct any profit back into the trust. Rejecting the suggestion of Lord Shaftesbury, the director of the Society for Improving the Condition of the Labouring Classes, to donate £75,000 to this existing social housing enterprise (collective philanthropy), Peabody established his own social housing trust, because he wanted to be remembered in history for his own philanthropic endeavor.[29] Though Peabody enlisted the help of a committee in deciding how to use the money, he was the sole financier of this trust so as to maintain ultimate control over it. Since he possessed enormous financial resources,[30] he was also in a position to finance such a philanthropic enterprise on his own. Not every nineteenth-century philanthropist was as wealthy as Peabody and therefore was limited in his decision with regard to the extent and character of their philanthropic engagement.

Sydney Waterlow, on the other hand, founded a limited-dividend company in which the profits (limited to 5%) were distributed among the various shareholders. Both enterprises represent different strategies and views about how to solve the housing question. Peabody's housing project intentionally excluded capitalist methods (profit for the investor). Clearly, he was not convinced that the housing problem could be solved using capitalist means. It is an admission that the market cannot provide solutions to all problems. Conversely, Waterlow tried to resolve the housing problem using market forces. By allowing for profit, though substantially reduced, Waterlow attempted to combine market economy and social welfare.

THE TRANSATLANTIC ADMIRATION
FOR PHILANTHROPY AND 5 PERCENT

From the outset, Henry I. Bowditch remained very skeptical about the success of Peabody's housing trust. Although he recognized the successes of the Peabody Trust in elevating the social and moral conditions of their tenants, he concluded in his "Letter from the Chairman" that the Peabody buildings "are almost purely philanthropic" and therefore they do not represent a potential way to solve the housing problem. "The percentage for rents on the original outlays is so small that no capitalist would desire to employ his surplus funds without greater gain."[31] Bowditch, who believed that philanthropy was supposed to provide a net gain for both sides—the one who gives and the one who takes—and that the main function of model tenements was to spark imitation, concluded that "we must look in other directions as for plans and successful experiments in which philanthropy and capital join hands."[32] Disappointed about the perceived limited success of the Peabody endeavour, Bowditch quoted the critique of an anonymous London capitalist on the Peabody buildings:

> Excellent as they are, how much more good would have been done, and how many more families would have been placed in healthful homes if instead of building these large and expensive tenements, the fund had, in part at least, been spent in the purchase of suitable sites which might have been let at such low ground-rent as to induce capitalists to build houses according to certain specifications to be laid down by the trustees.[33]

Rejecting the concept of a housing trust and "pure philanthropy," Bowditch found his perfect solution to the housing problem in Waterlow's Improved Industrial Dwelling Company.[34] Although a similar undertaking had been organized in Boston during the 1850s, Bowditch remarked that "nothing has ever been carried out on so grand a scale as by the above named company in London."[35] In 1871, Bowditch convinced 163 wealthy Bostonians to form the Boston Co-operative Building Company (BCBC), which was capitalized at $200,000 and *limited to 7 percent dividends*. The $200,000 was divided into 8,000 shares at $25 a piece. Four thousand nine hundred fifty-two shares were immediately bought, and the remaining shares were sold within the subsequent four years. By 1873, the foundation had $182,000 capital stock, which increased to $207,000 by 1875. In 1900, twenty-nine years after the foundation of the BCBC, the capital stock was valued at $292,000.[36] It should be noted that by 1912, 204 individuals owned 6,211 shares, while 65 trustees held 5,008 shares (in addition to three firms that held 393 shares and one corporation holding 68 shares).[37] These figures are indicative of the large number of individuals active in the financing of the company and of the fact that the shares were not sold but passed onto trustees in the last wills and testaments of the original shareholders. By 1912, it owned five building complexes with a total of 332 apartments: the East Canton Street Estate had 154 tenements, the Clark Street estate 19, Thatcher Street Estate 54, Harrison Avenue Estate 84, Massachusetts Avenue Estate 21.[38]

The BCBC was not the only philanthropic housing enterprise that was founded in an American city using the model of Waterlow's "Philanthropy and Five Percent" model, but it was the first one. According to the twenty-third annual report of the BCBC, housing reformers and philanthropists from "New York, Philadelphia, and Baltimore, and one even from Europe, who all commended the general plan and construction of our houses and the facilities they afford for housing the poor,"[39] visited and studied this enterprise. Henry I. Bowditch and the BCBC served as a conduit for the translation of Waterlow's "Philanthropy and Five Percent" into the American social, cultural, and economic context. While the basic elements of Waterlow's model remained unchanged, the limitation on the dividends was *raised slightly to 7 percent*. This modified concept of the limited dividend company was copied in many American cities during the 1880s and 1890s. After Alfred Treadway White had followed in Bowditch's footsteps and travelled to London in 1872, he established the Home Buildings in Brooklyn in 1877. These buildings were in their architecture the "first literal translation of the Waterlow type."[40] Three years later, White was able to convince fellow wealthy New Yorkers such as Cornelius Vanderbilt to found the Improved Dwellings Association as a limited-dividend company. In 1896, White finally initiated the establishment of another limited-dividend company—the City and Suburban Homes Company. Headed by Elgin R. L. Gould, this company "was destined to become the largest builder of model tenements in the country."[41] Philanthropists and housing reformers in Washington and Cincinnati followed in these footsteps and created similar housing enterprises that were based on the Americanized version of Waterlow's project.[42]

The goal of the Boston Co-operative Building Company was to build "small houses that should contain suites of apartments isolated, so far as may be possible, under a common roof." The first project was the creation of ten small houses in which "the floors should be so arranged as to accommodate one family only, and thus, though the entrance and the stairway will be in common, there being only one set of occupants on each floor, a tolerable degree of privacy will be secured."[43] This first project is not only an economic translation of the Waterlow model to Boston but also a translation of

Waterlow's views on the ideal apartment structure (heightened levels of privacy for individual families). The founders of the BCBC acknowledged their indebtedness to Waterlow by naming two of the streets within the housing projects "Waterlow Street" and "Sydney Place."[44]

Like their American counterparts, German social reformers studied London's social housing models and introduced them into German cities during the second half of the nineteenth century. In contrast to the shipment of philanthropic models via the Atlantic, German social reformers and philanthropists had, however, not only a much shorter distance to overcome but also enjoyed the help of a member of the British royal family, who assumed the function of a transmitter in this transnational transfer. In July 1862, Alice, the second daughter of Queen Victoria, married Duke Ludwig of Hesse-Darmstadt and moved from London to the provincial city of Darmstadt.[45] In 1863, she began visiting hospitals and, influenced by Florence Nightingale, founded the Hülfsverein (Committee of Aid) and the Alice Society for Aiding the Sick and Wounded. It was her goal to establish a network of aid associations run by women for the entire duchy of Hesse-Darmstadt after the blueprint of Baden, Bavaria, and Prussia.[46] In addition to her engagement in the field of medical care, Alice also considered the education and professional training of women as an essential part of her reform agenda. After 1872, however, Alice dedicated her life to housing reform along the lines of Octavia Hill's house management system.

Octavia Hill advocated not the creation of new tenement buildings but the cleaning up of old ones and reeducation of the tenants. It was her fundamental conviction "that the poor needed example, tuition, inspiration and guidance in their everyday lives more than they needed charity."[47] However, Hill would never have been able to realize her ideas without the support of John Ruskin, who had been her employer and her friend. Ruskin, a fierce critic of capitalism, who felt "temperamentally unable to deal personally with poor people," encouraged Octavia Hill to develop her ideas about the improvement of living conditions for poor families.[48] After Ruskin inherited a considerable amount of money from his father in 1864, he approved Hill's plan of purchasing three houses "in one of the worst courts of Marylebone."[49] While Hill prepared a plan to clean up these apartment buildings and to implement her system of friendly rent collecting and close supervision and education of the tenants, Ruskin concerned himself with the financial aspects of this undertaking. Perhaps following Waterlow's idea of combining philanthropy with market mechanisms, he convinced Hill that "it would be far more useful if it could be made to pay; that a working man ought to be able to pay for his own house; that the outlay upon it ought, therefore, to yield a fair percentage on the capital invested."[50] Hill agreed and went ahead to purchase the three houses in her immediate neighbourhood for £750.

To manage the tenements in these three houses, Hill set up a management system that included weekly visits and contacts with the tenants, insistence of punctual payment of rent, and strict standards of cleanliness for the communal parts of the houses and the tenements. In order to avoid overcrowding of the apartments, Hill encouraged big families to rent two rooms instead of just one "and for these much less was charged than if let singly."[51] Subletting was strictly prohibited and tenants who did not follow the instructions of Hill and her lady visitors or damaged the building were evicted.

Hill, like Waterlow, was never interested in small-scale reform projects. She hoped to develop a model that could be followed by many others and would lead to a tremendous improvement of living conditions for London's poor. Therefore, Hill began publishing articles in several English journals to propagate her ideas and successes beginning already in 1866. The first article was published in the *Fortnightly Review* in November 1866 but was actually sent to this journal six month earlier—in May 1866 (only about one year after Hill had bought the three houses).[52] Many more articles followed in *Macmillan's Magazine* and the *Nineteenth Century*. These articles were later combined into the volume *Homes of the London Poor*, which was first published in London in 1875.[53] As a result of this publicity campaign, Hill found herself in charge of 5,000 to 6,000 houses after a couple of years. She had become an icon of housing reform, and she attracted visitors from all of continental Europe and North America. Hill's articles were reprinted in the *Journal de St. Petersbourg*, and Louisa Lee Schuyler, who had founded the State Charities Aid Association of New York (SCAA), organized the publication of Hill's *Homes of the London Poor* in New York in 1875. The copies of this 78-page work were sold by the SCAA for twenty-five cents each.[54]

During one of her visits to London, Alice arranged to meet Octavia Hill and to take incognito a tour of the social housing projects administered by Hill in 1876. Alice described her impressions from such a visit in a letter to her daughter: "With a charming excellent lady Miss Octavia Hill . . . I have been this morning in some of the very poor courts in London, garrets and streets . . . such quantities of little children and so many living in one dirty room. It was sad to see them—on one way, but beautiful to see how these ladies worked amongst them, knew them, did business with them. I have been trying to see as much and learn as much as possible of what is done for the poor in every way and have heard of such good and unselfish noble people . . ."[55] Impressed by the housing-management system of Octavia Hill, Alice entered into an exchange of letters with Hill to learn more about her concepts and visions. In late 1876, Alice finally inquired if Octavia Hill would give her permission to translate her book *The Homes of the London Poor* into German. Hill responded enthusiastically and even suggested that Alice should write an introduction to the German translation. With the arrangement of the translation of this book, Alice virtually occupied the position of a translator of Hill's methods into a German environment. This book appeared under the title of *Aus der Londoner Armenpflege* in 1878 in Wiesbaden and became quickly the most influential book on housing reform in Germany.[56] Housing reformers such as Wilhelm Schwab (Darmstadt) and

Gustav de Liagre (Leipzig) used the German translation of Hill's book as guidebooks in their attempts to establish social housing enterprises following her example.[57]

In 1883, Gustav de Liagre, inspired by the "tremendous success of Octavia Hill's endeavors in London,"[58] purchased, together with eleven friends, two buildings with 240 rooms in Leipzig. Like Hill, Liagre did not construct new buildings but purchased run-down buildings close to the inner city of Leipzig. He convinced eight men and three women to each contribute 5,000 marks to this enterprise by promising them a 4 percent return on their invested capital. He chose a building he was already acquainted with from his time as a friendly visitor (Armenpfleger) during the 1870s. After acquiring these tenement houses, Liagre insisted, like Hill, on basic improvements but did not add any new appliances. His goal was to provide healthy and affordable small tenements for poor families who had shared much larger apartments with other families before they entered his housing complex. Liagre insisted on weekly rent collection by lady visitors, compliance to certain cleanliness standards among the tenants, and the ban on subletting parts of these tenements. His enterprise received much attention among housing reformers in Leipzig (Emma Hasse, Therese Rossbach, and Herrmann Julius Meyer) and in other German cities. In his history of the *Verein zur Verbesserung der Kleinen Wohnungen* in Berlin (Association for the Improvement of Small Tenements in Berlin), Paul Felix Aschrott pointed out that it even influenced the housing reform in Berlin.[59] According to several sources, Liagre (Leipzig) and Schwab (Darmstadt) were probably the first German housing reformers to replicate Hill's management system in Germany. In contrast to Schwab, however, Liagre gave several public talks in many German cities and published accounts of his enterprise, thus publicly showing that it was possible to integrate Hill's method into the German social and economic environment.[60] Therefore, it was not Schwab but Liagre who was soon regarded as the expert on Hill's concepts. While Alice remained anonymous—she signed the introduction to the German translation of Octavia Hill's book just with "A"—Liagre became a public figure who gained extensive influence among philanthropists and housing reformers.

A few years later, German housing reformers began to travel to London to study Peabody, Waterlow, and Hill's projects firsthand. In 1884, Wilhelm Ruprecht published the first German scholarly account of housing reform in London under the title *Die Wohnungen der Arbeitenden Klassen in London* (*The Tenements of the Working Classes in London*).[61] Ruprecht, who aspired to take over his father's publishing company Vandenhoeck & Ruprecht,[62] went to London in October 1883 because an old friend of his father, Nikolaus Trübner, offered to employ Ruprecht for a year in the Oriental department of his London publishing house. However, after just a few weeks, Ruprecht was bored by the monotonous work in this enterprise. Therefore, he chose to dedicate much of his time during his one-year stay (1883–84) to the study of the housing conditions of London's working class instead. For this reason, Ruprecht interviewed individuals who were involved in the housing reform; he studied government publications such as reports and laws, as well as books such as *The Homes of the London Poor* and newspaper and journal articles (*Nineteenth Century, Times, Pall Mall Gazette, The Contemporary Review*, etc.). The result of this research became his aforementioned book, which was positively received by fellow social reformers and led directly to the formation of the *Göttinger Spar- und Bauverein* (Göttingen Building and Savings Society), which dominated social housing in Göttingen after 1900.[63]

In his work, Ruprecht provided an exhaustive overview over the housing problem in Great Britain's capital, the English laws concerning working-class housing, and the steps taken by Peabody, Waterlow, and Hill to improve the housing situation of working-class families. Writing for a German public, Ruprecht hoped that his descriptions of housing reform would convince politicians and philanthropists alike to tackle this social problem back home. Arguing that there were many parallels between London and Berlin's problems with regard to the housing of the urban poor, he intended to provide an account of possible solutions that had withstood the test of time.[64]

Ruprecht called for close collaboration between state and philanthropists—the state was expected to set up certain standards of housing (regulation regarding overcrowding, architectural standards, etc.) and the philanthropists were expected to follow in Peabody, Waterlow, and Hill's footsteps by financing affordable and hygienic apartment buildings. Believing that workers did not have the necessary financial means to found cooperatives, Ruprecht rejected the creation of housing cooperatives as unsuitable to solve the housing problem. Instead, Ruprecht argued in favour of philanthropic help for the poor in the realm of social housing. He further rejected the provision of housing by employers since not all of the urban poor worked in factories but in other sectors of the economy. The absence of factory housing in London confirmed his suspicion that factory villages could be created only in a rural setting and not in highly urbanized industrial centers.[65] Subsequently, Ruprecht felt that the Peabody Foundation, Waterlow's limited dividend company, and Hill's housing-management system offered the best ways for the housing of the working classes. By describing these three different approaches, Ruprecht highlighted the economic aspects of these enterprises, their architectural specifications, the intentions of the founders, and the outcome of these projects. The picture created in his account depicted Peabody, Waterlow, and Hill's enterprises as shining examples of what could be done if wealthy bourgeois would be willing to tackle the housing problem. While Ruprecht admired the sheer quantitative success of the Peabody Trust—24 million marks capital, about 4,400 tenements, and about 18,000 inhabitants by 1883—he shared the doubts of Bowditch and favoured Waterlow's Improved Industrial Dwellings Company.[66] However, his admiration was not unlimited since he pointed out that most of the people living in both the Peabody Trust and the Waterlow Company did not belong to the lower parts of the working class. He credited Hill with accomplishing exactly what Peabody and Waterlow's enterprises did not achieve.[67] In his eyes, only the combination of all three forms of philanthropy, with a dominance of the investment philanthropy model, would provide a viable social system to end the housing crisis of modern urban society. Like Bowditch, Ruprecht argued that causing imitation was to be the main task of philanthropic housing enterprises. Offering a limited annual return of about 5 percent seemed to provide an incentive that potentially would attract German investor-philanthropists to participate in such enterprises.

In the same year that Ruprecht's account of London philanthropic housing was published, Paul Felix Aschrott embarked on one of his study tours to London to collect information on the topic of housing reform in the British metropolis. Aschrott, a Prussian jurist with extensive interests in the housing of working-class families, went to London in July 1884 and remained there for more than a year.[68] The result of this research trip was the publication of his report, "Die Arbeiterwohnungsfrage in England" ("The Question about How to House the Working Class in England"), which was included in the already discussed volume *Die Wohnungsnoth der Ärmeren Klassen in Deutschen Großstädten und Vorschläge zu deren Abhülfe* published by the *Verein für Socialpolitik* in 1886. In 53 pages, Aschrott described the horrible living conditions of the London poor, focusing on the overcrowding of tenements, the existence of basement tenements, and the percentage of workers' incomes spent for rent. Using statistical methods, Aschrott pointed out that more than 88 percent of the working-class families paid more than one-fifth of their income in rent and that 46 percent of all tenants paid between 25 and 50 percent of their wages in rent.[69] He continued to analyze the causes of the crisis in working-class housing and the reactions of parliament and government towards this social problem. Discussing the Labouring Classes Lodging-Houses Act (1851), the Artizans' and Labourers' Dwellings Act (1868), and the Artizans' and Labourers' Dwellings Improvements Acts from 1875, 1879, and 1882, Aschrott pointed to the inherent flaws, especially in the last two legislations, which actually encouraged landlords to worsen the living conditions in their tenement buildings instead of improving them. Positively mentioned are the government loans for building societies that provide healthy tenements for working-class families and the introduction of workmen's trains, which were to transport workers from the suburbs into the city for affordable fares, thus exporting the problem of housing the poor from the city to the suburbs (Cheap Trains Act of 1883).[70]

After briefly discussing building societies, which enabled their members to purchase the houses in which they lived, Aschrott focused on the Peabody Trust, the Metropolitan Association for Improving the Dwellings of the Industrious Classes, the Improved Industrial Dwelling-Company, and the management system of Hill. His description of the Peabody Trust includes important observations of the paternalistic regime over its tenants. The majority of tenants were, according to Aschrott, trained workers and artisans who had steady jobs and a secure income. However, applicants with a weekly income of more than 30 shillings were not accepted as tenants.[71] The families living in the Peabody Buildings were not allowed to sublet rooms and had to comply with a certain set of rules. Every night at 11 p.m. the gas light would be turned off and the entrance gate to the building complex closed. Tenants possessed their own house keys, but they had to enter the building through one main entrance and thus were spotted, controlled, and noted by the doorman. Showing up drunk after 11 p.m. during the week and even on weekends resulted in immediate cancellation of the rental contract.[72]

After the Peabody Trust, Aschrott went on to discuss what he called the *Baugesellschaften mit humanitärem Charakter* (building societies with a humanitarian character). These building societies, the Metropolitan Association for Improving the Dwellings of the Industrious Classes and the Improved Industrial Dwelling-Company, differed from the Peabody Trust in that they expected an annual divided of 4 to 5 percent. Aschrott, however, considered them to be of humanitarian character since they were founded to improve the living conditions of the working poor and the dividend for the investors was limited. Aschrott concluded his report by suggesting that German housing reformers should consider the English experiences. He also pointed out that housing reform was the necessary basis for any other far-reaching social reform, thus mirroring the common assumption about the family as the basic cell of society and the home as the place where every social change has to begin.[73]

However, Aschrott was not only a prolific writer who resorted to theoretical discussions of what could be done; he was also a passionate practitioner who engaged in housing reform. In June 1888, Aschrott, together with the architect Alfred Messel and the banker Valentin Weisbach, founded the *Verein zur Verbesserung der Kleinen Wohnungen in Berlin* (Society for the Improvement of Small Tenements in Berlin). This housing society closely followed Waterlow's "Philanthropy and Five Percent" model since the bylaws stated the investors should receive an annual return of maximal 4 percent on their invested capital. Beginning in 1891, a number of bourgeois women joined the society and, following the example of Octavia Hill, took over the responsibility of weekly rent collecting and friendly visiting.[74]

From these examples it should become clear that American and German social reformers favoured collective philanthropy over individual philanthropy. Although Henry I. Bowditch and Wilhelm Ruprecht praised the Peabody Trust for its successes, they also pointed out that it was unsuitable for imitation. Only limited dividend companies, which promised a 5 percent return on the invested capital, were considered a viable tool for providing hygienic and affordable housing for working-class families. Ruprecht and Aschrott attempted to prove to their German audience that "Philanthropy and Five Percent" worked successfully. It is interesting to note that while Susannah Morris argues that they rarely reached a 5 percent dividend,

German nineteenth-century observers always argued that these companies reached their intended goal of guaranteeing a 5 percent annual return.[75] These views of German social reformers were echoed by American social reformers such as Marcus T. Reynolds. In his study *The Housing of the Poor in American Cities*, Reynolds pleaded for the improvement of the housing conditions of the poor by adapting "Philanthropy and Five Percent." Arguing from an economic point of view, Reynolds remarked that wealthy citizens could only be persuaded to invest their money in such housing enterprises "if it is clearly demonstrated that a dividend of at least five per cent. will be forthcoming." Housing reform, in Reynolds's interpretation, was not about charity but about the provision of healthy and affordable living space for a fair rent which would allow for a limited return on the invested capital. The guarantee of a 5 percent return would set an example and attract other wealthy citizens to participate in these enterprises or to set up their own social housing projects.[76]

Housing reformers on both sides of the Atlantic hoped to create a network of housing companies that would attract philanthropists and investors alike. However, most of the individuals who bought shares in limited-dividend companies, such as the Boston Co-operative Building Company or the Leipziger "Ostheim," a philanthropic housing enterprise founded by Therese Rossbach in 1898, behaved like philanthropists and not like capitalists. By behaving too philanthropically, these philanthropists defeated the goals of "Philanthropy and Five Percent" advocates. Even though the returns of the BCBC rarely reached their stated goal of 7 percent, shareholders held on to their shares and did not sell them. A 7 percent return was paid only between 1871 and 1875, but between 1876 and 1889 "dividends were stopped or reduced to three percent and earnings were invested." In the 1890s, dividends reached between 5 and 6 percent.[77] It is telling that despite these lower returns the investors maintained their involvement in the enterprises. Obviously, making money was not their main concern. This point is confirmed by the fact that the stockholders in these philanthropic companies never sold their shares. In the case of the BCBC, shares were transferable but not available for purchase or sale.[78] Further, we have clear evidence that many of the shares (44%) were passed on from the original stockholder to trustees (through last wills and testaments).[79] There was a tacit agreement (and in the case of the "Ostheim," a written agreement) that the shareholders agreed never to withdraw their support, regardless of the financial success of the venture. The founding agreement of the "Ostheim" even gives the institution the right to decide when, if ever, they were to repay the stockholders.[80] This eradicated, in the end, the differences between the limited-dividend companies and the housing trusts. Philanthropists provided the necessary funding in both cases and seemed not to expect revenue from it. If one measures the success of the limited-dividend company by the lofty goals of its inventors, it must be considered a failure since it failed to achieve what its proponents had most hoped for: the solution of a social problem with market forces and the imitation and widespread acceptance of this model within society. However, limited-dividend companies attracted the attention of many American and German social reformers and philanthropists who advocated the creation of similar enterprises in their countries. Between the 1870s and World War I, several limited-dividend companies were founded in American cities such as Boston, New York, Philadelphia, and Washington. And even in Germany, social reformers succeeded in integrating elements of the limited-dividend company into the emerging model of the saving and housing cooperative.

LIMITED-DIVIDEND COMPANIES AND COOPERATIVES

Although German social reformers praised the advantages of limited-dividend companies, a pure "Philanthropy and Five Percent" model did not become as popular in Germany as in the United States. German social reformers nevertheless succeeded in integrating the British model of "Philanthropy and Five Percent" into the earlier English import: the model of cooperatives.[81] When in 1845 Saxon entrepreneurs purchased new machines for their spinning factories back in Chemnitz, they were also in need of specialists who could set up these machines. By bringing these English mechanics to Chemnitz, the owners of the Chemnitz Aktienspinnerei unknowingly caused a transfer of ideas, since these mechanics happened to be members of the Rochdale Society of Equitable Pioneers. Just one year earlier, in 1844, a group of weavers and Owenite Socialists had founded this cooperative, which is considered the beginning of the modern British cooperative movement. Inspired by conversations with the English mechanics, four employees of the Chemnitz Aktienspinnerei decided to establish a consumer cooperative. This cooperative served as a model for subsequent cooperatives of various kinds: consumer, productive, and housing cooperatives first in Saxony and later in other German states.[82]

About the same time, the university professor and conservative Victor Aimé Huber visited England and observed the developing cooperative associations. After his return to Berlin, Huber organized, together with C. W. Hofmann and G. S. Liedtke, the *Berliner gemeinnützige Bau-Gesellschaft* (Berlin Communal Building Society) in 1847 to provide housing for lower-class families of the Prussian capital.[83] In the following years, Huber published a large number of books, pamphlets and journals in which he provided detailed descriptions of English cooperatives.[84] For Huber, the exploitation of the workers by greedy shopkeepers and unscrupulous landlords was at the heart of the social question. To end this exploitation was to transform the dependent and exploited consumer and renter into an independent consumer and renter who co-owned the shops and tenement buildings by establishing consumer and housing cooperatives. Convinced that the workers would never be able to accomplish this on their own, Huber demanded that the state take a lead in this transformation of society by providing extensive subsidies to the prospective cooperative movement.[85] These ideas seem to have had a decisive influence on Ferdinand Lassalle, the founder of the General German Worker's Association (ADAV), which was the first political organization of the working class in the German states.[86] Hermann Schulze-Delitzsch shared Huber's and Lassalle's general enthusiasm and advocacy for the cooperative movement but as a Liberal insisted they would have to operate without any state interference and government subsidies. In 1867, Schulze-Delitzsch brought what was to become the first law regarding cooperatives before the parliament of the Northern German Confederation. This law recognized the cooperative as a legitimate form of business among other economic enterprises (like shareholder companies) and prepared the soil for the tremendous success story of cooperatives (producers, housing, savings, and agricultural cooperatives) in nineteenth- and twentieth-century German economic life.[87]

In 1889, the German Reichstag passed the law about limited liability of cooperatives.[88] This law ended the fear that in the case of bankruptcy the members of a cooperative would be held responsible with all their property and savings. The 1889 law decreed that the members of a cooperative were liable only up to the amount of their share (200–300 marks) in this enterprise. This law encouraged the combination of self-help with philanthropy, since German housing and savings cooperatives were often combined into one cooperative, which allowed not only its members but also outsiders (mostly wealthy middle-class citizens who wanted to become involved in philanthropy and housing reform but did not have sufficient financial means to establish their own housing enterprise) to open an account with this institution.[89] This situation may appear odd to those who associate cooperatives with self-help organizations. Their original constitution, though, was such that wealthy people took the initiative in creating cooperatives. In most cases, lawyers, architects, or civil servants initiated and administered the cooperatives. The lower classes were involved as members but did not have any say over the development of the cooperatives. The *Dresdner Spar und Bauverein* (Dresden Savings and Building Cooperative), founded in 1898, demonstrates this mixture of collective philanthropy and cooperative self-help.[90] Each member had to buy one share (300 marks) and, at the same time, this cooperative received financial support from leading members of Dresden's bourgeoisie and nobility, and from several enterprises. King Albert of Saxony contributed 1,500 marks, the distinguished businessman Carl Eschebach gave 10,000 marks, and Villeroy and Boch 2,000 marks each year for a period of ten years. The cooperative was, obviously, not financed by the shares sold to its members alone but also by donations from wealthy bourgeois of Dresden.[91]

Of equal importance was the linking of housing cooperatives with credit unions, first practised in Hanover, which integrated the "Philanthropy and Five Percent" concept with the concept of "Cooperation" and "Self-Help."

The *Hannover Spar und Bauverein* (founded in 1885) differed from earlier cooperatives in three ways: (1) It did not produce housing units that could be bought by its members over time. Instead, the buildings remained permanently in the possession of the cooperative; (2) it combined self-help with financial assistance from wealthy citizens by merging the housing cooperative with a credit union; (3) it adopted the legal provision of limited liability. This latter provision encouraged middle- and upper-class citizens to invest money into housing cooperatives since they were assured that they did not risk their entire fortunes in case the enterprise defaulted.[92] It was this legal change that allowed for the successful combination of "Philanthropy and Five Percent" with "Self-Help" in Germany. The Hanover housing cooperative established a credit union which guaranteed a 4 percent annual return on all deposits. These deposits, however, were considered loans not savings and provided the housing company with the necessary financial support to build affordable and hygienic apartment buildings for working-class families.[93] The merger of housing cooperatives with credit unions sparked imitation in Berlin, Göttingen, Leipzig, Dresden, and many other German cities.[94]

This unique German model of social housing allowed socially concerned citizens with limited resources to participate in the housing reform by simply depositing their money with the credit unions attached to housing cooperatives and purchasing shares of these enterprises. In contrast to British and American limited-dividend companies, these credit unions were, at least until the Second World War, even more successful in guaranteeing a steady return of 4 percent and, furthermore, underwent a democratization process in which they "freed" themselves from bourgeois domination. During the 1920s, German cooperatives slowly but surely evolved into self-help institutions, which were no longer dependent on bourgeois support and fell under the leadership of boards that were dominated by working-class and mostly Social Democratic members. These cooperatives received favourable loans and subsidies from local governments and state agencies (*Mietzinssteuer*) in order to produce apartments for low-income groups. In many cases, they aligned themselves closely with the Social Democratic Party and engaged in large-scale building projects, which were envisioned to reflect a socialist agenda.[95]

Before 1914, however, social reformers and proponents of building cooperatives, such as Wilhelm Ruprecht, rejected any state support for cooperatives. Arguing against Paul Lechler's suggestion of large-scale state support for the creation of housing cooperatives, Ruprecht suggested that the solution of the housing question could not be achieved by simply providing a large number of apartments.[96] Rejecting the idea that the housing question was only an economic issue, Ruprecht was convinced that it had also a social and cultural dimension. Although workers had to be in a position to afford the apartments built for them, they also needed, according to Ruprecht, education and guidance in how to maintain their apartments. In Ruprecht's view, many workers seemed not to care for keeping the apartments in good shape and therefore could not be entrusted with such improved housing conditions. These ideas closely reflect Octavia Hill's opinion on working-class housing. Only after working-class families were trained to maintain a certain level of cleanliness and care did Hill consider them worthy of better housing conditions. Both Ruprecht and Hill saw the housing question as a financial and educational project that could be accomplished only over a longer period of time.

Notwithstanding Ruprecht and Hill's arguments, indirect and to a certain degree unintentional state support for housing cooperatives in Germany began already during the 1890s. The creation of state-sponsored pension and accident-at-the-workplace insurance systems (Otto von Bismarck's Social Laws) produced an accumulation of capital from insurance contributions. The law, which established Germany's pension system in 1889, created thirty-one regionally organized insurance districts (*Landesversicherungsanstalten*, LVA), which were in charge of collecting the insurance contributions from employers and employees (each had to pay one-half of the state-mandated insurance fee). At the end of 1907, it has been estimated that all thirty-one insurance districts together had accumulated roughly 1,400 million marks.[97] According to the law, the insurance districts were required to invest the money so that it would benefit the insured workers. Section 129 of the law allowed investing the money in real estate and the construction of apartment buildings as long as it benefited the working classes.[98] It should be noted, however, that the lawmakers did not envision that this new law would result in state intervention into the housing market. It was an unintended and, from both sides (state and cooperative movement), unexpected outcome that derived from the simple need of investing the accumulated capital in a secure way.[99]

By 1900, the *Landesversicherungsanstalt Oberfranken und Mittelfranken*, for instance, invested one fifth of their capital in government and railroad bonds, about half of their capital in loans to municipalities and foundations, and the remaining amount in mortgages.[100] Initially, housing cooperatives were very reluctant to accept the loans offered by the regional insurance districts. Civil servants who were in charge of these new insurance districts toured the country and offered their financial support to the boards of housing cooperatives. In 1891, the Braunschweig housing cooperative was the first in Germany to accept such loans. Now that the ice was broken, housing cooperatives increasingly relied on the loans of the pension-insurance system. In 1894, housing cooperatives received about 2 million marks in loans. Only five years later, in 1899, this amount had climbed to 52 million marks at an interest rate of 2½ to 4¼ percent.[101] By 1907, about one-seventh of the total capital of the pension-insurance system, which stood at 195,752,982.08 marks, was loaned to housing cooperatives, foundations, employers and municipal housing companies for the construction of apartment buildings for working-class families.[102] Of over 195 million marks, housing cooperatives received 125 million marks (63.7 percent) at an average interest rate of 3.2 percent.[103]

The insurance districts intervened in housing production by formulating clear expectations with regard to the structure and the quality of the planned working-class housing projects and by offering loans with an interest rate that was about 0.5 percentage points below the interest rate charged by banks and savings cooperatives (according to Helmut W. Jenkis, the interest rate around 1900 was 3.75 percent).[104] The Landesversicherungsanstalt für Thüringen, for instance, made it a condition that apartments financed with its loans had to consist of at least one living room, two chambers of at least eight square metres, and a kitchen. The minimum size of such an apartment was to be at least 48 square metres. Lavatories and bathrooms had to be directly attached to the apartment and not to be shared with other tenants. Rooms were to have a minimum height of 1.75 metres.[105] If cooperatives were willing to comply with these requirements, the regional insurance district in Thuringia was willing to provide loans up to ninety percent of the estimated construction costs.[106]

Since the number of housing cooperatives increased tremendously after the law about limited liability was introduced, the antisocialist law lapsed in 1890, and the Social Democratic movement recognized cooperatives as an essential part of the working-class movement during the 1890s. The need for more funding led to a legal change in the law about pension insurance in 1899. Section 164 of the revised law permitted insurance districts to invest all of their accumulated capital in the construction of working-class housing. Furthermore, the new law no longer required that the loans should be used only for the benefit of working-class families but expanded the group of people who were to benefit from the funding provided by the insurance system.[107] By 1911, about 68 percent of the total capital used by cooperatives in the state of Saxony to construct apartment buildings came from the Landesversicherungsanstalt Sachsen. This financing scheme made the housing cooperatives the most important providers of social housing in the first half of the twentieth century.[108] Even after 1918, cooperatives and philanthropic housing enterprises produced a much higher number of apartments than the municipalities. And even after 1945, East German housing cooperatives remained an integral part of social housing provision. During the 1970s, about half of all apartment buildings (*Plattenbauten*) constructed in East German cities such as Dresden, Leipzig, and Halle were financed and built by housing cooperatives, and not the state, for budgetary reasons. Since the ambitious building program of the East German government strained the state budget, East Germany's economic planners looked for ways to maximize the output. Leaving a larger share of housing production to the housing cooperatives had the advantage that these cooperatives were required by law to provide 8 percent of the total construction costs of apartment buildings while the remaining part was to be financed by loans provided by the Central Bank of East Germany and subsidies handed out by the government.

Housing cooperatives accumulated their financial share by requiring their members to account for 15 percent of the construction costs of their prospective apartments. Cooperative members had to pay an entrance fee of at least 300 marks, and in their free time they had to work on the construction sites of their future homes for about 750 to 900 hours (valued at 1,250 and 1,900 marks). With the increasing mechanization of housing production, cooperative members increasingly chose to pay the equivalent amount of money instead of working at the construction sites.[109]

German housing cooperatives differed significantly from housing cooperatives in New York and Boston. The Boston Co-operative Building Company and similar undertakings in the United States were founded on the principles of "Philanthropy and Five Percent." They were in name only cooperatives since they excluded any form of self-help from the outset. Interestingly, it was not an American housing cooperative that attempted to combine both philanthropy and self-help for the first time in North America but a Canadian one. In February 1912, representatives of Toronto's Civic Guild, the Toronto branch of the Canadian Manufacturers' Association, the Board of Trade, the University Settlement, the National Council of Women, and the City Council announced their intention to create a limited-dividend housing company for Toronto. This company was to be founded upon the principles of "Philanthropy and Five Percent" as well as "cooperation." Furthermore, it was expected that the municipality would provide some support for this private company. In early 1913, the white-wear merchant and spokesman of Toronto's business community, George Frank Beer, announced the founding of the Toronto Housing Company (THC) to the public. The company was to build settlements inside the city limits but close to industrial centres. The apartments were to be rented to tenants who "would own a minimum of five shares (at $50 per share)."[110] Following the example of Henry Vivian's Ealing Tenants Ltd. in West London, the very first British copartnership housing scheme, outsiders were allowed and invited to purchase shares. The dividends were limited to 6 percent.[111] The initial plan of selling shares to tenants on a copartnership basis distinguished the THC from philanthropic housing companies in American cities but brought them closer to European models of social housing in both Great Britain and Germany. While many of the British and German housing cooperatives were in fact financed by tenants and outside investors alike, no such enterprises emerged in Boston, New York, or Philadelphia.[112] However, the copartnership/coownership idea was abandoned before construction of the first apartment buildings began. Shirley Campbell Spragge considers the quick dismissal of this innovative concept puzzling but points to the criticism voiced by the District Labour Council (DLC) in March of 1912. The DLC condemned "the project as useless to workers because few could pay the $250 down payment required . . ."[113]

After the idea of co-ownership was abandoned, Beer and his supporters engaged in a fund-raising campaign to secure CAD$100,000 before incorporation of the THC. One important supporter in this "Better Housing Campaign" was Lady Gibson, the wife of Lieutenant Governor Sir John Gibson. She organized a "large meeting of ladies" to advertise and sell the shares. Within a short period of time, CAD$104,000 had been subscribed by 170 individuals and companies.[114] All of the shareholders came from Toronto's most exclusive social circles. As Hurl pointed out: "The efforts of the promotion committee attracted a high calibre of supporters. The prominence of shareholders, by Beer's own admission, was such that a list of their names 'might almost be taken as a copy of *Who's Who* in Toronto.'"[115] Among its directors and company advisors were "influential businessmen and dedicated reformers" such as Alexander Laird (banker), Thomas Roden (manufacturer), Edward Kylie (professor of history at the University of Toronto), Sir Edmund Osler (president of the Dominion Bank of Canada), Joseph Flavelle (manufacturer), and Zebulon Lash (lawyer). The THC, however, was still in need of financial support from outside sources to finance its construction program.

Beer strongly believed that the provision of housing could not be considered a task of the state. In an article for the *Garden Cities and Town Planning Magazine*, Beer stated, "While town planning is essentially a matter for the action of governments, housing by its nature is a field in which private initiative should be most influential."[116] He continued to demand that "governments should remove obstacles to development, should direct aid and supervise but should not enter into competition in a matter which is so largely of individual choice and requirement."[117] While rejecting state intervention and state interference, Beer appreciated and welcomed governmental and municipal support for private actions to solve the housing problem. Therefore, he asked Lash to develop a bill that would guarantee financial support of the THC by the Ontario government. This draft "proposed that the provincial government should issue bonds to supply eighty per cent of the company's financial needs."[118] However, this bill did not win the support of Conservative Premier Sir James Whitney and was rejected. About one year later, in April 1913, the Ontario legislature passed the Act to Encourage Housing Accommodation in Cities and Towns, named the Hanna Act after Provincial Secretary William J. Hanna. The Hanna Act enabled companies incorporated to provide housing for the lower classes at moderate fees to petition municipal councils to guarantee its bonds up to 85 percent.[119] If such a company wanted to receive this support, it was obliged to allow the city council to appoint one board director. Furthermore, the city council would have to be consulted in the selection of land and the construction plans. The dividends of such a company had to be limited to 6 percent.[120]

After passage of the law, Beer petitioned the Toronto City Council for financial support. By 1913, the THC had sold a little over 2,000 shares and accumulated about CAD$104,000. This made the THC eligible for CAD$550,000 worth of bonds from the city of Toronto. In 1913, the city council "guaranteed CAD$550,000 of THC five per cent gold mortgage bonds, redeemable in forty years."[121] This move enabled the company to begin construction of its first project, Spruce Court. The Hanna Act, which followed very closely a similar provision enacted earlier in Nova Scotia, set Toronto apart from both its European and American counterparts, where a municipal guarantee of bonds was unknown until World War I.[122] The decision of Toronto philanthropists to ask for municipal financial support and the willingness of Toronto's city council to grant such support distinguishes Toronto's social philanthropy within the transatlantic world of philanthropy. While it was common that city councils granted financial assistance for the establishment of museums, art galleries, and libraries already before 1900, they were much more unlikely to extend their financial support into the field of social housing. After World War I, local and federal governments assumed partial responsibility for the provision of social housing for returning soldiers and working-class families. This transition was certainly not inevitable but the result of changing political circumstances and renegotiated social contracts.

CONCLUSION

London attracted social reformers and philanthropists from Europe and North America who came to observe and study philanthropic enterprises that provided affordable and healthy housing for working-class families. To these observers, Waterlow's "Philanthropy and Five Percent" model possessed great attraction since it represented a form of philanthropy that was based on the idea of mutual benefit for the giver and the receiver. German and American observers alike were fascinated by this idea and propagated these concepts in theory and practice in their home countries. However, neither American nor German philanthropists followed Waterlow's model to the letter. Americans insisted that a profit limited to 5 percent was too low to attract fellow citizens to invest in limited dividend companies, and Germans, facing an already emerging but largely still dormant cooperative movement, realized that the combination of the cooperative model with the "Philanthropy and Five Percent" model would produce a powerful instrument in the battle against social destruction. Both countries which with an eye on the twentieth century often are considered diametrically opposed when it comes to the provision of social welfare, were not so far apart in the nineteenth century as the admiration for the synthesis of philanthropy and market mechanisms shows.

Furthermore, German and American social reformers and philanthropists shared an admiration for Octavia Hill's house-management system. In both countries, Octavia Hill's writings were published and widely distributed. As a result, Octavia Hill associations emerged in various cities, and the majority of housing companies and housing trusts adopted Hill's method of "friendly visiting and rent collecting" as a standard practice in the administration of these housing projects. In sum, housing reformers on both sides of the Atlantic saw the housing question not as a purely economic problem but rather as a problem with a social and cultural dimension. Supervision and guidance for the working-class tenants, therefore, had to go hand in hand with the improvement of the living conditions by providing better and affordable housing for the deserving poor.

NOTES

1. Daniel T. Rodgers, *Atlantic crossings: Social policy in a progressive age*, Cambridge, MA: and London, UK: The Belknap Press of Harvard University Press, 1998, p. 2.
2. Wolfgang Ismayr, "Cultural federalism and public support for the arts in the Federal Republic of Germany," in Milton C. Cummings and Richard S. Katz, eds., *The patron state: Government and the arts in Europe, North America, and Japan*, New York/Oxford: Oxford University Press 1987.
3. Thomas Adam, "Transatlantic trading: The transfer of philanthropic models between European and North American cities during the nineteenth and early twentieth centuries," *Journal of Urban History*, 28, 328–51.
4. E. P. Hennock, *British social reform and German precedents: The case of social insurance 1880–1914*, Oxford: Clarendon Press, 1987; Günter Hollenberg, *Englisches Interesse am Kaiserreich: Die Attraktivität Preussen-Deutschlands für Konservative und Liberale Kreise in Grossbritannien 1860–1914*, Wiesbaden: Franz Steiner Verlag, 1974, pp. 222–42.
5. For the concept of cultural transfer, see Matthias Middel, ed., "Kulturtransfer und vergleich, "*Comparative*, 10(1), Leipzig: Leipziger Universitätsverlag 2000. For a very brief historigraphical overview on cultural transfer, see Florian Steger and Kay Peter Jankrift, "Einleitung," in Florian Steger and Kay Peter Jankrift, eds., *Gesundheit—Krankheit: Kulturtransfer medizinischen Wissens von der Spätantike bis in die Frühe Neuzeit*, Cologne/Weimar/Vienna: Böhlau, 2004, pp. 3–5. See also Stefan Berger and Peter Lambert, "Intellectual transfers and mental blockades: Anglo-German dialogues in historiography," in Stefan Berger and Peter Lambert, eds., *Historikeredialoge: Geschichte, Mythos und Gedächtnis im deutsch-britischen kulturellen Austausch 1750–2000*, Göttingen: Vandenhoeck & Ruprecht, 2003, pp. 11–18.
6. Paul Felix Aschrott, "Die arbeiterwohnungsfrage in England," in *Die Wohnungsnoth der ärmeren Klassen in deutschen Großstädten und Vorschläge zu deren Abhülfe: Gutachten und Berichte herausgegben vom Verein für Socialpolitik*, Leipzig: Verlag von Duncker & Humblot, 1886, pp. 97–146.
7. David C. Hammack, "Patronage and the great institutions of the cities of the United States: Questions and evidence, 1800–2000," in Thomas Adam, ed., *Philanthropy, patronage, and civil society: Experiences from Germany, Great Britain, and North America*, Bloomington: Indiana University Press, 2004, p. 80.; Thomas Adam, *125 Jahre Wohnreform in Sachsen: Zur Geschichte der sächsischen Baugenossenschaften (1873–1998)*, Leipzig: Antonym, 1999), pp. 37–39.
8. George Smalley, *The life of Sir Sydney Waterlow Bart., London apprentice, lord mayor, captain of industry, and philanthropist*, London: Edward Arnold, 1909, p. 68.
9. Volker Then, *Eisenbahnen und Eisenbahnunternehmer in der Industriellen Revolution: Ein preußisch/deutsch-englischer Vergleich*, Göttingen, Germany: Vandenhoeck & Ruprecht, 1997, pp. 315ff.

10. Lester Salamon and Helmut K. Anheier, "In search of the nonprofit sector. I: The question of definitions," *Voluntas* 3, 125–51.
11. Susannah Morris, "Changing perceptions of philanthropy in the voluntary housing field in nineteenth- and early-twentieth-century London," in Adam, *Philanthropy, patronage, and civil society*, p. 142.
12. Susannah Morris, "Market solutions for social problems: Working-class housing in nineteenth-century London," *The Economic History Review*, LIV(3), 529.
13. Bernard Harris, *The origins of the British welfare state: Society, state and social welfare in England and Wales, 1800–1945*, Palgrave Macmillan, 2004, pp. 60–61; Edward Palmer Thompson, *The making of the English working class*, New York: Pantheon Books, 1964; Thomas Mergel, "Die bürgertumsforschung nach 15 jahren," in *Archiv für Sozialgeschicht,e* 41, 515–38; Peter Lundgreen, ed., *Sozial- und Kulturgeschichte des Bürgertums: Eine Bilanz des Bielefelder Sonderforschungsbereichs (1986–1997)*, Göttingen, Germany: Vandenhoeck & Ruprecht, 2000.
14. Frank K. Prochaska, *Women and philanthropy in nineteenth-century England*, Oxford: Clarendon Press 1980; Anne M. Boylan, *The origin of women's activism: New York and Boston 1797–1840*, Chapel Hill and London: The University of North Carolina Press, 2002, p. 54; Kathleen D. McCarthy, *Noblesse oblige: Charity and cultural philanthropy in Chicago, 1849–1929*, Chicago and London: The University of Chicago Press, 1982; Thomas Adam, "Ein schritt in die bürgerliche öffentlichkeit? Frauen und philanthropische wohnprojekte im transatlantischen raum des 19. jahrhunderts," in *Ariadne*, 42, 24–31.
15. Helmut W. Jenkis, *Ursprung und Entwicklung der gemeinnützigen Wohnungswirtschaft: Eine wirtschaftliche und sozialgeschichtliche Darstellung*, Bonn: Domus-Verlag/Hamburg: Hammonia-Verlag, 1973, pp. 231–35.
16. Alfred Kelly, ed., *The German worker: Working-class autobiographies from the age of industrialization*, Berkeley/Los Angeles/London: University of California Press, 1987, p. 29.
17. Adelheid Popp, *The autobiography of a working woman*, Westport, CT: Hyperion Press, 1983, p. 10.
18. For New York, see Jacob August Riis, *How the other half lives: Studies among the tenements of New York*, New York: Charles Scribner's Sons, 1917. For Riis, see the introduction by Donald N. Bigelow in Jacob A. Riis, *How the other half lives: Studies among the tenements of New York*, New York: Hill & Wang 1957, pp. vii–xiv. For Leipzig, see H. Mehner, "Der haushalt und die lebenshaltung einer leipziger arbeiterfamilie," *Jahrbuch für Gesetzgebung, Verwaltung und Volkswirthschaft im Deutschen Reich*, 11, 301–34. See also Thomas Adam, "Wohnarchitektur und wohnalltag in Leipzig vom kaiserreich zur republik," in *Leipziger Kalender 2001*, Leipziger: Leipziger Universitätsverlag, 2001, pp. 92–94.
19. Ernst Hasse, *Die Wohnungsverhältnisse der ärmeren Volksklassen in Leipzig*, Leipzig: Duncker & Humblot, 1886. See also Ernst Hasse, *Die Stadt Leipzig in hygienischer Beziehung*, Leipzig: Duncker & Humblot, 1892.
20. *Die Wohnungsnoth der ärmeren Klassen in deutschen Großstädten und Vorschläge zu deren Abhülfe: Gutachten und Berichte herausgegeben im Auftrage des Vereins für Socialpolitik.* Zweiter band, Leipzig: Verlag von Duncker & Humblot, 1886.
21. Jan Palmowski, *Urban liberalism in imperial Germany: Frankfurt am Main, 1866–1914*, Oxford: Oxford University Press, 1999, p. 221; Nicholas Bullock and James Read, *The movement for housing reform in Germany and France, 1840–1914*, Cambridge/New York: Cambridge University Press, 1985, pp. 63–70.

22. *Entwerfen, Anlage und Einrichtung der Gebäude. Des Handbuches der Architektur* Vierter Teil. 2. Halb-band: *Gebäude für die Zwecke des Wohnens, des Handels und Verkehres.* 1. Heft: *Wohnhäuser.* Von Karl Weissbach, Stuttgart: Arnold Bergsträsser Verlagsbuchhandlung A. Kröner, 1902, pp. 223–80.
23. David M. Culver, *Tenement house reform in Boston, 1846–1898*, PhD thesis, Boston University, 1972, pp. 94–95.
24. Henry Ingersoll Bowditch, "Letter from the chairman of the state board of health, concerning houses for the people, convalescent homes, and the sewage questions," in *Second Annual report of the State Board of Health of Massachusetts January 1871*, Boston: Wright & Potter, State Printers, 1871, pp. 182–243.
25. Ibid., p. 191.
26. He compiled his observations of the London philanthropic housing scene in the already quoted "Letter from the chairman," pp. 182–243.
27. See Thomas Adam, "Transatlantic trading: The transfer of philanthropic models between European and North American cities during the nineteenth and early twentieth centuries," *Journal of Urban History*, 28, 328–51.
28. Morris, *Private profit and public interest*, pp. 60–61.
29. Morris, "Changing perceptions of philanthropy," p. 150.
30. During his lifetime, Peabody donated money to both American and English philanthropic causes. He gave $1.5 million to found the Peabody Institute at Baltimore, MD; $250,000 to establish the Peabody Institute in Peabody., MA; $150,000 to create the Peabody Museum of Natural History and Natural Science at Yale University; $150,000 to establish the Peabody Museum of Archaeology and Ethnology at Harvard University; $140,000 to found the Peabody Academy of Science in connection with the Essex Institute at Salem, MA; and $ 3.5 million (Peabody Education Fund) for the promotion of education in the South.
31. Bowditch, "Letter from the chairman," p. 198.
32. Ibid., p. 198.
33. Ibid., p. 199.
34. Ibid., pp. 201–10.
35. Ibid., p. 202. For this earlier housing experiment, see Charles Eliot Norton, "Model lodging-houses in Boston," *Atlantic Monthly*, 5, 673–80. Lawrence Vale mentions this project only briefly in his account of Boston public housing. See Lawrence J. Vale, *From the Puritans to the projects: Public housing and public neighbors*, Cambridge, MA/London: Harvard University Press, 2000, p. 63.
36. David M. Culver, *Tenement house reform in Boston, 1846–1898*, PhD thesis, Boston University, 1972, pp. 144–45; Robert Treat Paine, "The housing conditions in Boston," *The Annals of the American Academy of Political and Social Science*, XX, 125; *The first annual report of the Boston Co-operative Building Co. with the Act of Incorporation and By-Laws*, Boston, 1872, p. 3; *Third annual report of the Boston Co-Operative Building Company*, Boston, 1874, p. 10; *Twenty-Ninth annual report of the Boston Co-Operative Building Company*, Boston, 1900, p. 20.
37. *Forty-first annual report of the Boston Co-Operative Building Company*, Boston, 1912, p. 8.
38. *Forty-first annual report of the Boston Co-Operative Building Company*, Boston, 1912.
39. *Twenty-third annual report of the Boston Co-Operative Building Company*, 1894, p. 12.
40. Richard Plunz, *A history of housing in New York City: Dwelling type and social change in the American metropolis*, New York: Columbia University Press, 1990, p. 89.

41. Ibid., p. 101; *First annual report of the City & Suburban Homes Company; Four decades of housing with a limited dividend company*, Federal Housing Administration, Division of Economics and Statistics.
42. Eugenie Ladner Birch and Deborah S. Gardner, "The seven-percent solution: A review of philanthropic housing, 1870–1919," *Journal of Urban History*, 7, 403–38; Edith Elmer Wood, *Recent trends in American housing*, New York: The Macmillan Company, 1931, pp. 206ff.; Robert B. Fairbanks, "From better dwellings to better community: Changing approaches to the low-cost housing problem, 1890–1925," *Journal of Urban History*, 11, 321; Robert B. Fairbanks, *Making better citizens: Housing reform and the community development strategy in Cincinnati, 1890–1960*, Urbana and Chicago: University of Illinois Press, 1988, pp. 35–36.
43. *First Annual Report* (BCBC), pp. 3–4.
44. Christine Cousineau, *Tenement Reform in Boston, 1870–1920, philanthropy, regulation, and government assisted housing*, The Society for American City and Regional Planning History, the Working Paper Series 1990, p. 8.
45. Gerard Noel, *Princess Alice: Queen Victoria's forgotten daughter*, London: Constable, 1974); Eckhardt G. Franz, "Victorias Schwester in Darmstadt: Großherzogin Alice von Hessen und bei Rhein," in Rainer von Hessen, ed., *Victoria Kaiserin Friedrich (1840–1901): Mission und Schicksal einer englischen Prinzessin in Deutschland*, Frankfurt/New York: Campus Verlag, 2002, pp. 80–93; *Alice Grand Duchess of Hesse, Princess of Great Britain and Ireland: Biographical sketch and letters*, New York/London: G. P. Putnam's Sons, 1884.
46. For the emergence of these women's associations, see Jean Quartaert, *Staging philanthropy: Patriotic women and the national imagination in dynastic Germany, 1813–1916*, Ann Arbor: The University of Michigan Press, 2001.
47. Enid Gauldie, *Cruel habitations: A history of working-class housing 1780–1918*, London: Allen & Unwin, 1974, p. 214.
48. Nancy Boyd, *Josephine Butler, Octavia Hill, Florence Nightingale: Three Victorian women who changed their world*, London and Basingstoke: The Macmillan Press, 1982, pp. 107–08.
49. Octavia Hill, "Organized work among the poor; Suggestions founded on four years' management of a London court," *Macmillan's Magazine*, XX, 219.
50. Octavia Hill, "Cottage property in London," *The Fortnightly Review*, VI, 682.
51. Hill, "Organized work among the poor," p. 220.
52. Hill, "Cottage property in London," p. 681.
53. Octavia Hill, *Homes of the London poor*, 2nd ed., London: Macmillan and Company, 1883. For her other writings, see *The befriending leader: Social assistance without dependency. Essays by Octavia Hill edited and with an introduction by James L. Payne* (Sandpoint, ID: Lytton Publishing Co., 1997); *Extracts from Octavia Hill's "Letters to fellow-workers" 1864 to 1911 compiled by her niece Elinor Southwood Ouvry*, London: The Adelphi Book Shop, 1933; *House property & its management: Some papers on the methods of management introduced by Miss Octavia Hill and adapted to modern conditions*, London: George Allen & Unwin, 1921.
54. Octavia Hill, *Homes of the London poor*, New York: Publications of the State Charities Aid Association No. 8, 1875; Robert H. Bremner, "'An Iron Scepter twined with Roses': The Octavia Hill System of Housing Management," *Social Service Review*, 39, 227; Anthony S. Wohl, *The eternal slum: Housing and social policy in Victorian London*, London: Edward Arnold, 1977, p. 181. For the introduction of the Octavia Hill house-management system into the United

States, see Daphne Spain, "Octavia Hill's philosophy of housing reform: From British roots to American soil," *Journal of Planning History*, 5, 106–25.
55. Letter quoted after Noel, *Princess Alice*, pp. 221–22. See also Darley, *Octavia Hill*, pp. 161–62.
56. Darley, *Octavia Hill*, pp. 166–71; Noel, *Princess Alice*, pp. 222, 230; *Alice Grandduchess of Hesse*, pp. 358–59
57. For Schwab, see *Stadtarchiv Darmstadt: Schwab, Wilhelm 1816–1891*. For Liagre, see Thomas Adam, *Die Anfänge industriellen Bauens in Sachsen*, Leipzig: Quadrat Verlag, 1998, pp. 27–28.
58. Gustav de Liagre, "Ein versuch zur beschaffung guter wohnungen für arme in Leipzig," in: Ernst Hasse, *Die Wohnungsverhältnisse der ärmeren Volksklassen in Leipzig*, Leipzig: Duncker & Humblot, 1886, p. 95.
59. Felix Paul Aschrott, *25 Jahre gemeinnützige Tätigkeit für Kleinwohnungen: Zum 25 jährigen Bestehen des Vereins zur Verbesserung der kleinen Wohnungen in Berlin*, pp. 5–6.
60. Gustav de Liagre, *Wohnungen für Unbemittelte: Vortrag des Herrn G. de Liagre aus Leipzig gehalten am 4. mai 1888 auf Veranlassung Ihrer Majestät der Königin von Sachsen als Protektorin des Johannesvereins in Dresden*, Leipzig: Bibliographisches Institut, 1888; Gustav de Liagre, *Wohnungen für Unbemittelte: Vortrag von Gustav de Liagre. Öffentlicher Abend der "Sozial-Wissenschaftlichen Vereinigung" in Leipzig, am 21. November 1896*, Leipzig: Verlag von O. de Liagre, 1896; Gustav de Liagre, "Ein versuch zur beschaffung guter wohnungen für arme in Leipzig," *Die Wohnungsnoth der ärmeren Klassen in deutschen Großstädten und Vorschläge zu deren Abhülfe. Gutachten und Berichte herausgegeben im Auftrage des Vereins für Socialpolitik*, Leipzig: Verlag von Duncker & Humblot, 1886, pp. 383–88.
61. Wilhelm Ruprecht, *Die Wohnungen der arbeitenden Klassen in London: Mit besonderer Berücksichtigung der neueren englischen Gesetzgebung und ihrer Erfolge*, Göttingen. Germany: Vandenhoeck und Ruprecht's Verlag, 1884.
62. Wilhelm Ruprecht, *Väter und Söhne. Zwei Jahrhunderte Buchhändler in einer deutschen Universitätsstadt*, Göttingen, Germany: Vandenhoeck & Ruprecht, 1935.
63. Ibid., pp. 203–05; Wilhelm Ruprecht, "Der spar- und Bauverein, E.G.m.beschr. Haftpflicht in Göttingen," *Die Spar- und Bau-Vereine in Hannover, Göttingen und Berlin*, pp. 95–101; Ruprecht, "Gesunde Wohnungen," pp. 89–96.
64. Ruprecht, *Die Wohnungen der arbeitenden Klassen in London*, p. III.
65. Ibid., p. 100–01.
66. Ruprecht, *Die Wohnungen der arbeitenden Klassen in London*, pp. 102–06.
67. Anthony Wohl, in contrast to Ruprecht, argued that even though Hill reached a poorer class of tenants than the model dwelling companies and Peabody's housing trust, she failed to reach "the very poor who remained the hard core of the slum problem right into the twentieth century." Quoted after Harris, *The origins of the British welfare state*, p. 133.
68. Hauptstaatsarchiv Düsseldorf, Bestand Gerichte Rep. 11, No. 1474 vols. III, IV; Universitätsarchiv Leipzig, Phil. Fak. Prom. 4196.
69. Paul Felix Aschrott, "Die arbeiterwohnungsfrage in England," *Die Wohnungsnoth der ärmeren Klassen in deutschen Großstädten und Vorschläge zu deren Abhülfe: Gutachten und Berichte herausgegeben vom Verein für Socialpolitik*, Leipzig: Verlag von Duncker & Humblot, 1886, pp. 97–146.
70. Ibid., pp. 96–125.
71. The income limit of 30 shillings per week was somewhat above the contemporary estimates of poverty. In 1887, Charles Booth defined his "poverty line" in the following terms: "By the word "poor" I mean to describe those who

have a fairly regular though bare income, such as 18 to 21 shillings a week for a moderate family, and by "very poor" those who fall below this standard, whether from chronic irregularity of work, sickness or a large number of young children." Charles Booth, "The inhabitants of Tower Hamlets [School Board Division]: Their condition and occupations," *Journal of the Royal Statistical Society*, 50, 328. This regulation, by the way, is a very common arrangement in nineteenth-century philanthropic housing enterprises and trusts. Herrmann Julius Meyer's housing trust in Leipzig, for instance, accepted only those workers as tenants who had an income of 800 to 1,800 marks. If the tenants' income exceeded the maximum allowed under that rule, they were asked to move out from this housing trust. At the same time, Meyer and Bowditch were united in their opinion that it was not their task to house the poorest of the poor but only a "middle strata" of the working class. Heinrich Geffken and Chaim Tykocinski, *Stiftungsbuch der Stadt Leipzig*, Leipzig, Bär & Hermann, 1905, p. 686.

72. Aschrott, "Die arbeiterwohnungsfrage in England," pp. 130–32.
73. Aschrott, "Die arbeiterwohnungsfrage in England," p. 146.
74. [Paul Felix] Aschrott, *25 jahre gemeinnütziger Tätigkeit für Kleinwohnungen. Zum 25 jährigen Bestehen des Vereins zur Verbesserung der kleinen Wohnungen in Berlin*, n.p., n.d., pp. 5–10.
75. Morris, "Market Solutions for social problems," p. 538; Ruprecht, *Die Wohnungen der arbeitenden Klassen in London*, pp. 105–06; Paul Felix Aschrott, "Die arbeiterwohnungsfrage in England," p. 133.
76. Marcus T. Reynolds, *The housing of the poor in American Cities: The prize essay of the American Economic Association for 1892*, Baltimore: Press of Guggenheim, Weil & Co., 1893, p. 107.
77. Robert Treat Paine, "The housing conditions in Boston," *The Annals of the American Academy of Political and Social Science*, XX, 125.
78. *Sixteenth Annual Report* (BCBC), p. 22.
79. *Forty-First Annual Report* (BCBC), p. 8.
80. StadtArchiv Leipzig, Kap. 35 Nr. 748, Geschäftsbericht des Vereins Ostheim Leipzig für das Jahr 1904, p. 61.
81. Thomas Adam, "Der plagwitzer konsumverein (1884–1933): Die stellung des plagwitzer konsumvereins in der deutschen konsumvereinsbewegung,," *Leipziger Kalender 2002*, pp. 210–11; Carl Launer, *Die Konsumgenossenschaftsbewegung im Freistaate Sachsen*, Bad Dürrenberg, Germany: Drei-Kreis-Verlag, 1932, pp. 7–35.
82. Thomas Adam, "Der plagwitzer konsumverein (1884–1933): Die stellung des plagwitzer konsumvereins in der deutschen konsumvereinsbewegung," *Leipziger Kalender 2002*, pp. 210–11; Carl Launer, *Die Konsumgenossenschaftsbewegung im Freistaate Sachsen*, Bad Dürrenberg: Drei-Kreis-Verlag, 1932, pp. 7–35. For the Rochdale society, see Brett Fairbairn, "Self-Help and philanthropy: The emergence of cooperatives in Britain, Germany, the United States, and Canada from mid-nineteenth to mid-twentieth century," in Thomas Adam, ed., *philanthropy, patronage, and civil society: Experiences from Germany, Great Britain, and North America*, Bloomington: Indiana University Press, 2004, p. 56; Beatrice Webb, *Die britische Genossenschaftsbewegung*, Leipzig: Duncker & Humblot, 1893; Robert Wilbrandt, "Der sozialismus der redlichen pioniere von Rochdale," *Die Arbeit*, 1924, pp. 160ff.
83. Rudolf Elvers, "Huber, Victor Aimé," *Allgemeine Deutsche Biographie*, vol. 13, Leipzig: Duncker & Humblot, pp. 249–58. See also Rudolf Elvers, *Victor Aimé Huber: Sein Werden und Wirken* in two volumes (Bremen, 1872 and 1874); Ingwer Paulsen, *Victor Aimé Huber als Sozialpolitiker: Ein Beitrag zur*

Geschichte christlich-konservativer Gesellschafts- und Wirtschaftsauffassung, Leipzig: Hinrichs, 1931.

84. Elvers, "Huber," p. 257; Victor Aimé Huber, *Genossenschaftliche Briefe aus Belgien, Frankreich und England*, Hamburg: Rauhes Haus, 1854; Huber, *Über die kooperativen Arbeiterassociationen in England; Ein Vortrag veranstaltete von dem Central-Verein für das Wohl der arbeitenden Klassen, gehalten am 23. Februar 1852*, Berlin: Hertz, 1852; Huber, *Die Rochdaler Pioneers: Ein Bild aus dem Genossenschaftswesen*, Nordhausen: Förstemann, 1867; Huber, *Sociale Reisebriefe aus England*, Leipzig: Mayer, 1861. See also Wilhelm Treue, ed., *Victor Aimé Hubers Ausgewählte Schriften über Socialreform und Genossenschaftswesen*, Frankfurt am Main: Keip, 1990, reprint).

85. Elvers, "Huber," p. 256.

86. Helga Grebing, *The history of the German labour movement: A survey*, London: Wolff, 1969, pp. 34–35, 43–44; William Harbutt Dawson, *German socialism and Ferdinand Lassalle*, London and New York: S. Sonnenschein & Co., 1899, pp. 114–32.

87. "Gesetz, betreffend die privatrechtliche stellung der erwerbs- und wirthschaftsgenossenschaften vom 27. März 1867," in *Gesetzsammlung für die Königlich Preußischen Staaten* Nr. 34, pp. 67ff.

88. *Reichsgesetzblatt* Nr. 11, "Gesetz, betreffend die Erwerbs- und wirthschaftsgenossenschaften vom 1. Mai 1889."

89. Helmut W. Jenkis, *Ursprung und Entwicklung der gemeinnützigen Wohnungswirtschaft*, p. 206; Walter Vossberg, *Die deutsche Baugenossenschafts-Bewegung*, Halle a. S., 1905, p. 124.

90. For a historical account of the Dresdner Spar- und Bauverein, see Thomas Adam, *125 Jahre Wohnreform in Sachsen: Zur Geschichte der sächsischen Baugenossenschaften (1873–1998)*, Leipzig: Antonym, 1999, pp. 91–101.

91. StadtArchiv Dresden, Y 346: Dresdner Spar- und Bauverein, Geschäftsbericht für das Jahr 1899.

92. Wilhelm Ruprecht, "Gesunde wohnungen," *Göttinger Arbeiterbibliothek*, 1(6), 81–96; Adam, *125 Jahre Wohnreform*, pp. 37–39.

93. Ibid.; F. Bork, "Der spar- und bauverein, E.G.m.beschr. Haftpflicht in Hannover," *Die Spar- und Bau-Vereine in Hannover, Göttingen und Berlin. Eine Anleitung zur praktischen Betätigung auf dem Gebiete der Wohnungsfrage* (Schriften der Centralststelle für Arbeiter-Wohlfahrtseinrichtungen Nr. 3), Berlin: Carl Heymann Verlag, 1893, pp. 1–93.

94. Ibid.

95. See Adam, *125 Jahre Wohnreform in Sachsen*; Klaus Novy, *Wohnreform in Köln: Geschichte der Baugenossenschaften*, Cologne, Germany: Bachem, 1986.

96. Ruprecht, "Gesunde wohnungen," pp. 95–96; Paul Lechler, *Wohlfahrtseinrichtungen über ganz Deutschland durch gemeinnützige Aktiengesellschaften: Ein Stück sozialer Reform*, Stuttgart, Germany: W. Kohlhammer, 1892.

97. Rudolf Albrecht, *Die Aufgabe, Organisation und Tätigkeit der Beamten-Baugenossenschaften im Rahmen der deutschen Baugenossenschafts-Bewegung*, Stuttgart, Germany: Verlag von Ferdinand Enke, 1911, p. 44.

98. Walter Vossberg, *Die deutsche Baugenossenschafts-Bewegung*, Halle a. S., 1905, pp. 55–56; Jenkis, *Ursprung und Entwicklung der gemeinnützigen Wohnunsgwirtschaft*, p. 208.

99. A. Grävell, Die baugenossenschafts-frage: Ein bericht über die ausbreitung die ausbreitung der gemeinnützigen bauthätigkeit durch baugenossenschaften, aktienbaugesellschaften, bauvereine etc. während der letzten 12 jahre, Berlin: Selbstverlag des Centralverbandes städtischer Haus- und Grundbesitzer-Vereine Deutschlands, 1901, pp. 262–92.

100. *100 Jahre Arbeiterrentenversicherung in Oberfranken und Mittelfranken 1891–1991*. Eine Dokumentation der Landesversicherungsanstalt Oberfranken und Mittelfranken, p. 57.
101. Vossberg, *Die deutsche Baugenossenschafts-Bewegung*, pp. 56–59.
102. Albrecht, *Die Aufgabe, Organisation und Tätigkeit der Beamten-Baugenossenschaften*, p. 44.
103. Ibid.
104. Jenkis, *Ursprung und Entwicklung der gemeinnützigen Wohnungswirtschaft*, p. 209.
105. Thüringische Landes-Versicherungsanstalt, *Grundsätze zur Förderung des Kleinwohnungsbaues*, Weimar, Germany: Hof-Buch- und Steindruckerei von Diersch & Brückner, 1915, pp. 8–9.
106. Ibid., p. 16.
107. Vossberg, *Die deutsche Baugenossenschafts-Bewegung*, pp. 59–60; Thomas Adam, *Arbeitermilieu und Arbeiterbewegung in Leipzig 1871–1933*, Cologne/Weimar/Vienna, Böhlau, 1999, pp. 190–96.
108. Adam, *125 Jahre Wohnreform*, pp. 38–39, 50–51; Karl Eichhorn, *Die sächsischen Baugenossenschaften*, Engelsdorf-Leipzig: C & M. Vogel, 1929, pp. 129–31; Rolf Greve, *Wohnungsgenossenschaften und ihre Konzernstrukturen*, Institut für Genossenschaftswesen der Universität Münster, p. 31; Vossberg, *Die deutsche Baugenossenschafts-Bewegung*, pp. 55f.; Jenkis, *Ursprung und Entwicklung der gemeinnützigen Wohnungswirtschaft*, pp. 208ff.
109. Adam, *125 Jahre Wohnreform*, p. 107ff; Thomas Adam, *Die sächsischen Wohnungsbaugenossenschaften in der DDR*, Leipzig: Antonym, 1997, pp. 24–26.
110. Lorna F. Hurl, "The Toronto Housing Company, 1912–1923: The pitfalls of painless philanthropy," *Canadian Historical Review*, LXV(1), 35.
111. Ibid.; Shirley Campbell Spragge, *The provision of workingmen's housing. attempts in Toronto 1904–1920*, MA thesis, Queen's University Kingston, 1974, p. 117.
112. For a discussion of the overlap between philanthropy and self-help in the European co-operative movement, see Brett Fairbairn, "Self-help and philanthropy: The emergence of cooperatives in Britain, Germany, the United States, and Canada from mid-nineteenth to mid-twentieth century," in Adam, *Philanthropy, patronage, and civil society*, pp. 55–78.
113. Spragge, *The provision of workingmen's housing*, p. 118.
114. Spragge, *The provision of workingmen's housing*, p. 119; Paul Adolphus Bator, *"Saving lives on the wholesale plan": Public health reform in the City of Toronto, 1900 to 1930*, PhD thesis, University of Toronto, 1979, p. 204; Hurl, "The Toronto Housing Company," p. 37.
115. Hurl, "The Toronto Housing Company," , p. 37. A list of the THC shareholders can be found in City of Toronto Archives, *Better housing in Canada "The Ontario Plan" First Annual Report of The Toronto Housing Company, Limited 1913*, pp. 23–24.
116. Quote after Spragge, *The provision of workingmen's housing*, pp. 125–26.
117. Ibid., p. 126.
118. Hurl, "The Toronto Housing Company," p. 38.
119. Spragge, *The provision of workingmen's housing*, pp. 143–44. See also Hurl, "The Toronto Housing Company," pp. 40–41; Sean Purdy, "Class, gender and the Toronto Housing Company, 1912–1920," *Urban History Review*, XXI(2), 79.
120. Ibid., p. 144.
121. Hurl, "The Toronto Housing Company," p. 41.
122. Spragge, *The provision of workingmen's housing*, pp. 139, 158.

8 "New Alignments"
American Voluntarism and the Expansion of Welfare in the 1920s[*]

Andrew Morris

Union College

In early 1926, Linton Swift, head of the American Association of Organizing Family Social Work (AAOFSW), warned his board of directors that they needed to commission a study of their agencies' provision of material relief to poor people. Expenditures for relief were increasing and "the societies themselves were at a loss for an explanation." The economy had rebounded from the recession of the early 1920s, and there seemed to be no obvious reason for the rising applications and costs. A statistical study produced later that fall by Ralph Hurlin of the Russell Sage Foundation confirmed the reports from the field that Swift had been receiving. Ninety-six agencies in thirty-seven large cities showed a 215 percent increase in the amount of relief granted since 1916. Hurlin broke down the causes for the increase: the number of families receiving relief had increased 63 percent, the population of the cities had grown by 19 percent, the cost of living had increased 57 percent, and the average grants had increased by 24 percent. Swift wrote to Karl de Schweinitz, general secretary of the Family Society of Philadelphia (an AAOFSW member agency), "it appears from Hurlin's charts that the peak of ascending relief is not yet in sight. If it is impossible for family societies, particularly in chest cities, to obtain much greater resources, what are we going to do about it?"[1]

The financial pressure of increased relief needs would drive voluntary family agencies in the 1920s to reconsider their opposition to public welfare. While voices from the voluntary sector had sounded some of the loudest criticism of urban welfare practices in the late nineteenth century, by the early twentieth century many of its leaders began to see the public sector as critical to the survival of their own institutions. What is most notable is that this process began prior to the crumbling of many voluntary organizations in the early years of the Great Depression, when widespread unemployment

*Thanks to Olivier Zunz, Brian Balogh, and participants at panels at the Association for Research in Nonprofit Organizations and Voluntary Action conference and the European Social Science History conference for their thoughts on this chapter.

stripped their resources and created the political conditions for more extensive public social provision. Even before the desperate winters of the early
1930s, the leadership of voluntary agencies contemplated a variety of means
to shift cases and costs to public-sector institutions and to carve out more
specialized terrain of social service for themselves. This template, though
only implemented sporadically in the 1920s, would serve as the basis on
which the voluntary sector could reorganize following the expansion of
public welfare in the 1930s and 1940s.

The "family agencies" represented by the AAOFSW in the several hundred towns and cities where they existed in the United States in the 1920s
were prominent symbols of voluntary social welfare. In many cities, they
served as the most visible nonsectarian (though usually mainline Protes-
tant in orientation) source of monetary assistance in the voluntary sector.
They were also incubators of the emerging profession of social work; in the
1920s, they would have been one of the most likely places to find one of the
several thousand members of the American Association of Social Workers
(organized in 1921), the profession's national organization. Family agencies, along with hospitals, child guidance clinics, and mental hygiene clinics,
nurtured the profession. AAOFSW member agencies were almost synony-
mous with the professional subdivision of "family social work." Family
agencies, often known in this period as Associated Charities, forged the
link between the relief of poverty and the professional practice of social
work.

Using professional social workers to relieve poverty became unsustain-
able for the voluntary structures in which they operated. As many historians have noted, in the 1920s, as more and more social workers considered
themselves professionals, the individualized attention to their cases—cast
as "casework" by the profession's early codifier, Mary Richmond—became
central to their professional practice. As social workers stressed casework
as their primary "service," they became less satisfied with their day-to-day
practice of providing financial assistance or negotiating clients through the
tangle of social institutions in order to tend to their health, employment,
legal, and recreational needs. One reason for this tension was that social
work increasingly emphasized insights drawn from psychoanalysis. This
emphasis encouraged social workers to focus on the psychological and emotional roots of their client's "maladjustment" to society, which had manifested itself in unemployment, poverty, and misbehavior, and less on the
humdrum work of patching together meagre community resources for their
client.[2]

These professional changes would be central to the reconsideration of
public welfare by voluntary agencies. The shifting orientation of the profession, however, must be considered in tandem with the fiscal realities of
voluntary agencies in the 1920s as an explanation for this change in position. As I will demonstrate in the first half of this chapter, mounting expenditures on monetary assistance in the 1920s, even in a prosperous decade,

caused many social workers and agency executives to wonder if the public sector could shoulder part of the burden. The growing presence of community chests, centralized fund-raising organizations for voluntary agencies, introduced a new fiscal discipline in agencies. The fear that such discipline might sacrifice professional service in order to provide monetary relief made voluntary sector agencies consider the merits of public welfare. When family-agency social workers faced clients who were poor for reasons clearly out of their control, they often considered investing costly professional time unnecessary and a task suitable for public institutions. A handful of "model" public assistance agencies hinted that earlier fears of political meddling and indiscriminate giving could be assuaged by high standards of professional social work in public welfare. By the eve of the Depression, then, leaders of voluntary agencies were far more prepared to support public assistance than their institutional forebears had been in the late nineteenth century, or even in the early 1910s.[3]

The nascent support for public welfare also forced voluntary leaders to attempt to lay out the theoretical and practical basis for the coexistence of voluntary and public welfare. While coexistence in fact predated their attempts to grapple with it, acknowledging public welfare as a legitimate field required rationalizing the distinctiveness of public and voluntary ventures, if voluntary agencies were to continue to command financial support from donors. As the second half of this article shows, voluntary sector activists put forth models in the 1920s that stressed professional service and experimentation as the hallmarks of voluntarism in an age of expanded welfare. Voluntary agencies could also work to promote high standards in public programs. These would be the same cluster of ideas that the rank and file of voluntary agencies would turn to when the Depression and New Deal in the 1930s expanded public social services on a scale vaster than most imagined in the 1920s and would serve as the rhetorical staples of the defense of voluntarism in a welfare state in the post–World War Two era.

* * *

Increasing demands for relief in the 1920s were the root cause of the reconsideration of public welfare by voluntary agencies. The pressure of relief upon private family agencies was partly of their own doing. Many counted as their forebears the charity organization societies of the late nineteenth century, and they inherited the result of the effort to privatize "outdoor relief" or direct monetary assistance. The charity organization movement attempted to both rationalize and restrict the provision of material relief in large urban settings. In the United States, charity organization societies were created principally in urban areas in the East Coast and the Midwest that were expanding rapidly through industrialization and immigration. Conceived of initially as coordinating mechanisms for charity, they sought to practise a version of "scientific philanthropy" that would apply modern organizational principles such as efficiency to the distribution of social aid by centralizing the relief-giving process from the multitude of religious, ethnic, and philanthropic agencies that offered aid to the poor. At the same time, many charity organization societies worked to limit the amount of outdoor relief provided by public institutions, fearing the abuse by city political machines that might use the relief rolls to reward supporters. In several large cities, by the 1890s, notably Brooklyn, New York, and Philadelphia, the COS efforts were successful, and relief was privatized.[4] The legacy of opposition to public aid, and the contrasting claims of high standards and capacity in the private sector, had left private agencies as one of the more visible and best publicized sources of financial assistance in many cities. Despite providing less money than public sources, a critic of voluntarism noted, "private relief loomed large in the consciousness of the socially minded citizen. . . ."[5]

A similar phenomenon occurred in the effort to pass mothers' pension laws in the early twentieth century. By the 1920s, over forty states had passed mothers'-aid legislation. Such laws provided cash relief to single mothers, generally widows, to enable them to stay home to care for their children rather than go into the work force.[6] Charity organization societies were often the principal opponents of such measures, with criticisms similar to those against outdoor relief. To social workers such as Mary Richmond, casework's leading theorist in the 1910s, the prospect of the expansion of public welfare through mothers' pensions threatened to create an open-ended commitment to relief that politicians would move to exploit. Moreover, an entitlement to a pension eroded the central principle of casework, that aid should be proffered, denied, and tailored on the basis of the individual situation of the client. Public aid, freely given, in the eyes of some charity leaders, threatened the moral fibre of the recipient, who would learn dependency rather than self-sufficiency. Others thought that keeping the "deserving" poor out of the public-welfare system would help preserve their dignity. Gertrude Vaile, a professional pioneer in public welfare in the 1910s, recalled "heated arguments with private agency friends who thought an important part of their function was to save 'self-respecting people' from the 'humiliation of having to receive public relief.'" Critics of voluntarism also noted darkly that by ceding the care of perhaps the most "deserving" of the poor, widows with families, to the public sector, charities stood to lose one of their most powerful fund-raising appeals.[7]

The convergence of shifting professional interests with the institutional interests of voluntary agencies began to erode the strength of these attitudes against public welfare. The infusion of psychoanalytic theories into social work increased the emphasis on intense, individual relationships between caseworker and client, broadening the basis of the profession beyond the provision of relief. Immediately following World War I, the national conferences and publications of the family casework field began carrying articles by several scholars, primarily from the New York, Pennsylvania, and Smith

Schools of Social Work, exploring the relevance of new insights gleaned from Sigmund Freud's writing. Social work's interest in psychiatric and psychological knowledge had been conditioned by developments in other fields, notably, mental hygiene, child guidance, and the treatment of veterans from World War I. Practitioners in all these fields had been able to move the assessment of individual problems away from what they perceived as the moralistic judgments of the nineteenth century to seemingly scientific principles. For these workers, insights from psychiatry, and particularly Freud, helped explain the "maladjustment" of individuals as the specific results of a "psychic event" in the past, or of an unresolved inner conflict. The patina of scientific authority made such arguments attractive to caseworkers not only for use in their day-to-day work but as a means by which to bolster their professional standing and to distinguish themselves from the volunteers that had dominated social agencies through the early twentieth century. Moreover, the interest in the inner life of clients, as many scholars have argued, seem to shift the attention of caseworkers away from broader environmental problems that had preoccupied casework prior to the war, such as low wages or poor housing.[8]

Professional standards dictated a reasonable caseload so as to permit a real relationship between the caseworker and the client, or "intensive" casework. Leading private agencies attempted to provide these conditions, thus heightening the perception that voluntary agencies were singularly professional, particularly when compared to public agencies. As Gertrude Vaile recalled decades later, many social workers "simply could not understand how a social worker with case work ideals could go into a public agency." Such ideals, in the eyes of social workers in the private sector, required the careful and sustained attention of a social worker—not a political appointee or a clerk. A. A. Heckman, who led the St. Paul United Charities, recalled public welfare in that city in 1920s as consisting of, "a very fine, elderly lady, Nellie Van Duzen, sitting on a high stool behind a wicker screen passing out $5.00 and $10.00 grocery orders. That was it."[9]

Private agencies' embrace of a new model of social work led them to reconsider their attitudes toward relief. Karl De Schweinitz, general secretary of the Family Society of Philadelphia and a veteran of private social work from the charity-organization era, noted in 1927 that the general trend of family agencies was away from dealing with the relief of the impoverished and toward limiting the number of clients they accepted in order to allow for more intensive work with each person. The growing importance of therapeutic ideas in social work in general eroded the interest of voluntary-sector social workers in the provision of material goods. Grants without casework provided "no thrill of accomplishment" for the client, threatened self-esteem, and "add to our client's burden of inferiority." Some voluntary-agency workers did see possibilities for relief enhancing their work with clients; as one social worker from New York's Charity Organization Society wrote in 1930, relief, "because of the many ways in which it touches human emotions," could serve as a powerful tool in casework, with the adjustment of the client as the primary goal, and relief as a means to the end.[10] But focusing on the emotional aspects of relief made some people's needs less compelling to caseworkers. A committee of the AAOFSW studying the problem of the homeless, for instance, reported that transient men held little promise for casework, concluding that "the homeless are usually uninteresting and complicated cases to handle."[11] The elderly, whose needs were usually driven by their age and limited earning capacity, were viewed similarly. As relief was mounting as a function of family agencies, it was diminishing as a source of professional interest for some caseworkers—and made it seem more plausible that public agencies could assume this sort of routine, "uninteresting" work.

The community-chest movement that had accelerated in the 1920s also made relief giving problematic for voluntary family agencies. Initiated by businessmen who sought a more centralized and rationalized way to deal with the numerous charitable appeals they received, chests offered local voluntary social agencies, such as the Associated Charities, the Boy Scouts, the Young Men's Christian Association, or the local settlement house, a deal: in return for an agreement to forgo their own individual fund-raising drives, they would receive a portion of one large annual fund drive conducted by the chest. While the idea of "federated fund-raising" had been broached in the late nineteenth century, and had gained ground among Jewish social-welfare organizations in particular, the flood of appeals for foreign relief during World War I convinced many donors and agencies that some sort of mechanism was necessary to sort out charitable fundraising. In 1922, eighty cities had converted their "war chests" into community chests for peacetime fundraising, and by 1926 there were 251 chests; on the eve of the Depression, there were 315.[12]

The rise of community chests was not simply the result of businessmen seeking to reduce the annoyance of multiple appeals for donations. It was part and parcel of the "New Era" combination of voluntarism, coordination, and efficiency most closely associated with Herbert Hoover, Secretary of Commerce from 1921 to 1928 and then President. Chests served as a modernizing force within the charitable sector and offered agencies release from the time-consuming task of fund-raising to focus on their services. Moreover, the evidence suggested that in the initial years following the organization of a community chest, the total raised by its campaign often exceeded the combined efforts of the agencies prior to organization. Chests offered a chance to make voluntarism more streamlined and efficient. In exchange for participation in the chests, though, member agencies had to agree to review of their agency's budgets by the chest and thus sacrificed a significant degree of autonomy. Salaries and new programs were subject to chest approval. Chests also served as a legitimator of charities and generally excluded "controversial" agencies. While the emerging power of chests was a lively topic of discussion in social-welfare circles, most agencies that were offered the chance to join generally did so—with the significant exception of the Red Cross.[13]

The spread of community-chest fund-raising had the ironic impact of seeming to increase the awareness and expectations of relief, as Jeff Singleton has noted. Chests made the relief of the poor, particularly the "deserving" poor, a central element of their appeals for funds, thus publicizing the availability of relief. As one writer observed in 1929, the result of chest publicity had established "a tremendous contract with the community for meeting its relief needs" and had made family agencies the "relief pocket book" of the community. Linton Swift of the AAOFSW thought that chests had helped uncover new cases of need and increased demand for relief.[14] At the same time, chests were becoming wary of rising costs of relief within family agencies. Edward Lynde of the Cleveland Associated Charities complained in 1927 that "we have been challenged by prominent men, in community funds and elsewhere, to show results for our larger expenditure or to curtail our expenses radically both for service salaries and relief." Swift saw the combination of rising relief and chest oversight directly threatening the professional standards of voluntary agencies; in cities where relief expanded, Swift argued, agency relations with chests "were thereby made difficult and adequate or intensive case work seemed impossible."[15] Francis McLean, the executive director of the AAOFSW, reported in Little Rock, Arkansas, in 1927, that while the chest used the relief operations of the family society as a central element of its fund-raising appeal, "yet when the Society ran into an unemployment situation on a very limited budget, [the chest] was absolutely unsympathetic," and did not expand the agency's relief budget.[16]

One prominent example of the tensions that inhered in rising relief, standards of professional service, and the emergence of both public welfare and community chests was a controversy that flared up in Columbus, Ohio, in the early 1920s. Columbus, like a number of other cities, lacked a public-welfare department of its own and instead administered relief by granting appropriations to the private Family Service Society of Columbus, whose caseworkers handled administration. But in the post–World War I period, the FSS had been regularly overspending its annual grants from the city council, which the council then had to supplement. During the economic downturn of the early 1920s, the FSS's relief expenditures increased by 72 percent from 1921 and were over three times what the city had originally appropriated for that year. When the FSS requested an appropriation for 1923 that matched the 1922 request, the city balked and was further angered when, in the first months of the year, the FSS spent even more on relief than it had requested (and had been denied), despite the fact that its caseload had dropped by 25 percent.[17]

While the sharp increase in relief in 1922 was driven in part by economic conditions, several other factors were also at work in Columbus. The central issue was rising standards of professional conduct among social workers. "Adequate" relief, suitable to maintain the dignity of the family, was a central tenet of professional social work by the early 1920s, as opposed to the meagre allocations of politically appointed poor-law administrators. Observers commenting on the rise in relief costs in the early 1920s attributed it not only to economic problems but also to "a more liberal relief policy" on behalf of workers and agencies. In Columbus, the increase in expenditures as caseloads decreased in 1923 was seen as an effort by caseworkers to raise standards of relief—though the average grant of $17 in early 1923, an increase from $14 in the two years prior, was still low.[18]

The Family Service Society's desire for lower caseloads in order to permit more intensive work with clients was part of the complex conflict that ensued in Columbus. While the Columbus agency had averaged roughly sixty cases per worker in the late 1910s, the surge in cases in 1922 led the new executive of the agency, Walter West, to add additional staff in order to bring caseloads back in line. In response to this expansion of the private agency, the city cut off its subsidy and created a public agency to distribute relief. At the same time as the relationship between the city government and FSS was deteriorating, business leaders in Columbus were organizing its community fund (another common name for a community chest organization), which the FSS joined in 1923. But the relationship with the fund proved as rocky as that with public officials. Fund leaders were convinced that West had hired more staff on the eve of the fund's assuming the responsibility of providing income for the agency in order to lock in lower caseloads for his workers. Furthermore, the FSS continued to overspend the amount the fund appropriated for relief to supplement the public allowances. In the rancour that followed, FSS social workers and board members protested that "no self-respecting experienced worker" would work with such meagre amounts of relief "because she would be quick to realize how useless her work would be." A committee from the American Association of Social Workers determined that high caseloads and low relief would "break down the health and the professional morale" of the workers.[19] For its part, the community fund accused the agency of deliberately, unilaterally, and consistently spending above and beyond the amount granted. "However desirable it may be to provide funds to approximate ideal standards of work," the Fund wrote to the FSS, they nonetheless had to live within their means. Despite efforts at mediation on behalf of representatives of the national associations of both community chests and family agencies, the situation deteriorated to the point where the fund temporarily expelled the FSS from the federated fundraising organization.[20]

It was clear that the national leadership saw the future of voluntarism in maintaining high professional standards. The "Columbus controversy," which was widely discussed in social-work circles, raised an important point about the intermingling of relief and casework in voluntary agencies: how could the voluntary sector's orientation toward spending more time with clients be reconciled with increasing demands for relief and with more restrictions on agencies' freedom to meet those needs as they saw fit? While an investigation of the situation in Columbus, coauthored by the AAOFSW, had spread the blame for the situation between both the fund and the FSS, the AAOFSW went on to offer Walter West a job after he left the troubled agency. The job offer, said the AAOFSW, was to serve as evidence of the group's "support for the standards of work for which he and his Board of Directors had stood in the Columbus dispute." West, wrote another national social work leader, "actually suffered from the end results of big business control of social work. He has stood for liberty."[21] West's martyrdom for agency autonomy and high professional standards puts into sharp focus the fact that relief would be a thorn in the side of family agencies in the 1920s.

Relief continued as a major preoccupation of voluntary agencies beyond the recession of the early 1920s and persisted even in the boom years of the later decade. While the general awareness of an economic crisis would not dawn until late 1929, voluntary social agencies felt the ripples of instability well over a year earlier. In New York City, family agencies noticed an increase in applications for relief between 11 and 17 percent in early 1928, the Municipal Lodging House saw a rise of 15 percent in transient men seeking shelter, and employment services had a harder time placing people. *The Survey* noted reports in January 1928 of rising unemployment in cities across the country. But, as William Bremer has noted, "the veil of 1920s prosperity hung over" the agencies and most saw it simply as a recession along the lines of those of 1914–1915 and 1921–1922. But even that was bad enough. Linton Swift of the AAOFSW took the opportunity to call again for looking into public, rather than voluntary, financing of unemployment relief, in early 1929, months before the stock-market crash.[22]

In cities with a strong emphasis on voluntarism, charities felt the brunt of the increasing demand for relief in the late 1920s. In Wilmington, Delaware, the Associated Charities (a member agency of the AAOFSW) was one of the most prominent sources for relief. The board of directors of the agency, dominated by the du Pont family and the employees of the family's booming chemical company, had long embraced an ethic of voluntarism made even more plausible by their immense wealth in a small state. Pierre S. du Pont, the most active of the family, had almost single-handedly financed a school-building program that modernized the state's school system in the late 1910s and early 1920s; A. I. du Pont had started a system of old-age pensions out of his own pocket; while T. Coleman du Pont had helped sponsor a state road-building project. The board also boasted a living emblem of the power of voluntary action: Emily Bissell, who, as a Red Cross volunteer in 1907, in order to raise money to support a tuberculosis sanatorium, coined the idea of the Christmas Seals campaign that eventually grew into the fund-raising basis for the National Tuberculosis Association. The public welfare apparatus of the city and county was weak. The Trustees of the Poor for New Castle County distributed some outdoor relief in both Wilmington and the surrounding county, but it was meagre and lacked any "supervision" of the families receiving it. The city had no welfare department of its own but made small appropriations to the Associated Charities, $534 of the $2,842 the agency provided in relief in January 1929. The Associated had been the court of last resort for decades for the unemployed and destitute, occasionally in tandem with public authority. It had provided relief during the recession of 1914 and 1915, though the city had supplied some of the funds; on the other hand, during the 1921–22 recession, the Associated Charities and its du Pont sponsors had financed the make-work program run by the parks department.[23]

The agency was straining under increasing demands for relief in the late 1920s, and the agency executive began to push her board of directors to consider advocating for a broader public role in relief. Ethelda Mullen, general secretary of the agency and a member of the Mary Richmond–trained vanguard of professional social work, told her board in January 1928 that their figures for relief were higher than they had been in some time and that nearly half of the people they were aiding were employable heads of families who could not find jobs. In March, she observed that the unemployment problem ("which the Chamber of Commerce assures us is not acute," she added sarcastically) was throwing able-bodied wage earners, "Wilmington men with families," at the mercy of the Associated Charities—not the drifters assumed to be the main recipients of the charity's largesse. She remarked that she had heard a talk at the national conference of social work about the "unavoidable" cycles of unemployment, generating needs unconnected to the client's "maladjustment." She noted the example of Minneapolis, where the private society had limited its intake to specialized cases and let the public take over most of the relief, particularly of the aged and unemployed. Even when the burden of relief eased during the summer and fall of 1928, Mullen put the case to her board that much of the staff's time was taken up "tiding over and patching up" families. Other cities had found ways to lighten the burden of the voluntary society so the society's workers could be released for more intensive efforts. Was the Associated to be simply "the relief pocketbook of the community?" she asked, her language echoing Edward Lynde's criticism of community chests the year before. When the intake at the agency skyrocketed in January 1929 to the highest level since the early 1920s, with a large number of families the agency had never seen or had not seen since the depression of 1921–22, Mullen again suggested that unemployment might be the proper responsibility of public authorities.[24]

In Baltimore, similar signs of distress evidenced themselves at the Family Welfare Association of Baltimore (another AAOFSW member). The Baltimore agency had a distinguished history; some of the leading figures in late nineteenth-century social work had been involved with the agency in its original incarnation as the Charity Organization Society of Baltimore: John Glenn, who would direct the Russell Sage Foundation from its inception in 1907 until 1931, had chaired the executive committee of the COS from 1887 to 1907; Amos Warner, whose *American Charities* was a seminal text for charity reformers, served as its general secretary from 1887 to 1889;

Mary Richmond, the social-work theorist, who started her career at the agency in the early 1890s. In the 1920s, Baltimore gave no "outdoor" (cash or in-kind) relief, and the FWA, as the only citywide, nonsectarian agency, was the principal resource for organized assistance—though the Bureau of Catholic Charities and the Hebrew Benevolent Union dealt with most of their coreligionists. Though Baltimore's economy appeared relatively prosperous, with 103 new manufacturing plants opening in the city in the 1920s, demands on the agency due to unemployment "in the so-called prosperous years of the 1920s" had steadily mounted. In mid-1927, a slump in employment threw many people on the agency's resources, and the local community fund was forced to meet the agency's deficits. As relief spending mounted in early 1928, the fund, as had its counterparts in Columbus, Little Rock, and elsewhere, refused to appropriate any more money to the agency and told the agency to seek help from the city. Mayor William Broening also refused to help until all voluntary resources were exhausted, and for two weeks in late April and early May, the agency closed its doors and turned away 136 families seeking assistance for unemployment—whereupon the city's Board of Estimates granted the agency an emergency appropriation. In 1929, an FWA board of directors committee concluded that "it would certainly be inadvisable for the Association to hold itself out as providing a kind of unemployment insurance fund, that may be freely tapped in all cases of unemployment." The annual report of the FWA called for unemployment relief to be taken over by taxpayers.[25]

Thus, by the late 1920s, a number of factors combined to make relief a pressing issue for voluntary family agencies. The general increase in costs, driven by increased organization and publicizing of welfare services by community chests and by rising professional standards of "adequate" relief, was exposing the financial limits of family agencies. The Columbus agency's efforts to achieve higher levels of service, both in the amount of relief given and the numbers of clients workers dealt with, had been repudiated by the local chest, and suggested that, under the new regime of chest financing, relief might be more of an albatross than advantage to family agencies. More promising alternatives beckoned. The Family Welfare Association of Minneapolis, which over the 1920s had shifted much of its relief giving over to public bodies, used the mounting costs of relief in 1925 to experiment with a temporary transfer in *all* relief giving to the public bodies and using its caseworkers to work more intensively with their other clients. The success of this experiment led the agency's board to increase the number of social workers on the agency's staff.[26] These factors helped reduce the ideological and institutional resistance of voluntary family agencies to public welfare that had characterized them a generation earlier. As one participant in an NSWC forum in April 1930 observed, "Twenty years ago, of course, public outdoor relief was disliked intensely by all private agencies and apparently as far as I can make out the private agencies have now changed their position. They have reversed their position of twenty years ago."[27]

EMBRACING WELFARE

The financial limitations of voluntary agencies in the 1920s pushed leaders in the voluntary sector to begin to create an intellectual framework for a division of labour between public and private agencies, a framework that would be widely embraced when the Depression of the 1930s made the financial limitations of voluntarism evident to all. This process was encouraged in the 1920s by the expanding amount of public-welfare activity, even before the Depression. The engine of this expansion was the widespread passage of mothers'-aid laws, and the establishment of public-welfare departments, particularly at the state level—though the latter generally focused on child welfare and state institutions, such as mental hospitals or prisons. As the Executive Committee of the AAOFSW observed in 1920, "many of the societies, particularly in the west, are confronted with all sorts of plans involved in amendments to city charters, city and county ordinances, acts of state legislatures for the organization or reorganization of departments of charity or family welfare, boards of public welfare, etc., which often touch upon the field work of our societies." State welfare spending rose from $52 million in 1913 to $151 million in 1927, an increase of 290 percent, while the cost of living rose only 180 percent. Outdoor relief (noninstitutional aid, such as cash grants or commodities), the form of spending most criticized, remained a widespread phenomenon; 87 percent of cities over 30,000 appropriated funds for outdoor relief in 1925. Of those cities, their spending on outdoor relief rose from $2.2 million in 1911 to $16.4 million in 1928.[28]

Moreover, by the late 1920s, statistics confirmed the fact that in most cities public funds contributed the bulk of expenditures, even in "outdoor relief," even if private agencies were more visible. A study in Chicago revealed that in 1928, the Cook County Bureau of Public Welfare and the Mothers' Pension Division of the Juvenile Court distributed 63.7 percent of the relief funds, while private agencies handled 36.3 percent. A similar study in 14 midsized cities found a breakdown of 70.2 percent public and 29.8 percent private.[29]

The growth of public welfare and the increase in spending on relief by private family agencies convinced the national leadership of the family-service field that they needed to try to work with and improve public welfare and systematize their relationships with those institutions. Francis McLean of the AAOFSW had spent time as a charity administrator in Montreal and Chicago and had travelled extensively in areas of the country that lacked strong private agencies and thus had a more sober view of the limits of voluntarism than some of his colleagues from cities that enjoyed dense networks of voluntary agencies. He urged his colleagues to engage and promote the development of public-welfare departments. Gertrude Vaile recalled that McLean was "utterly undefensive in his attitude toward agency functions," that he was able, unlike some old-guard social workers, to envision legitimate spheres of operation for both public and private welfare.[30]

McLean was instrumental in arranging for Vaile—whose social casework credentials were impeccable, and under whose guidance the Denver Department of Welfare had become a model of social-work practice (outshining even its private counterpart)—to head a committee to research how voluntary and public agencies were actually interacting in the places where they coexisted.[31] Their survey of member societies elicited replies from agencies in 162 cities. Of these, eleven cities had no form of public outdoor relief. twenty-nine others had some sort of combination or subsidy plan, whereby private agencies administered public funds or were linked to public departments. Those lacking any outdoor relief were generally very large cities, such as Baltimore, which had abolished such relief in the late nineteenth century. The cities that combined departments tended to be small, eight having a population of less than 30,000. The remaining 122 cities had both private and public organizations, with no formal institutional links between them, but with varied patterns of interaction. About a third of the cities had an active social-service exchange, in which both private and public agencies exchanged information on the clients with whom they were working.[32]

Vaile discerned a trend toward private agencies shifting the most costly cases to the public. The Minneapolis Family Welfare Society (the agency singled out as an example by Ethelda Mullen to her board of directors in Wilmington, Delaware) reported that the city's Board of Public Welfare had, in the past three to five years, taken responsibility not only for the mothers'-aid cases but also for cases relating to unemployment and old age, "because the load was too heavy for the [private society] and they seemed best to turn over." Public departments were more likely to handle old-age-related poverty and cases with long-term need, while private societies tended to handle short-term cases. Vaile noted that "it is generally agreed that the public department should bear the heavy burden of relief." Faced with the challenge of increasing numbers of the "deserving" poor, private societies in practice tried to shift the most expensive, most routine, and least interesting cases into the public sector. In places like Worcester, Massachusetts, as the Associated Charities (an AAOFSW member) reported to Vaile, "the [Overseer of the Poor] takes all families falling into distress, who have lived in Worcester only a short time or have a pauper record acquired or inherited; they mean to leave us all young families, who are not paupers or pauper families." Other studies confirmed such patterns. In Chicago, in 1928, while the private agencies provided only 36.6 percent of the relief funds, they handled 72.2 percent of the cases, suggesting that they tended to deal with numerous cases needing only "minor relief." In Worcester, as in many places, the survey noted, "This div. of wk. just grew"—likely due to the financial constraints of the voluntary sector and the desire of its social workers to focus on more interesting, and perhaps more helpable, clients.[33]

Despite the lack of a clear pattern in actual practice, social-work leaders nonetheless reached for some sort of guiding principle. The most common rationalization for public-private collaboration was that private societies could act as a proving ground for public policy. Private agencies would try new techniques which then, if found effective, would gain public approval and be recognized as something worthy of public support. This was a position articulated two decades earlier by Amos Warner in his influential book *American Charities* (1894). As opposed to charity, Warner argued, "the state is not inventive, its agencies are not adaptive and flexible; but it is capable of doing a large, expansive work when the methods for it are sufficiently elaborated."[34] Charity, Warner and others held, could serve as the trailblazer for future expansion of public services. By the 1920s, some social-work leaders acknowledged that the government's resources, and at times its powers of coercion, made it more effective in applying the techniques that charity developed. As Ralph Barrow of the private Children's Aid Society of Hartford, Connecticut, wrote in 1925, private agencies could use their resources "as a laboratory," but the public would take over once the project had been "approved as good."[35] Dr. William Snow of the American Social Hygiene Association posited in 1925 that there was a natural continuum from the university to private agencies and then to the public sector: from research to demonstration to policy.[36] There were occasional examples where such a model was put into practice. In the small city of Petersburg, Virginia, for instance, city manager Louis Brownlow in the mid-1920s, en route to becoming a leading authority on public administration at the University of Chicago, used the local chapter of the Red Cross to "demonstrate" the efficacy of public-health nursing, whereupon the city then hired its own public-health nurse, while the Red Cross moved on to focus on child welfare. Brownlow saw this model applicable to social work as well; he helped organize an Associated Charities in Petersburg to demonstrate the utility of professional social work.[37]

This model had its limits in both theory and practice, however. When voluntary family agencies talked of demonstration and experiment in the 1920s, they usually meant experimenting with casework. The most common argument for family agencies to collaborate with public-welfare authorities was that it would relieve the financial burden of massive caseloads from the private agency in order to "limit its intake and do the intensive experimental work which is a very important contribution which only a private society can make."[38] As the theory went, once such intensive techniques were proven to have value, the private agencies would then be able to arouse public sentiment to support government provision of such service. But most family-service agencies at the time did not see themselves in the business of putting themselves out of business. The Vaile report made it clear that casework as a technique in public welfare would be a long time in coming and that certain cases "that primarily involve personality problems calling for especially intensive work" would probably remain the province of private agencies.[39] David Holbrook, secretary of the National Social Work Council, commented that even when government-sponsored social welfare was a "going concern," there would still remain work for voluntary organizations to do.[40]

Private agencies could act as gadflies on public-welfare programs in order to hold them to high standards. Voluntary agencies in other fields had embraced this role. Charles Chute, of the National Probation Association, which had over a decade of experience working with the court system, thought his organization played a dual role as "critic and promoter" of the government agencies it worked with. McLean agreed, arguing that "a public agency without considerable participation or without the presence of a private agency is in a very unprotected condition."[41] Ruth Taylor, a professional social worker and deputy commissioner of public welfare of Westchester County, New York, added that the "opportunity for the private agency lies in changing the direction of public opinion," to help support higher quality work in public welfare agencies.[42]

Here, the national leadership of the family agencies took the lead. The AAOFSW, through the prodding of McLean and Vaile, opened membership in the organization to public departments of welfare that were using professional social workers. Membership would bring to "good public departments the help and support which private forces should bring to public administration." Roughly a dozen departments joined in the next few years.[43] Similarly, McLean corresponded with a number of social workers in public mothers'-aid departments, most notably Mary Bogue, who headed Pennsylvania's Mothers' Assistance Fund, in an effort to encourage such agencies to join the AAOFSW.[44] The voluntary agency's reputation for supporting high-quality, professional work won it admirers from outside the field. Louis Brownlow, now at the University of Chicago, encouraged the use of the Family Welfare Association of America (as the AAOFSW had been mercifully renamed in the early 1930s) as a standard setter for public-agency practice.[45]

Finally, some agencies carried the role of demonstrator and gadfly directly into the political arena. Francis McLean wrote in the early 1920s that "my present belief is that the great function of family societies is to educate local groups of people so that they may act not only through our societies but through other agencies."[46] In some cities, voluntary agencies took his charge, not simply by finding constructive ways to coexist with public-welfare agencies but by actively promoting their creation and professionalism. In Providence and Boston, representatives of the family agencies actually helped lobby *for* mothers'-pension bills; in Chicago, private agencies worked with the mothers'-pension bureau to obtain competent staff; in New York, the New York State Charities Aid Association, a group of voluntary agencies, played a central role in helping draft and lobby for changes in the state's public welfare law that called for more preventative work in welfare and more rational administration of local poor relief. In Minneapolis, the Family Welfare Association pushed the county welfare board to reduce the waiting period for mothers' pensions and the city to provide supplementation for inadequate county funds, "thus reducing the percentage of the Family Welfare Association funds used for these purposes."[47]

All of these models—of experimentation, of gadflies, of lobbyists— would prove to be central to the reconsideration of the voluntary-public relationship after the New Deal. Why then, with all this new prepared- ness, did it make such marginal impact on actual public policy prior to the Great Depression and the New Deal? First, experimenting and demonstra- tion offered a vision of seamless cooperation between voluntary agencies and government, while leaving open-ended the question of what functions a public authority might adopt and when. But some doubted whether this accurately captured the public-voluntary dynamic. Frank Bruno, the for- mer executive at the voluntary Family Welfare Association of Minneapolis, moved on to teach social work at Washington University. His own work within the voluntary sector had made him wary of the grand claims of some charity promoters. He found in his own survey of thirty-five agencies that the "so called experimental activities of private agencies, if not entirely so, are mostly in the field of the imagination." One relationship that Bruno found prevalent was simply the practice of voluntary agencies supplement- ing the meagre allotments of public authorities—often necessary, but hardly a distinctive role. Voluntary agencies in other fields, such as those working with public-health and vocational-rehabilitation programs, testified to simi- lar patterns.[48]

Second, there remained an air of disdain among many social workers in private agencies for their public-agency counterparts, even as they rec- ognized the possibility for broader public involvement. Prominent volun- tary-agency leaders admitted that "there has been and still is great need for private agencies to be more cordial to public agencies."[49] Frank Bane, commissioner of public welfare in Virginia and an early activist in organiz- ing public-welfare administrators, recalled that at the national social-work conventions, the meetings for public-welfare officials "always had the back room." In his eyes, most social workers saw the task of public welfare as somewhere between corruptly political and unskilled labour, "people who have to handle the day-to-day routine dishwashing jobs," who had neither the time nor ability to do skilled casework.[50] As the Depression set in and public-welfare services began to expand, public-welfare professionals ulti- mately formed their own organization, the American Public Welfare Asso- ciation, which quickly played an important role in the organization of relief administration during the 1930s.[51]

Third, much of the discussion of these new relationships was by volun- tary leaders at the national level, not from the local institutions where vol- untarism was being practised. A frustrated McLean wrote in 1927,

> Despite the growing recognition that the participation of the public de- partments in the family field in an effective way is necessary and that one of the reasons for the crippling of our societies by overloads is the absences of such departments, we should not say that either the field reports or the correspondence with the office yet indicate the working

out of long-term plans for the realization of this on the part of many societies.[52]

McLean's own reports on agencies he visited across the United States further suggest that many voluntary family agencies, from the standpoint of the national office, would not be capable of performing the exemplary work that a new model of private-public collaboration might require. Throughout the 1920s, McLean reported back to New York City on his experiences with "primitive" voluntary agencies in "deep ruts," of "reactionary or slowed down societies," "backwards situations," and societies "organized early in the history of the movement [that] have not kept progress with it."[53]

Finally, even though the leadership, and some of the rank and file, of voluntary family agencies had changed their minds as to the advisability of some public-welfare programs, this did not translate into an embrace of a federal welfare state in the 1920s or even in the first few years of the Depression. Indeed, most of the public-private relationships envisioned and debated were at the local, or at most the state, level. Voluntary agencies, local in their organization and orientation, were keenly focused on activities in their back yard, not on those at the national level. Thus, Mrs. John Glenn, a lay leader of the voluntary family social-work movement, could admit in April 1930 that "I was one of those benighted people who opposed Mothers' Aid," while still harbouring doubts about the advisability of national unemployment insurance to deal with what was shaping up to be a major economic depression.[54] Linton Swift, executive director of the AAOFSW and a proponent of collaboration between public and private, also worried early in the Depression about the dangers of federal public relief. It would take the brutal winters of the early 1930s, as voluntary agencies staggered and in some cases folded under the weight of the needs of the unemployed, to translate the willingness to countenance a wider role and new relationship between public and private welfare to outright advocacy, in the case of Linton Swift, for federal relief by 1932.[55]

It is this localism and initial reluctance to embrace programs such as social insurance that coloured the debate about the voluntary agencies and public welfare in the late 1920s, and that has shaped subsequent histories. Isaac Rubinow, a prominent advocate of publicly funded social insurance, submitted an essay in 1929 to *The Survey*, a social work magazine, attacking the presumptions of private charities, and particularly the community chests, to stand in as a substitute for public authority. Titled "Can Private Philanthropy Do It?" Rubinow's essay argued that voluntary institutions simply lacked the capacity to deal with large-scale social problems such as unemployment. However, he believed that the relentless fund-raising by community chests had portrayed voluntarism as an adequate substitute for meeting the relief needs of communities. "In moments of stress, such as this," he wrote in September 1929, "it is the inefficient political machinery that has the power (though it sometimes lacks the will) of making emergency appropriations, making loans, and issuing bonds if necessary." The argument that voluntary methods were more intimate and individualized simply did not hold water, at least on the fund-raising side, said Rubinow. Centralized fund-raising had become as impersonal and businesslike as the government, although lacking the power to tax; "Voluntary self-taxation is picturesque, but infinitely less effective than the official tax collector." Government should be granted the power to provide relief and leave private agencies to try "new experiments, new approaches to old problems."[56]

Rubinow's critique angered many in the voluntary sector, but his last recommendation was actually in keeping with the direction that some within the private family agencies felt that their institutions needed to move.[57] In cities across the United States in the 1920s, voluntary agencies began to try to hold public officials and institutions more accountable for carrying the burden of the community's welfare needs. That city fathers more often than not evaded such responsibility, and that most voluntary agencies did not engage themselves politically to promote such institutions, much less a fully elaborated system of unemployment insurance, should not diminish the significance of the philosophical and programmatic shifts occurring within the voluntary sector. Linton Swift, executive director of the FWAA, wrote in 1934 that "many of us have long felt that the relief of such general social-economic ills as unemployment should not be primarily a matter of 'charity' at all, but an unescapable responsibility of society as a whole, expressed through various units of government." Swift went on to lay out a course for private agencies that involved "abandoning some old traditions, re-emphasizing others, and accepting the limitations as well as the ever-new possibilities of truly private effort," strategies that included experimenting with new techniques, reaching out to populations unreached by social programs, building public support for new social services, and focusing their casework expertise on "personal maladjustments" that were not primarily economic in nature.[58] All of these were practices embryonic in the 1920s and that would emerge as the core of private-agency programs in the post–New Deal era, though it took the economic and political shocks of the Depression and New Deal to bring them to the centre of the voluntary agenda.[59]

NOTES

1. Administrative Committee Minutes, American Association for Organizing Family Social Work, Jan. 30, 1926, Folder 5, Box 4; Linton Swift to Karl de Schweinitz, Aug. 4, 1926, Folder 10, Box 14; "How May the Private Family Welfare Agency Meet the Financial Dilemma Resulting from the Rising Tide of Relief Expenditures?" [1929], Folder 28, Box 32, all in Family Service Association of America Records (FSAA), Social Welfare History Archives (SWHA), University of Minnesota, Minneapolis, Minnesota.
2. On the professionalization of social work in the 1920s, see Clarke Chambers, *Seedtime of reform: American social service and social action, 1918–1933*, Minneapolis: University of Minnesota Press, 1963, pp. 91–106; Roy Lubove, *The professional altruist: The emergence of social work as a career, 1880–1930*,

New York: Atheneum, 1973; John Ehrenreich, *The altruistic imagination: A history of social work and social policy in the United States*, Ithaca, NY: Cornell University Press, 1985; Stanley Wenocur and Michael Reisch, *From charity to enterprise: The development of American social work in a market economy*, Urbana, IL: University of Illinois Press, 1989; Walter Trattner, *From poor law to welfare state: A history of social welfare in America*, 5th ed., New York: The Free Press, 1994, pp. 234–53.

3. Michael Katz, *In the shadow of the poorhouse: A social history of welfare in America*, New York: Basic Books, 1996, p. 161. I am indebted to Jeff Singleton, *The American dole: unemployment relief and the welfare state in the Great Depression*, Westport, CT: Greenwood Press, 2000, whose focus on the "rising tide of relief" in the 1920s informs my investigation of its impact on voluntary agencies; see Singleton, pp. 27–36.

4. Katz, pp. 47–54, 71–74. Such campaigns were not universally successful; see Adonica Y. Lui, "Political and institutional constraints of reform: The charity reformers' failed campaigns against public outdoor relief, New York City, 1874–1898," *Journal of Policy History*, 7(3):341–63.

5. Josephine Brown, *Public relief, 1929–1939*, New York: Henry Holt and Co., 1940, p. 159.

6. Theda Skocpol, *Protecting soldiers and mothers: The political origins of social policy in the United States*, Cambridge, MA: Harvard University Press, 1992, pp. 10, 425–28; Linda Gordon, *Pitied but not entitled: Single mothers and the history of welfare*, Cambridge, MA: Harvard University Press, 1994, p. 37.

7. Gertrude Vaile, "Contributions to Public Welfare," *The Family* (Mar. 1946): 33–34; Roy Lubove, *The struggle for social security, 1900–1935*, Cambridge, MA: Harvard University Press, 1968, pp. 101–06.

8. Ehrenreich, pp. 65–77; Lubove, *Professional altruist*, pp. 76–117.

9. Gertrude Vaile, "Contributions to public welfare"; A. A. Heckman Oral History, p. 8, A. A. Heckman Papers, SWHA.

10. Karl De Schweinitz to Walter West, July 6, 1926, Folder 11, Box 7, FSAA; Eleanor Neustadter, "Relief: A constructive tool in case work treatment," New York: Charity Organization Society, c. 1930, p. 9. A seminal work on the subject was Grace Marcus, *Some aspects of relief in family casework*, New York: Charity Organization Society, 1929.

11. Report of the Committee on the Homeless, AAOFSW, Apr. 1927, Folder 14, Box 13, FSAA.

12. Homer Borst, "Community chests and councils," *Social work yearbook, 1929*, New York: Russell Sage Foundation, 1929) p. 95; John Dawson, "Community chests," *Social work yearbook 1947*, p. 104; Vaile, "Contribution to public welfare"; John R. Seely et al., *Community chest: A case study in philanthropy*, Toronto: University of Toronto Press, 1957, pp. 17–21; Lubove, *The professional altruist*, pp. 183–219.

13. Dawson, p. 105; Lubove, *Professional altruist*, p. 184; Singleton, pp. 41–44.

14. "How may the private family welfare agency meet the financial dilemma. . . ."; Swift, "The relief problem in family social work," [1929], Folder 10, Box 15, FSAA (a draft of the article which came out in *The Family* in March, 1929); Singleton, pp. 41–43. See also Minutes, National Social Work Council, Mar. 2, 1928, Folder 3, Box 4, National Social Welfare Assembly Records (NSWA), SWHA for a discussion of worries about the influence of chests.

15. Edward Lynde, "The significance of changing methods in relief giving," *The Family* (July 1927): 135; Administrative Committee Minutes, AAOFSW, Jan. 30, 1926.

16. Francis McLean, "Field policies and trends, 1927–1928," p. 22, [1928], Folder 8, Box 11, FSAA.

17. [Allen Burns and David Adie], "Report on the break in working relations of the community funds and family service society of Columbus, Ohio and on efforts at securing a new working agreement," 1926, folder, Columbus, OH, 1926, Box 75, FSAA; "What happened in Columbus," *The Survey* (May 15, 1926): 261–63. Daniel Walkowitz has also explored this incident, with an emphasis on how the American Association of Social Workers perceived the issues at stake. Daniel Walkowitz, *Working with class: Social workers and the politics of middle class identity*, Chapel Hill: University of North Carolina Press, 1999, pp. 81–85.

18. "Statement of relief figures for three month's period," Apr. 30, 1922, Folder 28, Box 32; John B. Dawson, "A study of relief giving with special relation to increased costs," June 1922, Folder 29, Box 32; Dawson, "Comment on report of Columbus situation," Aug. 12, 1926, folder, Columbus, OH, 1926, Box 75, all FSAA. On the relationship between rising relief standards and professionalism, see Singleton, pp. 35–39.

19. Philip King, Gardiner Lattimer, Cecil North to Board of Family Service Society of Columbus [Oct. 1933], in "Report on break in working relations"; "Report of the Subcommittee of the American Association of Social Workers on the Break in the working relations between the community fund and the family service society of Columbus, Ohio" [1926], folder, Columbus, OH, 1926, Box 75, FSAA.

20. J. H. Franz to Frank Howe, Sept. 8, 1925, in "Report on break in working relations."

21. AAOFSW Administrative Committee, Apr. 10, 1926, Folder 5, Box 4, FSAA; David Holbrook to Howard Braucher, Feb. 25, 1928, Folder 43, Box 6, NSWA Supplement 1, SWHA. In his analysis of the Columbus situation, Walkowitz sees a division between "largely female caseworkers and male supervisors and executives." While the female caseworkers had articulated their discontent with their conditions of work, the increase in staff in 1922 happened with West's support, and the stance of the caseworkers had the support of a majority of the board and the agency's president—at least until West was apparently encouraged to resign as a result of the final agreement with the fund in early 1926. It suggests that the agency had a commitment to professional standards and agency autonomy shared by both executives and caseworkers, and that in this case, the divide along gendered lines is not so neat. West would go on to head the American Association of Social Workers. See Walkowitz, pp. 81–84.

22. William W. Bremer, *Depression winters: New York social workers and the New Deal*, Philadelphia: Temple University Press, 1984, p. 28; Linton Swift, "The relief problem in family social work," *The Family* (Mar. 1929): 7.

23. Board of Directors, Associated Charities of Wilmington, Mar. 21, 1922; "The first fifty years: Records and reminiscences of the personalities and activities to which Wilmington owes its progress in family relief work," Wilmington, DE: The Family Society, 1934, both in Children and Families First Library, Wilmington, Delaware. The "Reminiscences" claims that 1914 to 1915 was the only time the organization received public funds, though the directors minutes show it was administering public funds in the late 1920s; Carol Hoffecker, *Corporate capital: Wilmington in the twentieth century*, Philadelphia: Temple University Press, 1983, p. 101.

24. Board of Directors Minutes, Associated Charities of Wilmington, Jan. 17, 1928; Feb.21, 1928; May 15, 1928; Nov. 20, 1928; Feb. 19, 1929.

25. Board of Managers, Family Welfare Association of Baltimore, June 29, 1927; Sept. 8, 1927; Feb. 17, 1928; Mar. 23, 1928, May 25, 1928; "The Family Welfare Association report of the committee on unemployment," May 1929,

all Folder 27, Box 2, Baltimore Family and Children's Society (BFCS) Records, Special Collections, Milton Eisenhower Library, Johns Hopkins University; Anna Ward, "A century of family social work," p. 6, Folder 9, Box 1, BFCS; Grace Sperrow, "History of the Baltimore Family and Children's Society" [n.d.], Folder 26, Box 1, BFCS; Jo Ann Argersinger, *Toward a new deal in Baltimore*, Chapel Hill: University of North Carolina Press, 1988, p. 5.

26. Family Welfare Association of Minneapolis, *The Family Welfare Association in action, 1917–1926* (Minneapolis, 1927), pp. 20–22.

27. NSWC Monthly Meeting transcript, Apr. 4, 1930, Folder 53, Box 6, NSWA.

28. Morton Keller, *Regulating a new society: Public policy and social change in America, 1900–1933*, Cambridge, MA: Harvard University Press, 1994, p. 87; Mary Phlegar Smith, "Municipal expenditures for family relief," *Social Forces* (Mar. 1933): 370; AAOFSW Executive Committee Agenda, Oct. 30, 1920, Folder 11, Box 6, FSAA.

29. Helen Jeter and A. W. McMillen, "Some statistics of family welfare and relief in Chicago, 1928," *Social Service Review* (Sept. 1929): 448–59; "Receipts and expenditures of social agencies during the year 1928," *SSR* (Sept. 1930): 363; Katz, p. 159.

30. Vaile, "Contributions to public welfare," p. 34; Margaret Rich, *A belief in people: A history of family social work*, New York: Family Service Association of America, 1956, pp. 70–72.

31. Vaile, "Principles and methods of outdoor relief," *Proceedings, National Conference of Charities and Corrections*, 42 (1915): 480–81; Jim Stafford, "Gertrude Vaile," in Walter Trattner, ed., *Biographical dictionary of social welfare in America*, New York: Greenwood Press, 1986, pp. 723–25.

32. *Division of work between public and private agencies dealing with families in their homes*, New York: AAOFSW, 1925.

33. AAOFSW, "Memorandum regarding division of cases," 1924, pp. 14–16, Pub. Depts. Comm., Box 12, FSAA; *Division of work*, p. 10; Jeter and McMillen.

34. Amos G. Warner, *American charities: A study in philanthropy and economics*, Boston: Thomas Y. Crowell and Co., 1894, pp. 304–05.

35. Ralph Barrow, "Interpreting child welfare work to the community—the private agency," *Proceedings of the National Conference of Social Work, 1925*, pp. 132–36.

36. "Minutes of meeting of National Social Work Council," December 4, 1925, Folder 9, Box 2, NSWA.

37. Louis Brownlow to Josephus Daniels, May 10, 1921, "Associated Charities" Folder; Brownlow to I. Malinde Havey, December 20, 1922, "Red Cross" Folder, both Box 4, Louis Brownlow Papers, Special Collections, Alderman Library, University of Virginia.

38. "Division of work between public and private agencies," p. 16.

39. Ibid., p. 18.

40. NSWC Monthly Meeting transcript, Dec. 5, 1925, Folder 9, Box 2, NSWA.

41. Charles Chute to Holbrook, Nov. 18, 1925; "Minutes of meeting of National Social Work Council," Dec. 4, 1925, both in Folder 9, Box 2, NSWA; McLean, "Field policies and trends, 1927–1928," p. 29.

42. Frank Bruno, "The integration of effort in theory and practice by private and public agencies for the common good," *NCSW 1927*, pp. 240–46; Ruth Taylor, "The integration of effort in theory and practice by private and public agencies for the common good," *National Conference of Social Work, 1927*, pp. 246–52.

43. AAOFSW Executive Committee Minutes, Oct. 31, 1921; May 15, 1923, Folder 11, Box 6; "Report of Committee on Alignment of Socialized Departments" [July 5, 1921], Committee on Public Depts., Box 12, FSAA.

44. Mary Bogue to McLean, May 24, 1927; Ruth Edward Winch to McLean, Apr. 19, 1929, Folder 12, Box 16, FSAA.
45. "Special conference," May 25, 1931, Folder "Membership Departments," Box 17, FSAA.
46. Francis McLean to Edwin Elkund, Jan. 23, 1923, Folder 21, Box 13, FSAA.
47. Leah Feder, "The relation of private case working agencies to programs of public welfare," *Social Forces* (June 1931): 518; Elsie Bond, "New York's new public welfare law," *Social Service Review* (Sept. 1929): 415–16; Family Welfare Association of Minneapolis, *The Family Welfare Association in action, 1917–1926*, p. 26.
48. Bruno, pp. 242, 245; Charles Hatfield, "Relative function of agencies, viewpoint of the non-official agency," Dec. 1920, Folder 9, Box 2, NSWA; R. C. Branion, "Correlation of public and private work for the handicapped," *NCSW 1925*, pp. 325–27; Keller, pp. 191–95. As noted above, Bruno, while leading the FWA of Minneapolis, had pushed for public agencies to supplement public funds. Nonetheless, many voluntary agencies frequently supplemented mothers' pensions; see, for instance, Evelyn Hyman Goldman, "A history of the family consultation service of Rockford, Illinois, 1877–1947," MSW, Tulane University, 1948, and Singleton, p. 33. Jewish agencies made a practice of ensuring that needy Jews who received public assistance received supplementary assistance to allow them to live in a more dignified manner than possible on public allowances. Harrie Lurie, "Character of relationships of Jewish agencies with public or non-sectarian agencies in the field of family welfare," National Conference of Jewish Social Service, *Proceedings* (1927), reprinted in Robert Morris and Michael Freund, eds., *Trends and issues in Jewish social welfare, 1899–1952*, Philadelphia: Jewish Publication Society of America, 1966, pp. 196–97.
49. David Holbrook to Margaret Rich, July 11, 1928, Folder 30, Box 4, NSWA.
50. Bane would go on to direct the American Public Welfare Association in the early 1930s, and moved to become the first executive director of the Social Security Board in 1935. Frank Bane, "Public administration and public welfare," oral-history interview with James Lieby (University of California Regional Oral History Office, 1965), p. 93.
51. Narayan Viswanathan, "The role of the American Public Welfare Association in the formulation and development of public welfare policies in the United States, 1930–1960" (DSW, Columbia University, 1961).
52. McLean, "Field policies and trends, 1927–1928," p. 27.
53. McLean, "A special summary for the executive committee of the field work, Sept. 1920–Feb. 1921"; "Field policies and trends, 1927–1928"; "Situations and objectives of field work, season 1924–1925," all Folder 7, Box 11, FSAA.
54. National Social Work Council, Monthly Meeting, April 4, 1930, pp. 57–58, Folder 53, Box 6, NSWA, SWHA.
55. David Holbrook, "Federal action on unemployment," March 18, 1933, Folder 32, Box 4, NSWA Supplement 1, SWHA; Joanna C. Colcord, "Social work and the first federal relief program," *The Compass* (Sept. 1943): 17–23; Singleton, pp. 45–46.
56. Isaac M. Rubinow, "Can private philanthropy do it?" *Social Service Review* (Sept. 1929): 361–94.
57. *The Survey*, closely aligned with the voluntary sector, agonized for months over whether to publish Rubinow's article, sent it out for comments, and finally decided it was too incendiary after protests from community-chest leaders and several voluntary organizations. It was accepted at the *Social Service Review*,

published by the University of Chicago's School of Social Service, which was making a practice of illustrating the limits of voluntarism. See Bremer, p. 28.

58. Linton Swift, *New alignments between public and private agencies in a community family welfare and relief program*, New York: Family Welfare Association of America, 1934, pp. vi, 1, 12–13.

59. I explore the post–New Deal "new alignments" at length in Andrew Morris, "Charity, therapy, and poverty: private social service in the era of public welfare," PhD, University of Virginia, 2003.

9 Voluntary Failure, the Middle Classes, and the Nationalisation of the British Voluntary Hospitals, 1900–1946[*]

Paul Bridgen

University of Southampton

Voluntary hospitals began to be set up in Britain in the mid-1700s. They were to have a long and distinguished history, with their achievements recognised even by those who were not their most committed supporters. The period between 1861 and 1938 was a time of particularly rapid expansion. From the former date to 1891, bed numbers in Britain doubled to 35,500; by the latter date they had tripled to 101,300[1] provided in 1200 voluntary hospitals.[2] In some areas (e.g., Norfolk) they remained the only form of secondary health care in the prewar period.[3]

The hospitals were voluntary in the sense that traditionally they were financed by philanthropy, and the medical practitioners who worked in them provided their services on an honorary basis. Their traditional role was to offer free medical care to the "sick poor." In the post–1914 period, major changes began to occur in the financing and utilisation of the hospitals,[4] but the fact that they received virtually no peacetime state funds up to 1939 meant they maintained their place as the "flagship of the voluntary movement."[5]

However, this long and distinguished history did not protect the voluntary hospitals from nationalisation in 1946. As part of the establishment by the postwar Labour government of the National Health Service (NHS), the hospitals became funded almost entirely by taxation and an undifferentiated part of the state system, alongside the old municipal hospital system, which was similarly incorporated into a centralised administrative structure. All important vestiges of their former voluntary status were dispensed with.[6] As a result, in postwar Britain, voluntarism has played very little part in the provision of acute health care.[7]

---

*Acknowledgments: This chapter owes much to the work in this area of others. I am particularly grateful to Bernard Harris, Martin Gorsky, and John Mohan for their generosity in sharing their work and ideas and for their insightful comments on earlier drafts.

Until relatively recently, this major change in the sectoral status of British hospitals has not been the primary concern of historians investigating the reforms of 1946. Rather, the first wave of historians interested in the establishment of the NHS were mainly concerned to explain the respective influence or otherwise of the Labour Party; the medical profession; health bureaucrats; and/or medical ideas.[8] Reflecting a generally Whiggish orientation, these approaches tended to be based on the assumption that "the internal weaknesses of the inter-war voluntary hospitals had hastened the onset of state intervention," but this process was not investigated in any great detail.[9] This was despite the fact that in the reform process that led to the 1946 NHS Act, nationalisation had actually only been seriously considered quite late on, with the survival of some form of voluntarism appearing likely up to the mid-1940s. It is only more recently that the assumption of the inevitability of the voluntary sector's demise has been subjected to more rigorous scrutiny. This new work has shown that while the position and performance of the voluntary sector might not have been as bad as earlier historians had suggested,[10] the sector had in some regions at least nevertheless been significantly weakened by financial difficulties and the emergence of a rival municipal sector, and its performance was problematic in relation to coverage and the quality of care.[11]

On the basis of this new research, some commentators have continued to suggest quite straightforward links between the voluntary hospitals' interwar situation and their nationalisation in 1946. Thus, Waddington, for example, suggests: "[I]t gradually became clear that voluntarism was ill-suited to effective medical administration and that charity was unable to meet hospitals' financial needs without limiting provision and leading to widespread closure of beds . . . Under these conditions few avenues seemed open other than state funding and control . . . ."[12] Gorsky and Mohan are more circumspect. While emphasising the importance of the interwar weaknesses of voluntary hospitals as a reason for their ultimate demise, they also make plain that "[t]he coming of the NHS did not follow inexorably" from the weaknesses they identify.[13] Any assessment of "voluntary failure," they and Powell are careful to suggest, rests substantially on interpretation and perception; it is a product of the way in which the voluntary sector's performance was perceived and represented in the political debates of the time.[14] Such a view is consistent with recent developments in the theoretical literature on the voluntary sector, which has focused on the potential for voluntary bodies to become "embedded" within the social and political arrangements of the societies in which they exist.[15] Thus, their development, it is suggested, the nature of their role, and their relationship with the state are not determined solely by questions of rationality and efficiency; the voluntary sector does not immediately adapt to changing environments but can display "strong institutional inertia or historical inefficiency,"[16] with economic factors mediated by "prior patterns of historical development that significantly shape the range of options available at a given time and place."[17]

A focus on the more political aspects of the demise of the UK voluntary hospitals is thus welcome. While recent historical accounts of the voluntary sector's weaknesses in the 1930s are very strong in showing that there was a strong rational case for nationalisation by the 1940s, we still lack a clear sense of how this case interacted with—and was affected by—considerations of interest, power, and influence. The need for such analysis is strengthened by indications that evidence of significant popular support for the voluntary hospital during the immediate pre-NHS planning process could have secured voluntarism a greater role in the new health service, notwithstanding its weaknesses. "Effectively, government was challenging the voluntary sector to make good its claims to embody a genuine reservoir of public support," suggest Gorsky and Mohan.[18]

However, so far, in assessing why officials and politicians contemplating nationalisation were not overwhelmed by such a "reservoir of support," attention has focused mainly on contingent factors. Attention has been drawn to the destruction wrought on London voluntary hospitals during the blitz; the wartime growth of state intervention as part of the Emergency Medical Service (EMS); and the popular support for the 1942 Beveridge Report. These factors are undoubtedly important, as will be seen, but what has generally been ignored is any broader socially based explanation for reform. If such an explanation is evident at all, it is one that has emphasised the role of the Labour Party as an expression of working-class political power. What is missing is any real sense of the attitude of middle-class opinion to the threatened demise of the voluntary hospitals. This is an important gap, given that some leading commentators have identified the middle classes as an unambiguous source of support for the voluntary sector that can act to embed it into existing social and political arrangements.[19] Salamon and Anheier, using and adapting Esping-Andersen's typology of welfare regimes,[20] have suggested that where "middle class elements" are strong, the prospects for a liberal regime with a large voluntary sector are good.[21] So why in the liberal UK did the middle-class dog not bark with regard to the voluntary hospitals and the coming of the NHS? Salamon and Anheier suggest contingent factors: nationalisation occurred due to a temporary "postwar surge in working class support."[22] The middle classes remained supportive of voluntarism, but their views were disregarded when nationalisation was decided upon by the postwar Labour Government.

However, such an interpretation seems excessively reductionist and conflicts with work that posits a more differentiated social explanation for changes in welfare provision.[23] Thus, Baldwin in particular has shown that "class interests" cannot be categorised so simply in relation to social reform. They "cannot invariably be fitted into the binary logic of the labourist interpretation: working-class pressure confronting middle class resistance."[24] In fact, "because the middle-classes have not been immune from social risks they have often turned to the state to alleviate them,"[25] particularly, suggest Goodin and Dryzek, when their awareness of these risks has been heightened by traumatic events, such as war.[26] This more differentiated social approach is even more important, suggest Kuhnle and Selle, when the legislative outcome being referred to relates to the organisational rather than the distributive consequences of a reform proposal. They warn that because "there is no one-to-one relationship between who benefits from a given policy and the choice of organizational solution ... [t]he relationship between social interests and organizational model is very complex."[27] Significantly, Salamon's earlier work, which focused on the development of voluntary sector/state relationships, seemed to accept this situation and consequently was less categorical about middle-class support for voluntary provision.[28] In outlining the concept of voluntary-sector failure, under which certain inherent limitations of voluntarism (in relation to resources, expertise, and accountability) reduced its effectiveness, he indicated circumstances in which middle-class support for voluntary provision might not be guaranteed. Thus, state provision of collective goods might occur where "a majority of the community" becomes convinced that existing voluntary response is insufficient.[29] In other words, the middle classes might in some circumstances become the victims of voluntary insufficiency and/or particularism to the same extent as the working classes, so reducing their support for voluntary provision.

In tracing the development of the relationship between the UK middle classes and the voluntary hospitals from the late nineteenth century to the early 1940s, this chapter will argue that there is clear evidence to suggest that the middle classes were becoming victims of voluntary insufficiency by the beginning of the war.[30] It will suggest that the voluntary hospitals failed during this time sufficiently to respond to the growing demands of the middle class for hospital access and that as a result important elements in the middle classes—particularly those of "moderate means"—had little reason to defend them by the early 1940s. The failure of the voluntary hospitals in this regard will be shown to have been significantly related to the way in which the prewar health system was organised. Thus, the existing policy design (or policy legacy) and the position of established (or what Alford calls "structural") interests, as part of the institutional structure of these policy arrangements, shaped the way that the middle classes' interests were made manifest and constrained the voluntary sector's ability to respond.[31] In this regard, as will be seen, three issues are particularly important. The first relates to the limited understanding many voluntary hospitals had of their role, on the basis of their voluntarist ethos, which, together with financial constraints, meant that the demands of "ordinary," rather than middle-class, patients were often seen as the priority. The second concerns the possibility of a market response to middle-class demand, which, as will be seen, was made problematic by the existence of a well-developed voluntary system. The third relates to the main established interest in health politics, the medical profession, many of whom had good reason to obstruct middle-class entry into hospitals.

To be clear, the argument of the chapter is not that voluntary hospital insufficiency for the middle classes led directly to calls for nationalisation; consideration of this as an option arose for a range of reasons, some unrelated to the interests of the middle class. Rather, what the emerging interwar failings of the voluntary hospitals for the middle classes ensured was that officials and politicians, in proposing nationalisation, could be confident that it would receive some significant degree of cross-class support. The chapter will start by considering the rise of middle-class demand for hospital access. It will then assess the response of voluntary hospitals and explain why middle-class demand remained significantly unmet up to 1939. The chapter will conclude by considering how this general situation interacted with the contingent developments in health provision that occurred during the Second World War.

THE GROWTH OF A MIDDLE-CLASS
DEMAND FOR HOSPITAL ACCESS

Middle-class demand for hospital treatment in the UK only began to rise in the last decades of the nineteenth century. Before that, most middle-class patients preferred to be treated at home by the "family medical man"[32] or in private nursing homes.[33] Given the voluntary hospitals' charitable purpose, this situation suited the hospitals. Their role was to benefit "the sick poor."[34] Patients were generally granted access on the basis of a subscriber or governor's letter, which normally "guaranteed treatment or at least the attention of a doctor" in the hospitals to which the subscriber contributed.[35] As Gorsky and Mohan suggest, this allowed "active philanthropists the opportunity to appraise the deservingness of putative patients before they gave them the means of admission."[36] Most in the medical profession were also strongly supportive of this situation. They were anxious to prevent those who could afford to pay from "abusing" hospital charity, thus diminishing their private fees. GPs in particular had become increasingly concerned from the 1880s that patients who were not members of the "sick poor" were using hospital facilities (particularly outpatients) in an attempt to avoid having to pay a GP.[37] As will be seen, these GP concerns were to prove a persistent impediment to middle-class hospital access up to the Second World War.

The relatively small number of middle-class patients who did seek hospital entry in the mid-nineteenth century were nevertheless often able to slip through gaps in access procedures. Not all hospitals operated the "letter system," and many of those that did still allowed immediate access for accident and emergencies.[38] Moreover, where the letter system was in place, there is evidence that it was sometimes used by subscribers to gain access for their dependants or "to save their own pockets."[39] In other instances, individual doctors accepted middle-class patients as cases who "met their clinical interests or teaching needs," often using accident and emergency procedures or outpatient services to facilitate access.[40] In some hospitals (particularly cottage hospitals), middle-class patients could also pay for access, although this remained relatively uncommon up to the end of the nineteenth century.[41] Only 26 per cent of the 709 hospitals surveyed by Burdett's Hospitals and Charities in 1901 allowed admission on the basis of payment.[42]

In the early part of the twentieth century, the attitude of the middle classes to hospitals began to change, and consequently the ad hoc arrangements in existence to manage their access began to come under pressure. Improvements in hospital care as a result of significant medical advances and managerial reforms improved the standing of the hospitals among all sections of the population.[43] These changes were accompanied and supported by greater medical specialisation and the growth and utilisation of laboratory science.[44] At the same time, nursing standards also improved—ward sisters were better educated and training increased for all grades of nurse[45]—and "improvements in the physical fabric of many hospitals" led to a "reduction in post-operative mortality."[46] Managerially, voluntary hospitals also began slowly to modernise. Not without resistance from traditional voluntary elites and some in the medical profession, "an increasingly corporate system of medical management"[47] began to form in response to pressure from "agencies for charitable coordination" (e.g., the Charity Organisation Society and King Edward's Hospital Fund for London[48]) and as some hospitals established closer links with business and industry.[49] A greater concern for efficient and productive practice developed as the new professional middle classes asserted their claims to be involved in running of hospitals, suggest Sturdy and Cooter.[50]

The effect of these changes was not immediate. As Waddington suggests, "contemporary attitudes" to voluntary hospitals "lagged behind institutional and medical developments."[51] However, by the beginning of the twentieth century the perception of hospitals as merely "gateways to death" was disappearing.[52] Demand for hospital provision increased among all sections of the population. "By the 1880s," observes Pickstone, "they were beginning to appear as medical facilities necessary to most of the population. They provided standards of nursing and cleanliness which were unattainable in most homes."[53] They also compared more than favourably with conditions found in private nursing homes—the only alternative site for the institutional medical care of the middle classes. The development of these up to the mid-1920s was far less marked in comparison with the voluntary hospitals: many had no "room set aside as an operating theatre," no resident medical officer and no lift.[54] One leading consultant concluded in 1927 that it was only "in the best and therefore most expensive" that "the facilities afforded even distantly approximated to what is normally found in a first class hospital."[55] Increasingly, on this basis, medical professionals encouraged their private patients to avoid private nursing homes and seek hospital access, a development that was further prompted by evidence that nursing-home fees were too high for many moderate earners.[56] Overwhelmingly, it was the voluntary hospitals that were the focus of this new demand. While the municipal system was steadily improving up to 1939, this improvement was patchy, and its continued association with the Poor Law limited its attractiveness to the middle classes.[57]

These developments were not peculiar to Britain. Middle-class demand for hospital care in France, for example, increased, if anything, more rapidly than in Britain in the early part of the twentieth century, stimulated to a large extent by the greater number of casualties in the First World War and the conflict's more general effect on the civilian population.[58] In France, as Smith has shown, the voluntary hospitals were unable to respond to this new demand; and, as a result, the state became more substantially involved in the provision of hospital care. How well did the British hospital system cope with a similar, if less rapid, change of circumstances?

VOLUNTARY HOSPITALS AND MIDDLE-CLASS DEMAND

There is no doubt that change did occur. As was seen at the start of this chapter, voluntary hospitals expanded their bed numbers to cater for ever-increasing numbers of inpatients with admissions in London increasing from 39,931 in 1873 to 68,319 in 1893.[59] Outpatient admissions also rose. This led to a rise in the costs of staffing, provisions, medical supplies, and domestic maintenance, which was particularly rapid in the interwar years. In London alone, total voluntary hospital expenditure at current prices rose from £2.5 million in 1920 (112 hospitals) to £4.8 million in 1938 (146 hospitals).[60]

However, increased capacity in voluntary hospitals was of limited use if impediments other than supply restricted access to hospital provision; and, in this regard, as has been seen, access to those other than the "sick poor" had been restricted up to the end of the nineteenth century by hospitals' charitable ethos and the desire of the medical profession to preserve its fee base. To what extent were the voluntary hospitals willing or able to adapt their ethos and procedures in the face of these new demands?

On this matter, previous commentators have disagreed. Contemporaries sympathetic to voluntarism spoke of significant change, such that the hospitals had become by the 1930s "a co-operative effort in which all the classes of the community, including the Hospitals' patients themselves, combine as their means permit, to provide Hospital services which produce benefits for all classes."[61] More recently, Smith has suggested that recourse to private insurance allowed the middle classes reasonable access, thus forestalling the pressure that developed in France in favour of state intervention.[62] Other commentators are less sanguine. Prochaska concludes negatively: there was, he suggests, "a failure to satisfy middle-class demand for hospital treatment," which meant the "better-off" . . . were "unable to take advantage of ordinary hospital beds, and without sufficient pay-beds at their disposal" had "to enter expensive nursing homes."[63]

However, these conclusions are all somewhat impressionistic. Thus, the aim of the rest of this chapter is to look in more detail at the question of middle-class hospital access in the early part of the twentieth century. It will suggest that, while there is no doubt that significant changes took place in the UK voluntary hospital system, which significantly broadened and made easier hospital access, this process was often the unintentional consequence of changes made to secure other ends, most particularly the financial well-being of hospitals in the face of declining charitable subscriptions, and was not always directly aimed at the middle classes. As a result, tensions and controversy still surrounded the issue of middle-class access with questions (which had first arisen in the previous century) about its implications for the voluntarist basis of hospital provision and the economic situation of doctors still largely unresolved. These in turn placed limitations on the hospital capacity made available to middle-class groups. Thus, while access improved for middle-class patients, significant difficulties remained, a situation that was thrown into sharper relief by the generally more positive effect of access developments with respect to working-class patients.

There are two developments in the voluntary-hospital field in the early twentieth century that are of most importance in this regard. The first is the development of hospital contributory and provident schemes. The second is the introduction of patient payments and pay beds. With regard first to the growth of hospital contributory schemes, these were largely a working-class phenomenon for much of the interwar period, but their development nevertheless had important implications for middle-class access. The schemes had begun to develop in the early part of the nineteenth century but only became more general from the 1870s.[64] By the 1930s, most hospitals were involved with a scheme of some sort. This development was largely initiated by the hospitals themselves as a means of raising resources as expenditure rose and charitable subscription declined. It was strongly encouraged by the government-established Cave Committee in 1921.[65] The schemes were not generally established as a form of insurance, and there was no expectation that they would fundamentally alter the purpose of the voluntary hospitals. However, as Gorsky and Mohan suggest, "the new funding mechanisms gradually undermined the social hierarchies implicit in the administrative and operational procedures of the voluntary hospitals."[66] In particular, they altered the basis on which access to the voluntary hospitals was determined. From a charitable system designed to cater for the needs of the sick poor, the system gradually became one, with the growth of the contributory schemes, that granted access of some sort on the basis of entitlements built up—or perceived to have been built up—by the payment of a contribution. This development remained highly contested, and the extent to which contributory schemes granted their members an entitlement to hospital treatment remained a source of dispute up to the Second World War.[67] However, there is no doubt that in many cases contributory schemes eased hospital access for their members.[68] Partly as a result, the number of patients reliant on the letter system to gain hospital access declined.[69]

As was suggested earlier, most contributory schemes had working-class roots and were targeted at this group. Some originated within the friendly society or guild movement; others were set up by hospital or middle-class elites as a mechanism for raising funds from working-class sources and/or promoting working-class self-help. Most by the early twentieth century placed income caps on contributors such that those earning over a specified income could not join the scheme (see following). Thus, for example, the Hospital Savings Association (HSA), set up in London in 1922 at the instigation of the King's Fund, operated an upper-earnings limit of between £250 and £300 during the 1920s and 1930s.[70] Nevertheless, as many contemporaries realised, the working-class contributory schemes offered a model on which increased middle-class hospital access could be developed. Indeed, as Smith suggests, to some extent this is a development that did occur.[71] Hospital savings and provident schemes for the middle classes were developed (notably the British Provident Association), and some existing working-class schemes opened their doors to a broader social mix.[72] There is evidence of local middle-class schemes operating in Bath, Birmingham, Bristol, Buckinghamshire, Coventry, Manchester, Merseyside, Oxford, Sheffield, and Sussex in the 1920s and 1930s; and schemes were also offered by professional organisations, such as the Civil Service Whitley Council.[73] These schemes began to become more organised in the mid-1930s, mainly on the initiative of the BMA, which, as will be seen, wanted to control their development.[74] A series of conferences were held and "a loose federation of Provident Associations" was formed in 1937.[75] In London in 1943, after much delay (see following), a city-wide provident fund aimed at the middle classes, London Association for Hospitals, was incorporated. It was formed on the initiative of the King's Fund and extended hospital coverage above the limits set by the HSA.[76]

Some contemporaries, particularly in the medical profession, urged that this development should be part of a market-based solution to middle-class demands with the development of private pay hospitals, perhaps on the basis of the existing nursing-home network.[77] However, the existing institutional arrangements of health provision acted as an impediment on a development of this type. Thus, as has been seen, nursing homes were substantially inferior to the voluntary hospitals, and significant capital investment would be required to improve them or even build new hospitals for the middle class. The cost of this investment would raise patients' fees, which, it was feared, would limit market size.[78] Given the uncertainty that anyway surrounded the future of health-care provision, and indications that voluntary hospitals were slowly opening their doors to middle-class patients, few entrepreneurs were prepared to risk such a venture. Very few pay hospitals opened and those that did often struggled to stay afloat.[79]

Thus, with the market unable to react, it was the voluntary hospitals that responded to demands from middle-class patients generally on the basis of payment for service. As has been seen, in 1901 only 26 per cent of hospitals granted access on this basis. By 1928, however, this figure had increased to 43 per cent.[80] Within these hospitals the popularity of means-tested payment systems rose even more rapidly. Thus, while only 16 per cent of hospitals, providing access on the basis of payment in 1901, had means-testing arrangements in place, by 1928 this figure had risen to 54 per cent.[81] This increased role for payments did not by itself signify a new openness to middle-class patients: it was at least partially related to the growth of working-class hospital contributory schemes, with many hospitals asking for additional payments from "ordinary" contributory patients on a means-tested basis.[82] Pay beds, however, were a direct response by voluntary hospitals to middle-class demand. These beds were established in many hospitals specifically to facilitate access for those who were outside the limits of the contributory system but who were nevertheless of "moderate means" and unable to afford the fees of private nursing homes.[83] Thus, in London, in 1928, seventy-five of the 148 hospitals surveyed by the King's Fund provided pay beds;[84] by 1939, 114 out of 146 hospitals did so.[85] As a consequence, the overall number of pay beds provided increased from 552 in 1921[86] to 969 in 1928.[87] There were further rises to 1510 by 1931[88] and 2511 by 1939.[89] Outside London, a similar increase in pay-bed provision appears to have occurred. Whereas a 1930 BMA survey of 813 hospitals found that less than a quarter of the larger hospitals had private beds,[90] by 1938 the Nuffield Hospital Trust Survey found that 72 per cent of the 611 general and cottage provided pay beds.[91]

However, if progress was undoubtedly made in facilitating middle-class access to hospital care in the interwar period, was the development of middle-class provident schemes and the opening up of working-class schemes, in combination with the growth of pay beds, a sufficient response? There is strong evidence that it was not. Overall, the scale of middle-class provision remained comparatively small up to the early 1940s, and even this level of provision was very slow to develop. With regard first to middle-class provident funds, these remained very limited in terms of size and coverage. Thus, the BPA had only 2500 members by the late 1920s[92] and, on this basis, was described by the King's Fund as an "experiment . . . still on a small scale."[93] By the beginning of the 1940s, membership had only climbed to approximately 5000.[94] The Birmingham Extended Benefits Scheme—with 11,600 members by 1945—was bigger, but overall the scale of middle-class provident movement by the late 1930s was minute in comparison with those provided for working-class contributors. Thus, while twenty associations were represented at a BMA-organised conference in the mid-1930s, there were by this date over 400 working-class contributory schemes, representing close to 11 million members.[95] The 1941 edition of the *Voluntary Hospital Year Book* recorded forty-nine schemes in total, but twenty-seven of these were small-scale schemes associated with individual hospitals.[96] Moreover, while progress was undoubtedly made in the mid to late 1930s in expanding middle-class provident schemes (with, as has been seen, for example, the formation of the London Association for Hospitals), this came too late to embed the practice of middle-class health insurance before the Second World War put developments on hold.

An important reason for the slow pace of these developments were concerns among scheme administrators that insufficient accommodation existed for privately insured patients. Thus, Sir Alan Anderson, chairman of the BPA, argued in 1928 that "before any general propaganda [about the organisation] is started, there should be a sufficient number of beds placed at the disposal of subscribers to the British Provident Association to make it worth their while to join the scheme."[97] As has been seen, some argued that it should be the market (i.e., the provision of private pay hospitals) rather than the voluntary sector that should respond to this demand. However, because this did not occur, the development of middle-class provident funds became inextricably linked to the number of voluntary hospital pay beds—if this did not expand, neither could the provident funds.

In this regard, progress was also slow up to the war, notwithstanding the rise in the number of beds outlined above. Let us start with London. Here, developments began from a very low base figure, with the 969 pay beds provided by King's Fund-listed hospitals in London in 1928 amounting to only 6 per cent of the total number of beds. Neither the major hospitals nor the King's Fund were under any illusions that this figure was sufficient. St Mary's Hospital, for example, which provided no pay beds in the late 1920s, reported "almost daily" applications, and reported the existence of "a great unsatisfied demand."[98] Similarly, St Thomas's, which did provide pay beds, told the King's Fund that their "experience" was that "there is urgent need" for more beds.[99] The fund's 1928 pay-beds report concluded that "a material extension of this provision is urgently required to meet the existing demand." It sought to quantify this demand on the basis of a BPA estimate of middle-class requirements, calculated using the incidence of illness among its subscribers. It thus suggested that 5500 beds were immediately required, although the BMA thought this figure had been set too low.[100] As has been seen, even by the late 1930s the number of pay beds had only reached less than half this figure, and there is good reason to believe that in the interim demand among the middle classes had risen, particularly given the large-scale closure of nursing homes during this period.[101]

Moreover, many of the new beds that were supplied in London were aimed at the "well-to-do"—whose demand the King's Fund was later to report was growing to "an ever-increasing extent"—rather than those of moderate means.[102] Thus, while in London between 1927 and 1936, there was a 12 per cent increase in pay beds costing three guineas per week and a 70 per cent increase in those costing four to five guineas, the increase in beds costing six guineas was 126 per cent with a 424 per cent increase in beds costing seven guineas or more.[103] On this basis, the King's Fund concluded in 1937 that "there is a serious likelihood that the supply of pay beds for the well-to-do will outrun demand," and that "there is room for considerable growth in the moderate class."[104] Thus, many pay beds in London were expensive. However, this flat-rate fee was not the only cost incurred by middle-class patients. Many consultants charged additional fees, and there were also charges for X-rays, pathology, and laboratory work.[105] These additional costs often caused particular problems because, as the King's Fund found in the early 1940s, patients were not always told beforehand the size of the total bill they might be expected to pay. Patients were sometimes "shocked and surprised when they receive their account and see what extras have amounted to," a fund memo reported in 1944.[106] Where opportunities for provident scheme membership were limited, middle-class patients were unable to manage these costs in a way that lessened the burden of lump-sum payments. Some found themselves after discharge from hospital in a state of "considerable hardship."[107] Overall, therefore, contemporary observers were in no doubt that pay-bed provision in London was insufficient to meet middle-class demand. On this basis, the King's Fund spoke in 1936 of growing dissatisfaction with voluntary hospitals as a result of its "failure ... to adjust itself on an adequate scale to the growth of the middle classes. In London at any rate, the middle classes however defined represent a very large proportion of the population which proportion [sic] is not reflected in the provision of hospital accommodation."[108]

Outside London, the situation appears to have been similar. While, as been seen, most general and cottage voluntary hospitals surveyed by the Nuffield Hospitals Trust in 1938 provided pay beds, for 40 per cent of this group pay-bed provision constituted 10 per cent or less of total bed provision. Overall, only 13 per cent of bed provision in the surveyed hospitals was pay-bed provision. Although the situation was not the same everywhere, the inspectors who undertook the Nuffield Hospital surveys in the early 1940s reached similar conclusions on the basis of these figures to those at the Kings Fund. One reported: "We have generally been informed that the number of pay beds is totally inadequate for the requirements of the area, even where the largest provision has been made. We conclude therefore that the demand for this service is greater than the supply."[109]

THE OBSTACLES TO THE DEVELOPMENT
OF MIDDLE-CLASS PROVISION

Given this substantial evidence in the early part of the twentieth century of unmet middle-class demand for hospital access and the encouragement, on this basis, of greater provision from a wide range of sources sympathetic to the voluntary-hospital movement, why wasn't more progress made? The answer to this question lies in important ideological and institutional impediments that limited developments. The ability of voluntary hospitals to respond to middle-class demand was constrained, sometimes by the continuing salience of the voluntarist ethos amongst hospital authorities, which restricted moves to accommodate better-off patients at the expense of the sick poor, but also by the continuing resistance to such developments from general practitioners, and sometimes consultants, who feared for their own economic security and made their views known through the BMA (see preceding).

With regard to the first problem, the voluntarist ethos of hospitals placed a constraint on the developments in formal and informal ways. Formally, many hospitals were bound legally to concentrate their resources and provision on the sick poor, generally as part of their trust arrangements, which formed the basis for their charitable status.[110] If lost, this would affect the hospitals' income-tax exemption and favourable assessment for local rates.[111] This impediment should not be exaggerated. The charity commissioners were prepared to negotiate with individual hospitals about pay-bed development.[112] However, there is no doubt that it inhibited the development of pay beds and frustrated some hospitals' attempts to increase their number. The King's Fund sought to remove this impediment in 1934 by sponsoring a bill in the House of Lords.[113] This would have largely removed the restrictions placed on hospitals as a result of their charitable status. As the Treasury Solicitor's office commented in reading the bill, it was framed "mainly from the point of view of supplying public need, namely the provision of beds for paying patients."[114] However, government was not prepared to go this far. Concerns had been expressed in Cabinet about the effect of such a measure on provision for "ordinary" patients and, despite assurances that the charity commissioners would have the power to stop schemes that threatened this principle, the attorney general insisted on "fairly stringent restrictions" in the bill. "The Hospitals really wanted much more powers," a charity commissioner later conceded, but the attorney general was anxious "to make certain that buildings and endowments given for the very poor were not diverted to the benefit of the rich."[115] Largely as a result, only a relatively few hospitals applied to use their new powers in the late 1930s.

There were also less formal reasons for this reluctance. Many hospital authorities were quite simply unprepared to use any resources to cater for middle-class needs at a time when they were unable to deal with the demands of their "ordinary patients." One voluntary hospital official complained in 1927: "[A]ll the hospitals which I know of are more than full today; that is to say that the accommodation which they are providing is not sufficient to meet the wants of the class of persons whom they are today catering for. As a result all hospitals have long waiting lists."[116] Similarly, St George's Hospital reported that, while it had set up pay beds in 1913, it had closed them shortly after because "the demand for ordinary beds was so great." It also complained that middle-class patients wanted more "personal attention," which took up more staff time than was available.[117] Often for this reason, forty-one hospitals, including ten general hospitals, surveyed by the King's Fund in 1928 had no plans to provide pay beds.

As Prochaska suggests, the King's Fund itself was sympathetic to such concerns. It had "never taken the view that the charitable status of hospitals was incompatible with paying patients" but remained wary of a general orientation of voluntary hospitals towards the middle classes, given the needs of their primary constituency. For example, it refused a request from a member of the BMA in 1929 to provide money to assist the establishment of pay beds. "[T]he Fund's primary aim was for the voluntary hospitals," suggested the Earl of Donoughmore, a chairman of the Management Committee, "and not pay beds."[118] It was also reluctant to take the lead in the establishment of a middle-class provident fund for London (although it eventually did so) and offered only tacit support to the British Provident Association in its attempts to expand, despite repeated attempts by the association to establish a more formal tie.[119]

There were also more pragmatic financially based reasons for hospitals taking such a stance or at least placing very definite limits on middle-class access. These were related to the continuing, if declining, importance of charity and subscriber donations as a source of funds for the voluntary hospitals, which still made up one-third of hospital income in 1936.[120] These donations rested, it was felt, on the continued association of the voluntary hospitals with provision for "necessitous patients" and could be put at risk if access for this type of patient became regarded as a "secondary principle."[121] A similar effect was feared if hospitals became too strongly linked with insurance-based schemes. For this reason, as Gorsky and Mohan have shown, voluntary hospital authorities made concerted efforts to present working-class hospital contributory schemes as a form of self-help philanthropy.[122] However, it was far more difficult to present commercially based middle-class provident funds on this basis.

The second main obstacle to greater middle-class access to the voluntary-hospital system was the established interest of the medical profession, most especially general practitioners, in the existing health system. As has been seen, general practitioners had resisted the growth of paying patients in hospitals in the late decades of the nineteenth century as a threat to their private fee base. The changes that took place in the voluntary sector in the interwar period "revived" and "fanned" this "historic conflict between general practitioners and voluntary hospitals."[123] The increasing use of hospitals by the "nonpoor," including some in the middle class, who financed their treatment by direct payments or hospital insurance funds (see preceding), again raised the prospect of a declining private-patient base for general practice. For some GPs, who had access to hospitals, this development was less of a problem, but for most it was. For this reason, the British Medical Association (BMA),[124] while accepting that there was little that could done to reverse the general phenomenon, tried to ensure that it occurred in a way that preserved, so far as was possible, the position of GPs. It was at least partially for this reason, for example, that income limits were maintained on hospital-insurance schemes (see preceding)—to prevent the middle classes using them to pay for hospital treatment.[125] With regard to pay beds, the BMA's concerns were part of the reason why prices were kept high. The BMA tried to ensure that the beds were not subsidised by hospitals from their charitable funds but that hospital fees "fully cover every cost to the hospital," including capital cost.[126]

The BMA's efforts were not always successful. Thus, some of the biggest contributory schemes (e.g., the London-based Hospital Saving Association and the Birmingham Hospitals Contributory Association), while operating income limits, also included higher paid contributors on the basis of an additional charge.[127] The HSA thus became known among some in the BMA as "charity at the expense of the medical profession."[128] Other schemes imposed no income limits at all.[129] Nevertheless, there can be little doubt that medical opposition in combination with the other impediments served to delay and limit the scale of hospital provision for the middle classes.

MIDDLE-CLASS VOLUNTARY FAILURE AND NATIONALISATION

To summarise, while the voluntary hospitals did adapt to the changing demands of the middle classes in the interwar period, there were clear constraints on these developments, which meant that few contemporary commentators believed middle-class demands were being met. Importantly, some of these constraints were inherent to the voluntary-hospital system. They were a product of voluntarism. Thus, while the hospitals began to grant access to many patients beyond their traditional "sick-poor" constituency, the voluntarist ethos that dictated that the hospital existed mainly to serve the least well off remained very influential, both among some hospital administrators and, importantly, within government. This significantly slowed down the extent to which the hospitals could respond to the requirements of the middle classes. By the end of the interwar period there was a clear sense that the middle classes were victims of voluntary insufficiency and particularism.

This does not mean that the difficulties experienced by the middle classes in gaining access to hospitals in the interwar period were fed directly into the political process as a demand for fundamental reform of the voluntary system before the war. Middle-class hospital access was certainly, as has been seen, a subject that engaged policymakers, but most assumed that solutions to the problem could eventually be found within existing arrangements. Likewise, those who argued strongly for the nationalisation or municipalisation of the voluntary hospitals in the prewar period rarely did so explicitly on the basis of their problems in catering for the middle classes. They based their arguments more on the possibilities for planning and rationalisation it was thought nationalisation would create and because of ethical objections to the reliance placed on charity in the provision of a public good.

Nationalisation arose on the political agenda partly as a result of the greater salience of the former argument in wartime conditions and because of the growing influence of those who supported this type of approach. There is no doubt also that the establishment of the Emergency Medical Service was an important development.[130] Moreover, as the reform process began to gain momentum after the publication of the Beveridge Report, nationalisation also came gradually to be seen as the only way of overcoming the obstacles to reform posed by the existing policy legacy (i.e., the uncoordinated nature of prewar hospital arrangements) and the institutional interests of the medical profession. The former made some form of coordination a prerequisite; the latter prevented this from occurring on the basis of local authority-run health service.

However, an understanding of why nationalisation came seriously to be contemplated in the early 1940s can only be partial if consideration is not also given to the question of its broader social acceptability. Baldwin's suggestion that important decisions about social policy are generally only taken "in accordance with the concerns of the most powerful social interests"[131] might be regarded as too sweeping, but it is nevertheless extremely unlikely that nationalisation of the voluntary hospitals would have been considered if politicians had felt it would provoke substantial popular opposition from the middle classes. Greater public support would have more firmly embedded the voluntary hospitals as a fixture in UK social provision and made nationalisation a more risky political undertaking notwithstanding its administrative advantages. Certainly, Labour politicians, including Bevan, were not immune from considering the electoral implications of their actions. There was no sense of political invulnerability within the Labour Party in the mid-1940s despite the "landslide" victory of 1945. Indeed, as contemporary politicians and commentators were aware, Labour's victory owed a lot to middle-class support in a number of key constituencies.[132] In these circumstances, clear evidence of middle-class opposition to the nationalisation of the voluntary hospitals would have made the proposal substantially more problematic.

In fact, the evidence that existed about middle-class opinion pointed in the reverse direction. A range of opinion polls conducted in 1944 and 1945 suggested, in the words of the *The Economist*, that nationalisation had attained "an almost middle class respectability."[133] The British Institute of Public Opinion, for example, found 90 per cent support for a national heath service among lower-middle-class respondents.[134] These results might have overstated the level of middle-class support for nationalisation of health services.[135] Small mass-observation surveys on this issue undertaken in 1943 suggest the picture was less clear-cut, with the middle classes particularly suspicious of nationalisation of general practitioner services. However, support for hospital nationalisation was stronger. Almost half of the middle-class individuals surveyed in April 1943 indicated a preference for administration of hospitals by state bodies, municipal, or central government, with voluntarism favoured by only a fifth.[136] In July of the same year, more than 50 per cent of those middle-class individuals who expressed a preference favoured "government control" of hospitals.[137] Summing up the general picture on the basis of a larger and broader ranging survey undertaken at the end of 1943, one mass-observation surveyor suggested: "Many people who were otherwise moderately satisfied with available medical facilities felt, often very strongly, that the time was ripe for some changes on the hospital front . . . Many suggest that all hospitals should be financed by the state, not through voluntary contributions . . . Some who are more doubtful about the wisdom of nationalising medicine, all the same want to see state control of the hospitals."[138] It is difficult to be sure of the reason for this greater openness among the middle classes to hospital nationalisation, but it seems likely that it reflected in part the problems experienced in the prewar period in gaining hospital access. These had been thrown into sharper relief by the setting up of the EMS, which, despite problems of its own,[139] changed in important ways the procedures by which hospital entry was granted. Thus, access became less a product of income status, contributory scheme membership, or payment and more related to need. Initially, this focused on wartime casualties, who were granted immediate access, but as Webster suggests the "services . . . initially intended for casualties became available on an increasingly liberal scale to civilians."[140] As an experiment in greater state control, it compared favourably with the prewar system it had replaced, suggesting that the middle classes had little to lose from movement in this direction. Thus, consideration of nationalisation in the context of the voluntary hospitals became a relatively safe political option. This was certainly the view of Bevan. In proposing a nationalised hospital service to the Labour Cabinet in 1946, he confidently predicted: "I do not believe we need fear the political consequences. That there will be opposition, even violent opposition in some quarters, I do not deny. That it will lose us votes . . . I doubt."[141]

NOTES

1. Steven Cherry, "Before the national health service: Financing the voluntary hospitals, 1900–1939," *Economic History Review*, L(2), 305–26, at p. 306.
2. Martin Powell, *Evaluating the National Health Service*, Buckingham, UK: Open University Press, 1997, p. 22.
3. Steven Cherry, "Beyond National Health Insurance. The voluntary hospital and hospital contributory schemes: A regional study," *Social History of Medicine*, 5, 455–82; D. M. Fox, *Health polices, health politics: The British and American experience, 1911–1965*, Princeton, NJ: Princeton University Press, 1986.
4. On either basis they would certainly qualify as "voluntary" organisations under Salamon and Anheier's 1997 definition of the sector. See Lester Salamon and Helmut Anheier, *Defining the nonprofit sector: A comparative analysis*, Manchester: Manchester University Press, 1997.
5. Cherry, "Before the National Health Service," p. 315; see also Cherry, "Beyond National Insurance," p. 465.

6. The only element of voluntarism that remained under the NHS was that hospitals were allowed to raise supplementary income through voluntary fund-raising campaigns and the teaching hospitals were allowed to keep their endowments. See Martin Gorsky and John Mohan, *Medicine and mutual aid: British hospital contributory schemes in the twentieth century*, Manchester, UK: Manchester University Press, 2006.
7. Jeremy Kendall and Martin Knapp, *The voluntary sector in the United Kingdom*, Manchester, UK: Manchester University Press, 1996. The voluntary sector has continued, however, to play a significant role in the provision of palliative health care and social care. The provision of health and social care—the definitional boundary between which has always been ambiguous—has since 1946 been administratively and financially separate.
8. See, e.g., H. Eckstein, *The English health service: Its origins, structure and achievements*, Cambridge, MA: Harvard University Press, 1964; Charles Webster, "Conflict and consensus: Explaining the British health service," *Twentieth Century British History*, 1, 115–51; Daniel Fox, *Health policies, health politics: the British and American experience, 1911–65*, Princeton, NJ: Princeton University Press.
9. Martin Gorsky and John Mohan, "London's voluntary hospitals in the interwar period: Growth, transformation, or crisis?," *Nonprofit and Voluntary Sector Quarterly*, 30, 247–75; see also Frank Prochaska, *Philanthropy and the hospitals of London: The Kings Fund, 1897–1990*, Oxford: Clarendon, 1992. Certainly, Abel-Smith, who provides the fullest account of the political and administrative developments leading to the nationalisation of the voluntary hospitals, stresses these inherent weaknesses as the primary cause for the voluntary hospitals' demise. Brian Abel-Smith, *The hospitals 1800–1948: A study in social administration in England and Wales*, London: Heinemann, 1964, pp. 405–23.
10. Prochaska, *Philanthropy and the hospitals of London*, p. 104.
11. Cherry, "Before the National Health Service"; Martin Gorsky, John Mohan, and Martin Powell, "British voluntary hospitals, 1871–1938: The geography of provision and utilization," *Journal of Historical Geography*, 25, 463–82; Gorsky and Mohan, "London's voluntary hospitals in the interwar period: Gorsky and Mohan, *Medicine and mutual aid*.
12. Keir Waddington, *Charity and the London hospitals, 1850–1898*, London: Woodford, 2000, p. 216; my italics. See also Steven Cherry, "Accountability, entitlement and control issues and voluntary hospital funding *c*1860–1939," *Social History of Medicine*, 9, 220–21; and Steven Cherry, *Medical services and the hospitals in Britain, 1860–1939*, Cambridge, Cambridge University Press, 1996, p. 77.
13. Gorsky and Mohan, "London's voluntary hospitals in the interwar period," p. 269.
14. Gorsky, Mohan, and Powell, "British voluntary hospitals."
15. W. Seibel, "Government-nonprofit relationship: Styles and linkage patterns in France and Germany," in S. Kuhnle and P. Selle, eds., *Voluntary agencies in the welfare state*, Berkeley: University of California Press, 1992; see also S. Kuhnle and P. Selle, "Meeting needs in a welfare state: Relations between government and voluntary organizations in Norway," in A. Ware and R. Goodin, eds., *Needs and welfare*, London: Sage, 1989; and Lester Salamon and Helmut Anheier, "Social origins of civil society: Explaining the nonprofit sector cross-nationally," *Voluntas*, 9, 213–48.
16. J. G. March and J. P. Olsen, *Rediscovering institutions: The organizational basis of politics*, London: Macmillan, 1989; W. W. Powell and P. J. Di Maggio,

eds., *The new institutionalism in organizational analysis*, Chicago: University of Chicago Press, 1991.

17. Salamon and Anheier, "Social origins of civil society," p. 226.
18. *Medicine and mutual aid*, p. 155.
19. Salamon and Anheier, "Social origins of civil society."
20. Gosta Esping-Andersen, *The three worlds of welfare capitalism*, Cambridge: Polity Press, 1990.
21. The only circumstance in which middle-class support for a more statist approach to welfare provision is suggested is in alliance with a strong working class in social democratic regimes. However, the reasons why this might occur are not explained. Salamon and Anheier, "Social origins of civil society," p. 17.
22. L. M. Salamon, S. Wojciech Sokolowski, and H. K. Anheier, "Social origins of civil society: An overview." Working papers of the Johns Hopkins Comparative Nonprofit Sector Project, 2000, 19. Available online at http://www.jhu.edu/~ccss/pubs/pdf/cnpwp38.pdf.
23. E.g., Peter Baldwin, *Politics of social solidarity: Class bases of the European welfare state 1875–1975*, Cambridge: Cambridge University Press, 1990; C. Ragin, "Social origins theory: A comment on Salamon and Anheier," *Voluntas*, 9; and Hugh Heclo, *Modern social politics in Britain and Sweden : From relief to income maintenance*, New Haven, CT: Yale University Press, 1974.
24. Baldwin, *Politics of social solidarity*, p. 290. See also R. E. Goodin and J. Le Grand, *Not only the poor: The middle classes and the welfare state*, London: Allen and Unwin, 1987.
25. Baldwin, *Politics of social solidarity*, p. 289.
26. R. E. Goodin and J. Dryzek, "Risk-sharing and social justice: The motivational foundations of the post-war welfare state," in Goodin and Le Grand, *Not only the poor*. Their point is slightly different from that of Baldwin in its emphasis on the morally transforming effect of periods of uncertainty leading the middle classes to appreciate the interests of others. Baldwin, in contrast, suggests the middle classes are merely acting in their own interest and that this can sometimes be consistent with greater state provision.
27. ***Kuhnle and Selle, "Meeting needs in a welfare state," p. 17.
28. On voluntary sector/state relationships, see R. Kramer, *Voluntary agencies in the welfare state*, Berkeley: University of California Press, 1981; Jane Lewis, *The voluntary sector, the state and social work in Britain*, Aldershot, UK: Edward Elgar, 1995; Geoffrey Finlayson, *Citizen, state, and social welfare in Britain 1830–1990*, Oxford: Clarendon Press, 1994; Kuhnle and Selle, "Meeting needs in a welfare state"; Adalbert Evers, "Part of the welfare mix: The third sector as an intermediate area," *Voluntas*, 6, 159–82.
29. Lester Salamon, *Partners in public service: Government-nonprofit relations in the modern welfare state*, Baltimore, MD: Johns Hopkins University Press, 1995, p. 39.
30. In this regard, "middle class" is understood as it was at the time to include those people who had incomes above the limits set by National Health Insurance and/or hospital contributory schemes (see following).
31. Paul Pierson, "When effect becomes cause: Policy feedback and political change," *World Politcs*, 45, 595–628; S. Steinmo, K. Thelen, and F. Longstreth, eds., *Structuring politics: Historical institutionalism in comparative analysis*, Cambridge, Cambridge University Press, 1992.
32. G. Rivett, *The Development of the London hospital system 1823–1982*, London: King Edward's Hospital Fund for London, 1986, p. 121.
33. Prochaska, *Philanthropy and the hospitals of London*, p. 6; Rivett, *The development of the London hospital system*, p. 102; Keir Waddington, "Unsuitable

cases: The debate over outpatient admissions, the medical profession and late-Victorian London hospitals," *Medical History*, 42, 26–46, at p. 32.

34. This, according to *The Lancet*, meant they should assist "suitable cases for charity . . . whilst they are unable because of sickness or accident to follow their normal pursuits." Quoted in Rivett, *The development of the London hospital system*, p. 28; see also J. Pickstone, *Medicine and industrial society*, Manchester: Manchester University Press, 1985, p. 67; and Prochaska, *Philanthropy and the hospitals of London*, pp. 6 and 55; Waddington, *Charity and the London hospitals*, p. 8.

35. Waddington, *Charity and the London hospitals*, p. 33.

36. Gorsky and Mohan, *Medicine and mutual aid*, p. 19; see also Cherry, "Beyond national health insurance."

37. Waddington, "Unsuitable cases"; Waddington, *Charity and the London hospitals*; F. Honigsbaum, *The division in British medicine: A history of the separation of general practice and hospital care 1911–1968*, London: Kogan Page, 1979; Rivett, *The development of the London hospital system*.

38. Pickstone, *Medicine and industrial society*; Gorsky and Mohan, *Medicine and mutual aid*; Rivett, *The development of the London hospital system*.

39. Waddington, "Charity and the London hospitals," p. 33; also Waddington, "Unsuitable cases"; Rivett, *The development of the London hospital system*; Pickstone, *Medicine and industrial society*.

40. Gorsky and Mohan, *Medicine and mutual aid*, p. 19; see also Waddington, "Unsuitable cases"; and Rivett, *The development of the London hospital system*.

41. Cherry, "Beyond National Health Insurance"; Cherry, "Before the national health service."

42. Gorsky and Mohan, *Medicine and mutual aid*, p. 32.

43. With regard to the former, Sir George Newman, the chief medical officer in the Ministry of Health between 1919 and 1935, spoke of "four great ideas"—vaccination, anaesthesia, antisepsis, and understanding of causes of infectious diseases—developed or implemented in hospitals during this period that laid the basis for the development of Western biomedicine and, eventually, the new respectability of hospitals. Cherry, *Medical services*, p. 17; see also Prochaska, *Philanthropy and the hospitals of London*; Waddington, *Charity and the London hospitals*.

44. See also Cherry, *Medical services*; and S. Sturdy and R. Cooter, "Science, scientific management and the transformation of medicine in Britain *c.* 1870–1950," *History of Science*, 36, 421–66.

45. Rivett, *The development of the London hospital system*, p. 103.

46. Cherry, *Medical services*, p. 19.

47. Sturdy and Cooter, "Science, scientific management," p. 429; and Waddington, *Charity and the London hospitals*.

48. Prochaska, *Philanthropy and the hospitals of London*, p. 4

49. Ibid.

50. Sturdy and Cooter, "Science, scientific management," pp. 424–5.

51. Waddington, *Charity and the London hospitals*, p. 13.

52. Ibid.

53. Pickstone, *Medicine and industrial society*, p. 51; see also Abel-Smith, *The hospitals*; Cherry, "Beyond national insurance"; Fox, *Health policies, health politics*; Waddington, "Unsuitable cases"; Gorsky and Mohan, "London's voluntary hospitals in the interwar period."

54. Kings Fund Archive, London Metropolitan Archive (henceforward King's Fund), A/KE/168.

55. King's Fund, A/KE/168. Concerns about conditions in some nursing homes led to the passage of the 1927 Nursing Home Registration Act . See Abel-Smith, *The hospitals*, p. 342.
56. This was mainly, the Royal College of Physicians argued, because of the cost of accessory investigations (X-rays, laboratory tests, etc.). A/KE/52/2.
57. Powell, *Evaluating*; see also King's Fund, A/KE/184.
58. Timothy R. Smith, "The social transformation of hospitals and the rise of medical insurance in France, 1914–1943," *The Historical Journal*, 41, 1055–1087.
59. Waddington, "Unsuitable cases"; p. 29.
60. Gorsky and Mohan, "London's voluntary hospitals in the interwar period," p. 256.
61. Quoted in Prochaska, *Philanthropy and the hospitals of London*, p. 105; see also Abel-Smith, *The hospitals*.
62. Smith, "The social transformation of hospitals."
63. Prochaska, *Philanthropy and the hospitals of London*, p. 131; see also Eckstein, *The English health service*.
64. Gorsky and Mohan, *Medicine and mutual aid*.
65. Ibid.
66. Ibid., p. 31.
67. Gorsky and Mohan, *Medicine and mutual aid*; see also Cherry, "Beyond National Health Insurance."
68. Cherry, "Beyond National Health Insurance"; Gorsky and Mohan, *Medicine and mutual aid*.
69. Gorsky and Mohan, *Medicine and mutual aid*. This was also caused by the growing role of medical professionals in determining access.
70. Prochaska, *Philanthropy and the hospitals of London*.
71. Smith, "The social transformation of hospitals."
72. See King's Fund, A/KE/169; and Charles Webster, *Health services since the war*, London: HMSO, 1988.
73. Arthur Bryant, *A History of the British United Provident Association*, London: British United Provident Association, 1968; Gorsky and Mohan, *Medicine and mutual aid*; King's Fund, A/KE/169.
74. Abel-Smith, *The hospitals*, p. 399.
75. Bryant, *British United Provident Association*, p. 7.
76. Abel-Smith, *The hospitals*, p. 401; Bryant, *British United Provident Association*, p. 7.
77. King's Fund, A/KE/172 ; see also Abel-Smith, *The hospitals*, p. 343.
78. King's Fund, A/KE/172.
79. Abel-Smith, *The hospitals*, pp. 346–7; and King's Fund, A/KE/172.
80. A survey of 813 voluntary hospitals by the BMA in 1930 found that 60 per cent of small provincial hospitals admitted private patients . See also Abel-Smith, *The hospitals*, p. 345.
81. Gorsky and Mohan, *Medicine and mutual aid*, p. 32.
82. Gorsky and Mohan, *Medicine and mutual aid*. See also Steven Cherry, "Regional comparators in the funding and organisation of the voluntary hospital system *c.* 1860–1939," in Martin Gorsky and Sally Sheard, eds., *Financing medicine: The British experience since 1750*, London: Routledge, 2006, pp. 59–76; and J. Reinarz, "Charitable bodies: The funding of Birmingham's voluntary hospitals in the nineteenth century," in Gorsky and Sheard, *Financing medicine*, pp. 40–58.
83. King's Fund, A/KE/164 and 166.
84. King's Fund, A/KE/52/3.
85. King's Fund, A/KE/52a.

86. Gorsky and Mohan, "London's Voluntary Hospitals in the Interwar Period, p. 260
87. King's Fund A/KE/52/3.
88. King's Fund, A/KE/358.
89. King's Fund, A/KE/52a.
90. The survey included London.
91. I am grateful to John Mohan for access to this data.
92. Abel-Smith, *The hospitals*, p. 339.
93. King's Fund, A/KE/169.
94. Bryant, *British United Provident Association*.
95. Gorsky and Mohan, *Medicine and mutual aid*, p. 1.
96. The National Archive, Kew (henceforward The National Archives), MH 80/34.
97. King's Fund, A/KE/310a.
98. King's Fund, A/KE/166.
99. King's Fund, A/KE/52/1.
100. King's Fund, A/KE/168.
101. King's Fund, A/KE/52/4; see also Abel-Smith, *The hospitals*, p. 395.
102. King's Fund, A/KE/52/4.
103. King's Fund, A/KE/184.
104. Ibid.
105. King's Fund, A/KE/52/4; see also Eckstein, *The English health service*, p. 38; and Prochaska, *Philanthropy and the hospitals of London*.
106. King's Fund, A/KE/52/4.
107. Ibid.
108. King's Fund, A/KE/184.
109. The National Archives, MH 80/34.
110. Prochaska, *Philanthropy and the hospitals of London*, p. 131.
111. Gorsky and Mohan, *Medicine and mutual aid*.
112. King's Fund, A/KE/166; King's Fund, A/KE/52/1.
113. The National Archives, CHAR 3/123; see also King's Fund, A/KE/166, 168.
114. The National Archives, CHAR 3/123, 23/4/34.
115. The National Archives, CHAR 3/123; see also King's Fund, A/KE/52a.
116. King's Fund, A/KE/172.
117. King's Fund, A/KE/167.
118. King's Fund, A/KE/168.
119. King's Fund, A/KE/310a and 310b.
120. Gorsky and Mohan, *Medicine and mutual aid*, pp. 48–49.
121. Gorsky and Mohan, *Medicine and mutual aid*, p. 108; see also Prochaska, *Philanthropy and the hospitals of London*, p. 104.
122. Gorsky and Mohan, *Medicine and mutual aid*.
123. Abel-Smith, *The hospitals*, pp. 334–5.
124. As Honigsbuam has shown, after 1900 the BMA was mainly representative of the interests of general practitioners. See *The division in British medicine*.
125. King's Fund, A/KE/52/2; see also Gorsky and Mohan, *Medicine and mutual aid*; King's Fund, A/KE/52/2 and 3; and Abel-Smith, *The hospitals*.
126. King's Fund, A/KE/52/2; see also King's Fund, A/KE/52/4.
127. Gorsky and Mohan, *Medicine and mutual aid*.
128. Abel-Smith, *The hospitals*, p. 394.
129. Gorsky and Mohan, *Medicine and mutual aid*; see also King's Fund, A/KE/164.
130. See The National Archives, MH 80/29.
131. Baldwin, *Politics of social solidarity*, p. 49.

132. See Steven Fielding, "What did 'the people' want? The Meaning of the 1945 general election," *Historical Journal*, 35, 23–639, at p. 636.
133. Quoted in ibid., p. 634
134. Ibid., p. 636
135. University of Sussex Library, Mass Observation Archive (henceforward MOA).
136. MOA, File Report 1921A, Health; and Topic Collection 13, Health.
137. MOA, Topic Collection 13, Health.
138. Ibid.
139. See Bernard Harris, *The origins of the British welfare state: Society, state and social welfare in England and Wales, 1800–1945*, Basingstoke: Palgrave Macmillan, 2004, pp. 286–7.
140. Webster, *The health services since the war*, p. 24.
141. The National Archives MH 80/34.

Contributors

Thomas Adam is an assistant professor of German and modern transatlantic history at the University of Texas at Arlington since 2001. From 1999 to 2001, he taught at the University of Toronto while holding a Feodor Lynen Fellowship from the Alexander von Humboldt Foundation. He received his PhD from the University of Leipzig in 1998. Over the last seven years, he has published many articles, book chapters, and handbook entries on the topic of philanthropy in German and transatlantic history and German-American history, including *Traveling between Worlds: German-American Encounters* (coedited with Ruth Gross, published by Texas A&M University Press in 2006); the three-volume encyclopedia *Germany and the Americas: Culture, Politics, and Society* (ABC-CLIO, 2005); and *Philanthropy, Patronage, and Civil Society: Experiences from Germany, Great Britain, and North America* (Indiana University Press, 2004). He has recently completed a monograph, *Buying Respectability: Class and Philanthropy in American, Canadian and German Cities from the 1840s to the 1930s*, which is under review with Indiana University Press. Since 2005, he has been working on a research project about financing higher education in nineteenth- and early twentieth-century Germany.

Thomas M. Adams is a senior program officer at the National Endowment for the Humanities in Washington, DC. He is author of *Bureaucrats and Beggars: French Social Policy in the Age of the Enlightenment* (Oxford University Press, 1990) and related articles. He is currently working on a broad survey of Europe's welfare traditions.

Paul Bridgen has published widely on the history of British social policy, particularly in the areas of health and pensions. The chapter included in this volume reflects a particular interest in the politics of social policy-making, which is also reflected in a paper on the 1942 Beveridge Report and pensions published in *Twentieth Century British History* in 2005. He also has research interests in current social policy, particularly pensions and health promotion. He is currently working on an international project funded by the Anglo-German Foundation on recent developments in pensions policy in Britain and Germany.

Bernard Harris is Professor of the History of Social Policy at the University of Southampton, UK. His publications include *The Health of the Schoolchild: A History of the School Medical Service in England and Wales* (Open University Press, 1995) and *The Origins of the British Welfare State: Social Welfare in England and Wales, 1800–1945* (Palgrave, 2004), and he coedited *Race, Science and Medicine, 1700–1960* (Routledge, 1999). He has published a range of articles on different aspects of the history of height, health, and mortality. A coauthored study, entitled *Our Changing Bodies*, is due to be published by Cambridge University Press in 2008.

Peter Johansson has a PhD in history and is a researcher at the Institute for Futures Studies in Stockholm, Sweden. His previous publications in English on Swedish sickness-insurance policy include "Haunted by the Past: Continuity and Change in Swedish Sickness Insurance Policy from the 1880s to the 1930s" in E. Carroll and L. Eriksson, eds., *Welfare Politics Cross-Examined: Eclecticist Analytical Perspectives on Sweden and the Developed World from the 1880s to the 2000s* (Aksant, 2005). He is currently studying Swedish tax policy after the Second World War.

Marco H. D. van Leeuwen is senior researcher at the International Institute of Social History in Amsterdam and Professor of Historical Sociology at Utrecht University. His chosen field is social inequality from 1500 to the present. He has published on welfare (charity, mutual aid, insurance) and social mobility. His recent books are *Logic of Charity. Amsterdam, 1800–1850* (St Martin's Press, 2000), *HISCO: Historical International Standard Classification of Occupations* (Leuven University Press, 2002) (with I. Maas and A. Miles), as well as two volumes in Dutch on the history of risks in the Netherlands 16th–19th centuries. He coedited *Origins of the Modern Career* (Ashgate Publishers, 2004) and *Marriage Choices and Class Boundaries: Endogamy and Social Class in History* (Cambridge University Press, 2005).

Andrew Morris is an Assistant Professor in the Department of History at Union College in Schenectady, New York. He is currently revising a manuscript tentatively entitled *The Limits of Voluntarism: Charity and the Expansion of Welfare from the New Deal to Great Society*. An article derived from that study, "The Voluntary Sector's War on Poverty," *Journal of Policy History* (Fall 2004), won the Ellis Hawley Award from that journal in 2006.

Daniel Weinbren chairs the Friendly Societies Research Group, which is based at The Open University. His publications include work on friendly societies, on the history of the Labour Party, and on the armaments industries. He is a founding editor of *Family and Community History* and engaged in studying fraternal associations.

Index

Printed and bound by CPI Group (UK) Ltd, Croydon, CR0 4YY

01/11/2024

01782626-0009